BIRMINGHAM CITY
University

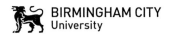

Please
remember to
return or
renew on time
to avoid fines

Renew/check due dates via
www.bcu.ac.uk/library

SHAPING HEALTH POLICY

Case study methods and analysis

Edited by Mark Exworthy, Stephen Peckham,
Martin Powell and Alison Hann

First published in Great Britain in 2012 by

The Policy Press
University of Bristol
Fourth Floor
Beacon House
Queen's Road
Bristol BS8 1QU
UK

Tel +44 (0)117 331 4054
Fax +44 (0)117 331 4093
e-mail tpp-info@bristol.ac.uk
www.policypress.org.uk

North American office:
The Policy Press
c/o The University of Chicago Press
1427 East 60th Street
Chicago, IL 60637, USA
Tel: +1 773 702 7700
Fax: +1 773 702 9756
e-mail: sales@press.uchicago.edu
www.press.uchicago.edu

British Library Cataloguing in Publication Data
A catalogue record for this book is available from the British Library.

Library of Congress Cataloging-in-Publication Data
A catalog record for this book has been requested.

ISBN 978 1 84742 757 1 paperback
ISBN 978 1 84742 758 8 hardcover

The right of Mark Exworthy, Stephen Peckham, Martin Powell and Alison Hann to be identified as editors of this work has been asserted by them in accordance with the 1988 Copyright, Designs and Patents Act.

Cover design by Robin Hawes
Front cover: image kindly supplied by istock.com
Printed and bound in Great Britain by Hobbs, Southampton
The Policy Press uses environmentally responsible print partners

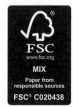

To Sarah, Dominic and Finnian

Contents

List of figures and tables

Figures

Tables

Contributors

Pauline Allen, London School of Hygiene and Tropical Medicine

Michael Calnan, University of Kent

Sue Dopson, University of Oxford

George Dowswell, University of Birmingham

David Evans, University of the West of England

Mark Exworthy, Royal Holloway, University of London

Ian Greener, University of Durham

Alison Hann, Swansea University

Stephen Harrison, University of Manchester

Joan Higgins, NHS Litigation Authority; Manchester University

David Hughes, Swansea University

Justin Keen, University of Leeds

Louise Locock, University of Oxford

Fraser Macfarlane, University of Surrey

Mike Marinetto, Cardiff University

John Mohan, University of Southampton

Adam Oliver, London School of Economics and Political Science

Calum Paton, Keele University

Stephen Peckham, London School of Hygiene and Tropical Medicine

Martin Powell, University of Birmingham

Marie Sanderson, London School of Hygiene and Tropical Medicine

David Wainwright, University of Bath

Micky Willmott, London School of Hygiene and Tropical Medicine

Abbreviations

ACE	Acting Chief Executive
AEG	area executive group
BBC	British Broadcasting Corporation
BMA	British Medical Association
BMI	Body Mass Index
BMJ	*British Medical Journal*
CASP	Critical Appraisal Skills Programme
CHC	Community Health Council
CMO	Chief Medical Officer
COHSE	Confederation of Health Service Employees
CQC	Care Quality Commission
DEG	district executive group
DF	development fund (in Chapter Twelve)/ Director of Finance (in Chapter Sixteen)
DGH	District General Hospital
DHSS	Department of Health and Social Security
EBM	evidence-based medicine
EMS	emergency medical services
FHSA	Family Health Service Authorities
GP	general practitioner; general practice
HA	Health Authority
HCAI	healthcare acquired infection
HSR	health services research
LDP	Local Delivery Plan
LINk	Local Involvement Network
LTC	long-term condition
MPC	Medical Planning Commission
MPR	Medical Planning Research
MRC	Medical Research Council
NHI	National Health Insurance
NHS	National Health Service
NHSLA	NHS Litigation Authority
NICE	National Institute of Clinical Excellence/National Institute for Health and Clinical Excellence
NPSA	National Patient Safety Authority
NUPE	National Union of Public Employees
PBC	practice-based commissioning
PCG	Primary Care Group
PCT	Primary Care Trust
PFI	private finance initiative

PRO   Public Records Office
QOF   Quality and Outcomes Framework
RAB   Resource Accounting and Budgeting
RCT   randomised controlled trial
RHB   Regional Hospital Board
RO   regional office
SAFF   Service and Financial Framework
SDO   Service Delivery and Organisation programme
SHA   Strategic Health Authority
SHARE   Scottish Health Authorities Revenue Equalisation
SHHD   Scottish Home and Health Department
SOP   standard operating procedure
TNA   The National Archives

Acknowledgements

We are grateful to the participants at the specially convened meeting of the annual Health Policy and Politics Network in Oxford in 2009. Organised by Alison Hann, this meeting enabled most of the authors to present and share their nascent ideas about case studies.

We would also like to acknowledge those in the health policy community with whom we have been lucky to collaborate. In addition to authors in this book, we include in this list Ewan Ferlie, Bob Hudson, Raymond Illsley, Rudolf Klein, Julian Le Grand, Ted Marmor, Nick Mays and Ray Robinson.

We thank Karen Bowler from The Policy Press for her ongoing support and encouragement.

Part One

one

Case studies in health policy: an introduction

Mark Exworthy and Martin Powell

Case studies have become, arguably, the predominant method by which much of social science is conducted. With its own long pedigree, health policy (allied to public and social policy) has not been immune to this trend. Yet, case study methods comprise inherent problems for designing and conducting research. They suffer from abuse and misuse, both in theory and in practice, in analysis and in application. In this book, we thus seek to recover and re-invigorate the case study as a valuable technique for researchers and practitioners. We do so in the context of health policy, a field which, sitting astride most social science disciplines, offers insights into the workings of the NHS and opportunities for the testing of theories and concepts. This book will explore the conceptualisation, design, practice and impact of case studies in health policy in the UK. Its aims are five-fold:

a. to raise awareness of case study as a technique for scholarly inquiry among researchers and students
b. to provide an accessible resource for use in education and training of students, academics and practitioners
c. to identify the value of exploring health policy in the UK using empirical case study methods
d. to reflect upon the value of case studies for contemporary health policy
e. to assess the ways in which case studies have enabled health policy learning.

This chapter is organised into three sections. First, we open the debate on case studies, rehearsing the principal arguments that will be examined in depth in later chapters. We tend to focus on health policy but are not limited to this field. The second section reviews our understanding of health policy. Third, we present the scope and rationale of the book (including its origins).

Case studies: a case of what?

What is a 'case'?

At the outset, it is important to examine the nature of the 'case' in policy analysis. Easton (1992) argues that the central function of case studies is to present solutions to 'complex unstructured problems' (p 4), but this begs a further question – what is the case?

Yin's (2009) definition of the case study is widely quoted and a useful starting point. He argues that it is

> An empirical study that investigates contemporary phenomena within a real life context, when the boundaries between the phenomenon and context are not clearly evident, and in which multiple sources of evidence are used. (p 18)

Marinetto (1999) offers a contrasting definition: the case study is a

> narrative-based account of a limited number of select instances which belong to a social or behavioural phenomena as it occurs in a natural setting. (p 63)

Locock et al (2006) claim that definitions of case studies invariably refer to the topics of inquiry and quote Schramm (1997) to highlight the fundamental role of a case study, which is to 'illuminate a decision or set of decisions; why they were taken, how they were implemented and with what result' (p 54). Others (such as Easton, 1992) highlight the learning potential of case studies.

Yin (2009, pp 16–18) writes that the most frequently encountered definitions of case studies have merely repeated the types of topics to which studies have been applied (such as a decision). However, citing a case topic is surely insufficient to establish the necessary definition of case studies as a research method. He produces a two-fold definition. The first part begins with the scope of a case study:

- a case study is an empirical inquiry that investigates a contemporary phenomenon in depth and within its real-life context and
- it is especially relevant when the boundaries between phenomenon and context are not clearly evident.

The second part includes other technical characteristics. The case-study inquiry:

- copes with the technically distinctive situation in which there will be many more variables of interest than data points
- relies on multiple sources of evidence, with data needed to converge in a triangulating fashion and
- benefits from the prior development of theoretical propositions to guide data collection and analysis.

Yin concludes that, in essence, the two-fold definition shows how case study research comprises an all-encompassing method, covering the logic of design, data-collection techniques and specific approaches to data analysis (p 18).

However, Yin (2009, pp 8–13) also sets out three conditions that determine when case studies should be used rather than other research methods such as experiments, surveys, archival analyses and histories. Case studies have a distinct advantage when a 'how' or 'why' question is being asked about a contemporary set of events over which the investigator has little or no control.

Finally, Yin (2009, pp 185–90) writes that 'exemplary' case studies should have the following characteristics: be significant, provide completeness, consider alternative perspectives, display sufficient evidence and be composed in an engaging manner. He presents, *inter alia*, six sources of evidence, three principles of data collection and five analytical techniques. In short, 'good case studies are still difficult to do' (Yin, 2009, p 16). Faced with such a counsel of perfection, it is likely that all case studies will fall short to some extent.

Moreover, Yin tends to focus on 'process' characteristics, but, in many ways, 'outcome' characteristics are more important. For example, the studies discussed in some of our chapters would probably not be termed 'case studies' by Yin (2009) because they do not satisfy all of his characteristics (see above). However, they have produced important empirical and conceptual contributions to knowledge and are well-cited standard sources (see, for example Chapters Three, Ten, Eighteen).

Unlike Yin, we tend towards a more minimalist definition of the case study, but one which incorporates rich, 'thick' descriptions that draw on multiple sources of evidence and on some theoretical insights. According to Marinetto (Chapter Two), the methodological value of the case study in policy analysis and public administration is that it embraces multiple research designs and sources, particularly those which are (though not exclusively) qualitative in nature. As such, the case method generates detailed, narrative-like description, which can be of interest in its own right. In intellectual terms, this methodological flexibility allows researchers to generate theoretical insights.

Recognising the definitional differences does not necessarily help with defining the 'case' as a unit of analysis. At a basic level, sociological definitions would suggest that a case study is a detailed study of a single social unit (see, for example, Chapters Two, Four, Twelve). However, this 'social unit' might comprise a person, an organisation, a policy, a social movement or even the NHS itself. Such breadth might not be helpful in surveying the field of case-studies health policy. Other common definitions focus on decisions or organisations. (for example, Chapter Nine). This has been termed 'intrinsic case analysis' (see Chapter Two). However, we agree with Yin (2009, p 35) that the role of theory development, prior to the conduct of any data collection, is one point of difference between case studies and related methods, such as ethnography. For case studies, theory development as part of the design phase is essential, whether the ensuing case study's purpose is to develop or to test theory. While we disagree with Yin (2009) on the need for a focus on 'contemporary events' and would therefore include 'historical case studies', this condition would exclude some of the narrative descriptions such as many of the individual accounts of creation of NHS (for example, Chapters Three and Four). However, examination of the accumulated studies does provide some theory development (for example, Chapters Seven and Twelve). Finally, we agree with Yin (2009) that case studies should be 'complete' and display sufficient evidence. Even if a case study drew on all six of Yin's (2009, pp 101–13) sources of evidence (documentation; archival records; interviews; direct observations; participant observation; and physical artefacts), it is unlikely that any study could be fully 'complete'. However, we feel that case studies should draw on more than one source of evidence. For example, we would not regard as a case study a study that drew solely on a single document.

Yin (2009, pp 46–60) sets out four types of design based on a 2 × 2 matrix. The two axes are single and multiple designs, and holistic and embedded designs. This gives four types: single-case/holistic; single-case/embedded; multiple-case/holistic; and multiple-case/embedded. He argues that single-case designs (with either single or multiple units of analysis) explore incidents which can be critical, extreme or unique or revelatory; these are common applications of case studies in health policy (for example, Chapters Six, Nine and Eleven). In summary, these approaches tend to categorise case studies rather than to define them.

A frequent concern (or complaint) about case studies is that they are not generalisable to wider groups or settings. Indeed, their design does not often enable empirical generalisation. This does not, however, detract from the need to ensure that case studies should achieve a high degree of validity (construct, internal and external). Yin (2009) does, however, argue that case studies can be valuable in aiding *theoretical* generalisation. This emphasises the way in which case studies can enable theories about policy to be tested empirically though inductive reasoning (Ham, 1981). Yin offers strategies by which generalisability may be enhanced:

- drawing on multiple sources of evidence
- generating a 'chain of evidence' (similar to programme theories)
- allowing informants to comment on the draft research report (triangulation)
- working with larger research teams and
- conducting comparative case studies.

However, it is the notion of 'replication logic' which offers particular methodological significance to case studies. Such a logic arises from theories about the case. Case selection becomes crucial so that it:

- predicts similar results (literal replication) or
- produces contrary results but for predictable reasons (theoretical replication) (Yin, 2009, pp 48–9).

In other words, generalisation involves 'replication logic' rather than 'sampling logic'. This relates to the theoretical framework, which needs to state the conditions under which a particular phenomenon is likely to be found (a literal replication) as well as the conditions when it is not likely to be found (a theoretical replication) (Yin, 2009, p 54). Although not discussed by Yin, this seems to fit with the search for context–mechanism–outcome (CMO) configurations advocated by Pawson and Tilley (1997) in 'realistic evaluation'. In other words, a rich description of 'context' is important in order to determine whether processes are universalistic or contingent. This contextualisation is also aligned with the work of Pettigrew and colleagues (see Chapter Thirteen), who championed the search for 'receptive contexts' through research that is historical, processual and contextual in character. Specifically, they emphasised the interaction between inner contexts (for example, of local organisational culture) and outer contexts (for example, of the socio-political environment). This replication logic shifts emphasis away from sampling issue per se and stresses the degree of external validity (Locock et al, 2006). It follows that case studies direct attention towards the significance beyond the case study itself and towards the potential transferability of findings to different contexts. Keen (Chapter Seven) argues that case studies conducted along the same lines as *Normal accidents* (Perrow, 1999) balance internal and external validity: they are sufficiently grounded in evidence to be credible, but also produce insights which can be applied generally.

Case studies – 'a striking paradox'

At the start of what has probably been the most influential book on case study research (cited 35,153 times, according Google Scholar, September 2010), Yin (2009) presents a 'striking paradox' about case studies:

> If the case study method has serious weaknesses, why do investigators continue to use it?

These weaknesses might include uncertainty about the definition of the 'case' (Ragin and Becker, 1992), misunderstandings about the generalisability of case study findings (Yin, 2009) (see above) and methodological controversies about how best to conduct case studies, among others. There has also, arguably, been a laxity in the execution of such research and the reporting of its findings on the part of the research community itself. Practitioners and policy makers, faced with an accumulating body of knowledge derived from case studies, may also be unsure how best to apply such research findings into their decision making (Easton, 1992). This concern is especially acute when evidence is diverse, the findings are unclear and the lessons are equivocal. How are they supposed to and how do they learn (if at all) from such case studies? What lessons have thus been learned?

Yet, case studies continue to be widely deployed (and, arguably, increasing) across most fields of social science and beyond (for example, education, engineering and architecture, see Easton, 1992). As one illustration of this, Table 1.1 presents the results of a search of the databases Zetoc and Google Scholar using the term 'case study health policy'. Results are presented in five-year periods (over the past 30 years). Although the two database results are constructed differently, they both show a significant rise in the scale of case study research in health policy, especially since the mid-1990s.

Table 1.1: The rise of case study research in health policy

Year	Number of hits	
	Zetoc	Google Scholar
1980–84	0	35,200
1985–89	1	76,200
1990–94	11	150,000
1995–99	61	356,000
2000–04	61	410,000
2005–10	354	417,000

Source: Zetoc and Google Scholar (searches conducted September 2010; search term: 'case study health policy')

What factors might explain this apparent trend in the use of case studies? It is hard to be precise, not least since the causes are likely to be a combination of interrelated factors. Three are noteworthy here. First, the rise of 'evaluation research' has been a long-term trend (Patton, 2002) and it has found expression in the 'evidence-based' movement (Davies et al, 2000; Locock et al, 2006; see also Chapter Seventeen, by George Dowswell and Stephen Harrison). Case studies have provided the setting for apparently discrete entities by which formative and summative evaluation can be conducted. Such evaluation has been particularly prevalent in health policy and health services research in the past decade or two. Second, the increasing contractualisation of university-based health-related research, particularly that funded by national governments, has also been instrumental in the sustained interest in case studies. One implication is that funding for case studies tends to be for shorter periods than might be the ideal, often with the hope of delivering 'quick answers'. For example, much of the National Institute for Health Research (NIHR) Service Delivery and Organisation programme might be classified as case-study research (Anderson et al, 2008); such research is, at best, three years in duration, though the empirical (data collection) phase is probably much shorter. This length of time might, nonetheless, be sensible in health policy, given the frequency of recent structural and organisational change in the NHS (Pollitt, 2009; see Chapter Twelve, by David Hughes). The inclination for empirical evidence helps to bolster the contractualised environment. Third, there has been a decline of book-length case study as the gold standard, in favour of journal articles (Hunter, 1980 is an example of the former; see Chapter Twelve). This is part of a wider academic trend towards journals, not least because of their apparent worth in research assessment exercises in UK universities. As a result, articles in journals report on case studies that are often shorter in length and cover shorter time periods (Locock et al, 2006). The trend towards shorter-term studies has reinforced a methodological perspective that has been descriptive and an approach that has tended to neglect theoretical developments (Crinson, 2009). Arguably, this further serves the needs of those who commission the research and makes the research more applied (and less theoretical). However, the longitudinal perspective that case studies are able to offer is one of their distinctive contributions, an aspect compounded by the length of time 'to prepare, write and test' such cases (Easton, 1992; see also Soulsby and Clark, 2011). Mike Marinetto explores the methodological provenance and application of case studies in policy research in Chapter Two.

The rise of the case study might be described in terms of methodological developments, too. Over, say, the 20 years since 1990, there has been a growing acceptance and use of qualitative methods in health policy, health services research and other fields (Pope and Mays, 2006, 2009). This acceptance has enabled methods such as in-depth interviewing, focus groups and participant observation to be more widely practised. Notably, the notion of 'policy ethnography' has gained particular traction (Glennerster et al, 1983; Strong and Robinson, 1990; Flynn et al, 1996). Additionally, qualitative case studies can be seen as an 'easy' methodology (cf quantitative methods) which may foster laxity in its execution.

Health policy: a 'chameleon concept'

Given that this book is explicitly concerned with health policy, it is important to delve into the scope and meanings of this field. What is policy and what issues does health policy encompass? Marinetto (1999) defines policy as the 'courses of action undertaken by public agencies and institutions under the authority of government' (p 3). Jenkins (1993) develops this definition by suggesting that policy is a set of interrelated decisions taken by political actors, focusing on a set of objectives. We tend to favour the inclusive approach of Hogwood and Gunn (1984), which stresses policy as behaviour and action, involves foreseen and unforeseen consequences, comprises purposive courses of action (which may be perceived retrospectively), process and outcome, involves public agencies and other stakeholders and is subjectively defined.

Central to the notion of 'policy' used in this book is that it is not a linear task:

> Policy is not a rational, objective, neutral activity devoid of values. (Hunter, 2003, p 18)

Several important consequences follow from Hunter's statement. The first is that individuals involved in policy (formulation and implementation) have many, often conflicting objectives. This prompts a concern with the (competing) values of interest groups and networks, and the ensuing 'conflicts about resources, rights and morals' (Klein and Marmor, 2008, p 892).

Second, the exercise of power is central to understanding and explaining the process and outcome of policy (Walt, 1994); there is thus a concern to answer Ham's (1981) questions:

> What approach to policy-making was adopted? Who was involved? How was the problem or issue defined? What was the policy response? How was the policy implemented? Who benefited? And whose will prevailed? (p 8)

We are also interested in countervailing issues relating to stifled interests: for example, who does *not* get services and which decisions are *not* 'made'?

Third, policy is beset with uncertainty, such that Heclo (1975) refers to policy as 'collective puzzlement'. This stimulates an interest in how policy is 'made', how its impacts are understood and how lessons are learnt. Such puzzlement prompts questions about policy makers' ability to learn from experiences (previously and elsewhere) and evidence.

Finally, implicit in the notion of the policy *process* is evolution over time. Wildavsky (1979) and Walt (1994) emphasise the need to view policy as a process as well as a product. Policy is not simply an end in itself but is also concerned with the means to such ends.

Moving from 'policy' in general to 'health policy' specifically, we propose a definition of health policy that is inclusive of both health (as it affects people's health) and healthcare (as it pertains to institutional systems, structures and processes). Gill Walt's (1994) definition of health policy neatly sums up our approach:

> Health policy embraces courses of action that affect the set of institutions, organisations, services, and funding arrangements of the health care system. It goes beyond health services, however, and includes action or intended actions by public, private and voluntary organisations that have an impact on health. (pp 4–5)

While there is a common tendency to focus on *healthcare*, our definition is broader. It therefore encompasses policy towards the promotion and maintenance of 'health', not simply sickness/illness services (Hunter, 2003). (Often, however, policy does not embrace this broader definition.) Thus, in this book our primary focus is on the NHS as the UK's most visible expression of public policy towards health, but it also addresses wider concerns: for example, with public health, health inequalities and health promotion (see Chapters Ten, Fifteen and Nineteen, by Evans, Hann, and Exworthy and Oliver, respectively).

The 'health policy' field is marked by a reasonably high degree of interdisciplinarity (Ham and Hill, 1993) and 'intellectual pluralism' (Klein, 1974). Studies draw on social and public policy, sociology, politics, organisation studies/public management (including public administration), and also anthropology, socio-legal studies, economics, geography, psychology, history and health services research. This diversity reflects the position where 'health policy' sits within the academy, across many of the boundaries of contemporary social science, and its characterisation as a 'chameleon concept' (Klein and Marmor, 2008, p 892). Though it owes much of its heritage to public/social policy, political science and sociology, it is increasingly encompassed by the title of 'health policy and management'; note, for example, academic positions with this title in management schools, medical schools and social science departments. Likewise, Paton and Bach's (1990) book is titled *Case studies in health policy and management*. This dualism (policy *and* management) is, arguably, a reflection of the ascendancy of 'new public management' across government and public services (Ferlie et al, 2005) and a reductionist approach which sees (policy) problems in terms of technical solutions (Hunter, 2003).

However, there is a strong danger that the distinctive contribution of 'policy studies' is subsumed within more generic approaches. Such approaches are perhaps illustrated by the balance between two key approaches: analysis *of* policy and analysis *for* policy (Gordon et al, 1977) (Figure 1.1). Likewise, Lasswell (1970) refers to knowledge *of* the policy process and knowledge *in* the process. Arguably, the balance between these has tilted from the former to the latter in recent years. The boundary between these two approaches is not clear cut and is invariably in flux. The reasons for this shift may appear similar to those that have encouraged the further development of case studies (see above), such as contractualised research in health policy (and related fields), government-funded evaluation of government-funded programmes and the (related) search for 'what works'.

Figure 1.1: Analysis of policy and analysis for policy

Policy studies ⟷ **Policy analysis**

| Study of policy content | Study of policy process | Study of policy outputs | Evaluation | Information for policy making | Process advocacy | Policy advocacy |

Knowledge of policy process ⟷ Knowledge in the policy process

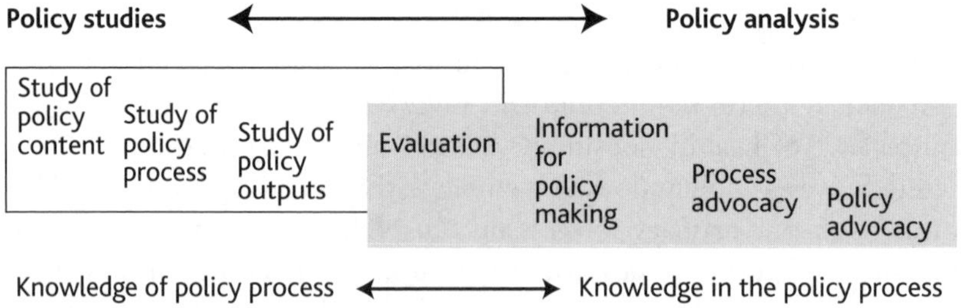

Source: Peckham and Exworthy (2003, p 26)

The scope and rationale of this book

This book is an attempt to explore Yin's 'striking paradox' of case studies in the 'chameleon' context of health policy. In what ways have the 'weaknesses' of the case study method shaped the conduct of health policy research in last decade or so? How has such research adapted to the wider changes in the social science research? Which case studies have been enduring in policy and academic communities? What lessons have been learned from them? In Paton and Bach's (1990) words, we are thus engaged in 'understanding the past and predicting the future' (p 3). Specifically, what does the experience of each of our case studies tell us about the dynamics of health policy and the evolution of the NHS (see Ham, 1981, p 4)? In answering these broad questions, we seek here to rediscover and reclaim the methods and theoretical approaches offered by case studies.

We thus aim to enhance the methodological rigour of case studies. However, we do not offer a comprehensive methodological account of how to design and conduct case studies in practice. For this, we would direct attention to Patton (1980), Ragin and Becker (1992), Ragin (1999), Dopson (2003) or Yin (2009). Instead, we aim to assess critically the value of the case study 'method' in terms of its ability to understand previous events and to explain emergent policy developments. To achieve this, we provide a collation of some key case studies that have been conducted in health policy and offer a synthesis of them.

In terms of a theoretical contribution, we also seek to demonstrate the current vitality of the field through the breadth and depth of health policy research. The book covers the key theories that have been and continue to be applied in health policy settings. They relate to three primary axes that have shaped health policy: public/private, state/profession and local/national (Exworthy and Freeman, 2009). However, this book does not delve into the explanations of concepts, theories and frameworks of health policy; it is not a health policy textbook. If this is of interest, we would direct attention to Abel-Smith (1994), Baggott (2000), Buse et al (2005), Baggott (2007) or Klein (2010). None of the chapters, in themselves, seeks to explain the range of theoretical contributions to health policy. Rather, the book takes many of these as already known and understood, and uses them to illustrate the case studies.

The 'shared vision' of health policy, which marked the NHS for much of its first 30 years, invoked a consensual approach to the welfare state. This vision was, however, somewhat illusory, according to Greener (2009), and recent health policy reforms have, arguably, undermined that impression further. At the start of the second decade of the 21st century, health policy (in the UK) is marked by continuity and change from previous research practices. On the one hand, as Greener argues (2009), the NHS is an organisation with 'considerable institutional memory' (p 4) that has, for the most part, resisted various attempts at reform. On the other hand, the NHS has undergone, in particular over the past 20 years, remarkable transformation that reflects not only the health policy reforms but wider social and demographic trends (Klein, 2010). (These reforms threaten such institutional memory, see Pollitt, 2009.) Klein's (2010) has proposed the analogy of the NHS as an opera in which the actors move position around the stage but melodies provide continuity. This analogy remains apposite; recent health policy might thus be seen as challenging both the actors and melodies of the NHS 'opera'.

Origins of the book

The origins of this book lay in our interest in synthesising the cumulative knowledge of case studies in health policy. What were the key case studies in health policy? Was there a consensus about such a list? What impact have these case studies had upon health policy and practice? What lessons could they offer for contemporary health policy? How might such learning take place or even be conceptualised?

The book was also inspired by the apparent reinvention and recirculation of familiar themes in health policy in frequent NHS reorganisations. It thus prompted further questions such as: How enduring were 'classic' case studies? What impact did they have upon (health policy) research? How were previous health policy reforms enacted? What can current reforms learn from the past?

In order to gauge the significance of case studies in health policy for the community of health policy academics, the editors sent an e-mail survey to academics in 2008. Over 30 UK-based 'health policy' academics responded to the survey. We sought views on what they considered to be the three 'most important/significant/interesting (published) case studies of UK health policy'. We were somewhat uncommitted as to the definition and selection of case studies. We did not define explicitly what we meant by a case study, nor did we confine ourselves to any single discipline; rather, we waited to see if consensus emerged about a definition. However, we did state our interest in collating a cross-section of case studies from different sectors (for example, primary and secondary care), different periods (that is, covering the life of the NHS) and different stages of the policy process (for example, agenda setting, policy formulation and implementation).

We received responses that cited 42 different case studies. The breadth of these 42 case studies, perhaps unsurprisingly, tended to focus on more recent case-study publications (mostly over the past 20 years or so), though some responses included examples from the 1960s and 1980s. More surprising was the lack of consensus among respondents, in terms of both the case studies themselves and their authors. Only three case studies were cited more than once, and these were only cited twice (that is, Alford, 1975; Hunter, 1980; Pettigrew et al, 1992; all three are included as chapters in this book by Stephen Peckham and Micky Willmott, David Hughes, and Louise Locock and Sue Dopson; Chapters Eight, Twelve and Thirteen respectively). Rudolf Klein was the only author who was cited more than once, with four citations (Klein, 1979; Day and Klein, 1989; Day and Klein, 1992; Klein, 1995).

Moreover, there was little consistency in the type of case study; responses included policy initiatives/programmes and publications (including books, book chapters, journal articles and research reports). There was also a range of sectors and different stages of the policy process. It is equally remarkable that some case studies were omitted. It is rather invidious to select such omissions, but they might include Ham (1981) on the Leeds hospital board, Korman and Glennerster (1990) on the closure of long-stay hospitals or Klein et al (1996) on rationing. There might also be observed omissions in terms of sectors, such as mental health or dentistry, and in terms of insights from *within* the policy-making process. Equally, there was an implicit tendency to focus on England. While devolution of health competencies is a relatively recent phenomenon (since 1999), it is rather surprising that studies from Wales, Scotland or Northern Ireland are largely absent. (Studies by Hunter, 1980 and Greer, 2009 are notable exceptions, for example.) The lack of insight from research of central government policy-making processes was also apparent. (Exceptions to this include Greer and Jarman, 2007, for example.) Likewise, there still remains (relatively) little policy research on public health issues or on the practices of the independent sector (including private healthcare and third sector activity). (Exceptions to this include Baggott, 2000 or Hunter, 2003 and Higgins, 1988, respectively.)

Among the case studies that were nominated in the survey there appeared to be two broad categories of 'case study'. One concerned what might be termed the 'policy' case study, while the other might be termed the 'academic' case study. Broadly speaking, the former refers to legislation, programmes and initiatives emanating from within the health system. The latter, however, refers to scholarly publications, which comprise mainly empirical studies of health policy in action.

Organising the book

The book is not intended to be a health policy textbook, nor a 'reader' in health policy. Instead, we present a set of reflexive case studies which, collectively and individually, offer perspectives across NHS history and across the policy process. Each author was asked to frame their chapter in terms of:

a. a brief description of the original case study to which it refers
b. discussion of the methods and approaches used in the analysis reflecting on the case study approach and
c. a commentary on the contemporary relevance to health policy of the original case study.

Our framing of health policy case studies was a binary division between the policy process and periods of NHS history. Others have deployed alternative frames. These include 'stages of the policy process and different levels of analysis' (Marinetto, 1999, p 78; see also Ham and Hill, 1984) and coverage of various substantive policy areas. We also sought a breadth of authors who are 'scholars with considerable expertise in policy areas' (Jenkins–Smith and Sabatier, 1993, p 6).

Policy process

While we would not defend the 'stages' model of the policy process per se, it does offer some value in this analysis. It does, for example, disaggregate the policy process into 'manageable segments', it emphasises the processual nature of policy and 'transcends any given institution' (Jenkins-Smith and Sabatier, 1993, p 2). However, it implies a top-down approach to the policy process and emphasises temporal dimensions. On balance, we would argue that division of the policy process into agenda setting, formulation, implementation and impact (evaluation) does offer a logical structure which can be aligned to most case studies.

Periodisation of the NHS

One of the primary values of the case study approach is its ability to provide lessons from history for current and future policy makers and researchers. Indeed, this has been the objective of some leading health policy case studies. With this purpose in mind, we have deliberately chosen case studies that span the 'broad sweep of development of the NHS as a major organisational innovation' (Ham, 1981, p 3). However, in order to achieve this, it is useful to provide a justification for the way in which NHS history has been viewed.

Defining the temporal dimension of the NHS is subject to interpretation and purpose, and is thus open to contestation. One might divide the life of the NHS (or parts of it) into key (legislative or decision making) 'moments' (Greener, 2004). Alternatively, Ham (1981), for example, divides the period 1948–74 into four periods (1948–53, 1953–60, 1960–67 and 1967–74). Klein (2010) offers a contrasting perspective across eight eras of NHS politics:

- creation
- consolidation
- technocratic change
- disillusionment
- value for money
- big bang
- third way and
- reinvention.

However, we present a shifting pattern of institutions, interests and ideas which, together, point towards three major eras:

a. creation, consolidation, disillusion (1948–80s)
b. 'safe in our hands' – conflicts and challenges (1980s and 1990s) and
c. New Labour, new NHS? – the NHS since the 1990s.

While appreciating that the boundaries of these periods are somewhat indistinct and reconciling the brevity and depth of analysis, we use this trilogy to frame the chapters in the book. This policy process and periodisation is illustrated in Table 1.2.

In short, case studies and ways of analysing them (here, by periods of the NHS and by stages of the policy process) are heuristic devices to aid our understanding and explanations. Combined, they seek to reveal and explain the patterns and outcomes of the interactions between health policy, institutions, interests and ideas. Case studies are, inevitably, partial interpretations of the ways in which health policy is shaped, but they provide insights that other methods are often ill equipped to deliver. This book presents such insights through the analysis of individual chapters, but also through the perspective that they collectively provide.

Table 1.2: Framing the book chapters

Periods of the NHS	Policy process			
	Agenda setting	Formulation	Implementation	Impact
1948–80s	• Keen	• Mohan • Peckham and Willmott	• Powell	• Greener • Higgins
1980s–1990s		• Evans • Hughes	• Wainwright and Calnan • Locock and Dopson	• Macfarlane et al
1990s onwards	• Hann • Exworthy and Oliver		• Peckham and Sanderson • Paton • Dowswell and Harrison	• Allen

References

Abel-Smith, B. (1994) *An introduction to health: Policy, planning and finance*, London: Prentice Hall.

Alford, R.A. (1975) *Health care politics*, Chicago, IL: University of Chicago Press.

Anderson, S., Allen, P., Peckham, S. and Goodwin, N. (2008) 'Asking the right questions: scoping studies in the commissioning of research on the organisation and delivery of health services', *Health Research Policy and Systems*, vol 6, no 7, www.health-policy-systems.com/content/pdf/1478-4505-6-7.pdf.

Baggott, R. (2000) *Public health policy: Policy and politics*, Basingstoke: Palgrave.

Baggott, R. (2007) *Understanding health policy*, Bristol: The Policy Press.

Buse, K., Mays, N. and Walt, G. (2005) *Making health policy*, Buckingham: Open University Press.

Crinson, I. (2009) *Health policy: A critical perspective*, London: Sage.

Davies, H.T.O., Nutley, S.M. and Smith, P.C. (eds) (2000) *What works? Evidence-based policy and practice in public services*, Bristol: Policy Press.

Day, P. and Klein, R. (1989) 'Interpreting the unexpected: the case of AIDS policy making in Britain', *Journal of Public Policy*, vol 9, pp 337–53.

Day, P. and Klein, R. (1992) 'Constitutional and distributional conflict in British medical politics: the case of general practice, 1911–1991', *Political Studies*, vol 40, no 3, pp 462–78.

Dopson, S. (2003) 'The potential of the case-study method for organizational analysis', *Policy and Politics*, vol 31, no 2, pp 217–26.

Easton, G. (1992) *Learning from case studies*, 2nd edn, London: Prentice Hall.

Exworthy, M. and Freeman, R. (2009) 'The United Kingdom: health policy learning in the NHS', in T. Marmor, R. Freeman and K. Okma (eds) *Comparative studies and the politics of modern medical care*, Yale New Haven, CT: University Press, pp 153-79.

Ferlie, E., Lynn, L.E. and Pollitt, C. (eds) (2005) *Oxford handbook of public management*, Oxford: Oxford University Press.

Flynn, R., Williams, G. and Pickard, S. (1996) *Markets and hierarchies: Contracting in community health services*, Buckingham: Open University Press.

Glennerster, H., Korman, N. and Marsden-Wilson, F. (1983) *Planning for priority groups*, Oxford: Blackwell.

Gordon, I., Lewis, J. and Young, K. (1977) 'Perspectives on policy analysis', *Public Administration Bulletin*, December, p 25.

Greener, I. (2004) 'The three moments of New Labour's health policy discourse', *Policy and Politics*, vol 32, no 3, pp 303–16.

Greener, I. (2009) *Healthcare in the UK: Understanding continuity and change*, Bristol: Policy Press.

Greer, S. (2009) *Territorial politics and health policy: UK health policy in comparative perspective*, Manchester: Manchester University Press.

Greer, S. and Jarman, H. (2007) *The Department of Health and the civil service: From Whitehall to department of delivery to where?*, London: Nuffield Trust.

Ham, C. and Hill, M. (1984) *The policy process in the modern capitalist state,* New York: Harvester Wheatsheaf.

Ham, C. and Hill, M. (1993) *The policy process in the modern capitalist state*, Brighton: Wheatsheaf.

Ham, C.J. (1981) *Policy-making in the National Health Service: A case study of the Leeds Regional Hospital Board*, Basingstoke: Macmillan.

Heclo, H. (1975) 'Social policy and policy impacts', in M. Holden and D.L. Dresang (eds) *What government does*, Beverley Hills, CA: Sage, pp 151–76.

Higgins, J. (1988) *The business of medicine: Private health care in Britain*, Basingstoke: Macmillan.

Hogwood, B.W. and Gunn, L. (1984) *Policy analysis for the real world*, Oxford: Oxford University Press.

Hunter, D.J. (1980) *Coping with uncertainty: Policy and politics in the National Health Service*, Letchworth: Research Studies Press.

Hunter, D.J. (2003) *Public health policy*, Cambridge: Polity.

Jenkins, B. (1993) 'Policy analysis: models and approaches', in M. Hill (ed) *The policy process: A reader*, Hemel Hempstead: Harvester Wheatsheaf.

Jenkins-Smith, H. and Sabatier, P. (1993) 'The study of public policy processes', in P. Sabatier and H. Jenkins-Smith (eds) *Policy change and learning: An advocacy coalition approach*, Boulder, CO: Westview Press, pp 1–9.

Klein, R. (1974) 'Policy problems and policy perceptions in the National Health Service', Policy and Politics, vol 2, no 3, pp 219–36.

Klein, R. (1979) 'Ideology, class and the National Health Service', *Journal of Health Policy, Politics and Law*, vol 4, no 3, pp 464–90.

Klein, R. (1995) 'Big bang health care reform: does it work? The case of Britain's 1991 National Health Service reforms', *Milbank Quarterly*, vol 73, no 3, pp 299–337.

Klein, R. (2010) *The new politics of the NHS: From creation to re-invention*, 6th edn, Oxford: Radcliffe Publishing.

Klein, R. and Marmor, T.R. (2008) 'Reflections on policy analysis: putting it together again', in M. Moran, M. Rein and R.E. Goodin (eds) *Oxford handbook of public policy*, Oxford: Oxford University Press, pp 892–912.

Klein, R., Day, P. and Redmayne, S. (1996) *Managing scarcity: Priority setting and rationing in the National Health Service*, Buckingham: Open University Press.

Korman, N. and Glennerster, H. (1990) *Hospital closure: A political and economic study*, Milton Keynes: Open University Press.

Lasswell, H.D. (1970) 'The emerging conception of the policy sciences', *Policy Sciences*, vol 1, no 1, pp 3–14.

Locock, L., Ferlie, E., Dopson, S. and Fitzgerald, L. (2006) 'Research design: upscaling qualitative research', in S. Dopson and L. Fitzgerald (eds) *Knowledge into action: Evidence-based health-care in context*, Oxford: Oxford University Press, pp 48–78.

Marinetto, M. (1999) *Studies of the policy process: A case analysis*, Hemel Hempstead: Harvester Wheatsheaf.

Paton, C. and Bach, S. (1990) *Case studies in health policy and management*, Parts I and II, London: Nuffield Provincial Hospitals Trust.

Patton, M.Q. (1980) *Qualitative evaluation and research methods*, 2nd edn, Newbury Park, CA: Sage.

Patton, M.Q. (2002) *Qualitative research and evaluation methods*, 3rd edn, Thousand Oaks, CA: Sage.

Pawson, R. and Tilley, N. (1997) *Realistic evaluation*, London: Sage.

Peckham, S. and Exworthy, M. (2003) *Primary care in the UK: Policy, organisation and management*, Palgrave Macmillan: Basingstoke.

Perrow, C. (1999) *Normal accidents: Living with high risk technologies*, Princeton, NJ: Princeton University Press.

Pettigrew, A., Ferlie, E. and McKee, L. (1992) *Shaping strategic change: Making change in large organizations*, London: Sage.

Pollitt, C. (2009) 'Bureaucracies remember, post-bureaucratic organizations forget?', *Public Administration*, vol 87, no 2, pp 198–218.

Pope, C. and Mays, N. (eds) (2006) *Qualitative research in health care*, 3rd edn, Oxford: Blackwell.

Pope, C. and Mays, N. (2009) 'Critical reflections on the rise of qualitative research', *British Medical Journal*, no 339, pp 737–9.

Ragin, C. (1999) 'The distinctiveness of case-oriented research', *Health Services Research*, vol 34, no 5, pp 1137–51.

Ragin, C. and Becker, S. (1992) *What is a case? Exploring the foundations of social inquiry*, Cambridge: Cambridge University Press.

Schramm, W. (1997) *Note on case studies of instructional media projects*, Working paper for Academy of Educational Development, Washington DC seminar no 4 (December).

Soulsby, A. and Clark, E. (2011) 'Theorizing process through punctuated longitudinal case-study research', in C. Welch and R. Piekkari (eds) *Rethinking the case-study approach in international business research*, Cheltenham: Edward Elgar Publishing Limited, pp 411-46.

Strong, P. and Robinson, J. (1990) *The NHS under new management*, Buckingham: Open University Press.

Walt, G. (1994) *Health policy: An introduction to process and power*, London: Zed Books.

Wildavsky, A. (1979) *Speaking truth to power: The art and craft of policy analysis*, Boston, MA: Little Brown.

Yin, R.K. (2009) *Case study research: Design and methods*, 4th edn, London: Sage.

two

Case studies of the health policy process: a methodological introduction

Mike Marinetto

Introduction

This introduction attempts to set the health policy case study within a general academic context, tracing methodological discussions and debates in relevant disciplinary fields. In particular, the use of case studies within the political sciences, as well as sub-disciplinary factions, has no small bearing. Initially, the case study was popularised by American academics working in specialist sub-fields of political science, especially in public administration (see Stein, 1952). By the 1970s, American political scientists were using the case approach to explore policy decision making. One notable example was Allison's (1971) *Essence of Decision*, which used the Cuban missile crisis of October 1962 as the basis for exploring decision making in political arenas. British political scientists, as well as students of policy process and public administration, have also come to rely on case analysis. This includes research into health policy and the institutional settings in which such policy is enacted.

The methodological value of the case study to policy analysis and public administration is that it embraces multiple research designs and sources, particularly those which are (though not exclusively) qualitative in nature. As such, the case method generates detailed, narrative-like description which can be of interest in its own right. In intellectual terms, this methodological flexibility allows researchers to generate theoretical insights. Such 'theory work' uncovers the complex influences that impinge on public bodies and the context-bound, event-driven nature of policy decisions. The methodological and intellectual import of the case method is particularly useful in researching health policy, the subject matter that forms the basis of this book. As a preface to the following chapters, this chapter aims to place health-based policy case studies in a disciplinary and methodological context. The first half of the chapter explores how case analysis has been adopted within political science and allied sub-disciplines such as public administration and policy analysis. After commenting on the general place of case-based research in the political and policy sciences, this introductory chapter focuses more specifically on the emergence and development of the case study within the field of health policy research.

The interdisciplinary origins of the case study

The methodological status of the case study is far from clear cut. Gerring observes how the case study is a 'research design best defined as an intensive study of a single unit ... where the scholar's aim is to elucidate features of a larger class of similar phenomenon' (2004, p 341). However, Robert Stake (2005) questions whether case-based analysis is a research methodology or a research design. Stake's concerns are well founded. The case study does not come with a discrete theory of how research should be conducted. By contrast, something like an experiment is accompanied by a clear and coherent set of methodological stipulations. Case analysis does not prescribe the methods that should be used and how or what type of data should be gathered. Neither does it privilege the use of certain research techniques or methods above others. That said, the case study is more often than not associated with qualitative research approaches – ethnography or semi-structured interviews. As Gerring observes: 'the traditional association of case work with qualitative methods is correctly regarded as a methodological affinity, not a definitional entailment' (2007, p 36).

If the case study is a research-based activity without a methodology or research design, what is it, exactly? When it comes to case analysis, argues Stake, it is 'not a methodological choice but a choice of what is to be studied' (2005, p 443). A variety of methods can be used to build up a case. Just to make the point, van Wynsberghe and Khan point out that several different types of case study exist. Exploratory, explanatory, longitudinal, deviant, instrumental, multi-site, exploratory, explanatory: the case study takes various forms but 'none of them require specific data collection procedures' (van Wynsberghe and Khan, 2007, p 82). But regardless of the method or type of case study being used, what is distinctive about case methodology is that researchers focus on *the case*. Researchers who choose to study a particular case may not even employ the term 'case study'. According to Stake, the term 'case study' is used by some researchers 'because it draws attention to the question of what specially can be learned about the single case' (2005, p 443). What is without question, however, is the fact that the study has become something of a mainstay within contemporary social science.

Historically, the intense study of a single or a select number of cases has been associated with clinical settings, particularly those linked to medicine and psychiatry. The clinical case history is synonymous with the name of Sigmund Freud, who endeavoured, his penchant for cocaine aside, to uncover the incestuous, psycho-sexual desires of psychiatric patients. He did this, essentially, by conversing with his patients. Rat Man, Dora, Wolf Man, Judge Screber and Little Hans were the aliases used by Freud for his most infamous patient cases. Overall, in Freud's writings you can find references to over 130 patient cases. That said, the case method has a long and significant presence outside the medical sciences. The case study has been sufficiently flexible and adaptable to have gained acceptance across a range of other intellectual and research endeavours. It has been particularly welcomed by disciplines outside the natural sciences – the so-called human sciences: psychologists, sociologists, anthropologists and even historians have made extensive use of the case approach.

Arguably, the figure responsible for popularising the case study in the social sciences is the 19th-century Frenchman Frederic Le Play, an itinerant, amateur sociological sleuth. As a mining consultant to companies and governments in the mid-1800s, Le Play travelled extensively. During his travels, he conducted research on working-class communities – studies that he began as an undergraduate student. To explore the living conditions of European workers, Le Play became a pioneer of the family case study. Travelling to different locations in his mining work, he would select a family in whatever location his travels had taken him to and would stay with it until he had gained comprehensive details about its way of life. Le Play used 57 family studies as the basis of his 1855 book *European workers*, which exposed the nascent social science to case research. Le Play, influenced by his scientific background, developed a systematic and rigorous approach to case research. According to Mogey: 'His training in the physical sciences sent him searching for a more exact mode of expression than mere subjective description and he soon developed a system of basing his notes upon a comprehensive outline of the material possessions, income, and occupations of the family' (1955, p 310). Le Play's search for a scientific form of case analysis presaged the development of the case study within the modern social and political sciences.

The emergence of the case study as a methodological mainstay in the 20th century is not linked to research. Rather, it owes more to its employment as a teaching method in rapidly expanding and professionalised university institutions. Enter Harvard Business School and the North American academic system. The paucity of business-related teaching materials became apparent in the years following the establishment of Harvard's business department in 1905. And, necessity being the mother of invention, the faculty went about developing teaching-focused case studies. The Harvard case teaching method pioneered a participatory, discussion-led teaching method which valued experiential learning (see Barnes et al, 1994). The rationale behind the Harvard case method was to teach students the value of critical thinking and problem solving. Using primary interview material, over the years, faculty members developed and used case studies in the Harvard MBA course. Sensing a good business opportunity (as you would expect from an institution that can count Lehman Brothers' Dick Fauld as one of its illustrious alumni), in recent years Harvard Business School has marketed these case studies. Literally hundreds, if not thousands, of business case studies are available to buy online. Christopher Grogan and Jeanne Brett, for instance, have devised a case study titled *Google and the government of China: A case study in cross-cultural negotiations*. This can be all yours for $6.95. North American academics were aware of the case study's inherent flexibility and it soon moved from the seminar room to the research field. What follows is a discussion of the rise to prominence of case analysis in the social sciences, focusing particularly on the American academy, which has been at the forefront in popularising the case study. In the discussion, I focus, in particular, on a field of disciplinary endeavour which is closest to health policy analysis, that is, political science and the sub-field of public administration.

American policy analysis and the Chicago School approach to case study research

Case analysis has surfaced with no little amount of prominence in political analysis. The employment of case studies in political science and allied disciplines has not been set in stone. Indeed, over time academic practitioners have come to redefine the role of the case study in political research. One reason for this is the spectre of disciplinary fragmentation. The field of political science is of course made up of distinct sub-disciplinary specialisms, such as international relations, political theory, domestic or national governance, comparative politics, developmental politics, public administration, policy analysis and so on. These various sub-fields, apart from that concerned with political theory, all draw on case analysis. There are distinct approaches and ideas as to what it means to do case research within the various disciplinary species that populate political science. Domestic-level political analysis, the study of British government, for instance, uses case analysis to focus on particular institutions, such as central government departments and local authorities. Comparative politics, on the other hand, has opted for a more macro level of case analysis, taking national contexts as the focal point. Comparative political analysis has also made extensive use of multi-site case studies to explore issues of diversity in politics and systems of governance. The advantage of the multi-site case study for comparative analysts is that the data can form the basis of grand thinking or propositions. For example, Robert Putnam's (1993) comparative study of governance in Italy attributed different levels of democratic engagement across Italian regions to the structural vitality of civic life within specific geographical locations.

There is a varied and rich history of case research in public administration and policy analysis; the specialist fields of interest are most closely related to the study of health policy. The public administration or policy case study is a multi-dimensional beast which can, potentially, operate at different ontological levels of analysis (see Marinetto, 1999). What policy case studies share with other sub-disciplines within the field of political science is a general agreement that case analysis is essentially qualitative in its methodological intent:

> Despite their distinctive histories and occasionally competing ontological and epistemological presuppositions, the discipline's [political science] sub-fields share a widespread agreement associating case studies closely with qualitative research. (Yanow et al, 2010, p 109)

Formative case studies examining policy and public administration, which were predominantly US-centred, relied on intense fieldwork within real settings. The dominance of qualitative research in early policy research owes much to the Chicago School approach (Yanow et al, 2010). In fact, if Harvard University Business School pioneered the use of case studies in teaching, the University of Chicago's sociology department helped to establish the case study as a research strategy in the North American academy.

Noteworthy sociologists from the University of Chicago conducted anthropological-like studies of urban city locations during the 1920s and 1930s, using participant and non-participant observation, semi-structured interviews and in-depth documentary analysis. Seminal case research within political research, and for that matter in public administration, was informed and predominantly fashioned by the research modus operandi of the Chicago School:

> Early case studies ... consist of largely single-site studies that allow researchers to immerse themselves in the uniqueness of real-life events in what might be called a traditional Chicago-School-type approach. The analysis is inductive and human-centred ... (Yanow et al, 2010, p 110)

The key characteristic of the Chicago School sociological approach to case analysis is the reliance on a single site or a highly specific case. Early efforts include Pendleton Herring's (1940) work on political leadership from the 1940s and Elmer Schattschneider's (1935) case-work on trade tariffs. Post-war, the stand-out policy case study was Graham T. Allison's *Essence of decision*, about the 1962 Cuban missile crisis. The 1970s saw the publication of other classic, in-depth American policy case studies: Derthick's *New towns in-town* (1972), Pressman and Wildavsky's *Implementation* (1973), Heclo and Wildavsky's *Private government of public money* (1974), Neustadt and Fineberg's *The* swine flu affair (1978). In many ways, this was a golden age for the policy case study, a time when book-length case analysis was valued and the journal article was not yet the absolute gold standard for academic success. Take, for example, Heclo and Wildavsky's (1974) ethnographic case study of the workings the UK Treasury. Although Heclo and Wildavsky's study is outdated in terms of current ideological proclivities within the Treasury, the study illuminated the practices and goings-on of an unexplored hinterland in British executive government. This predilection for thick sociological-style description also characterised early health policy case studies in the wake of the post-war welfare boom.

The intrinsic case study and the professional health bureaucracy

The academic profession is adept at following trends that occur beyond the walls of the academy. The history of health service provision in the industrialised world, particularly the in the United States, is a case in point. The expansion of health services as part of the post-Second World War welfare settlement was inevitably accompanied by growing academic research into health policy and its organisation. As part of the burgeoning interest, the case study became one research approach used to study health policy. The initial forays into health case research were predominantly, though not exclusively, American in terms of their setting. The case study, of course was already well established by the 1930s, both as a teaching tool at Harvard University's Business School and as a research method in the University of Chicago's sociology department. The lessons, especially from the latter, were not lost on early health policy researchers in the United States and elsewhere.

Formative case studies on health policy emulated the sociological approach of the Chicago School. The sociological emphasis can best be described, using Robert Stake's terminology, as 'intrinsic case analysis' (2005, p 445). The intrinsic case study has a concern for the detailed nuances of ordinary, quotidian existence, with abstract claims left to one side: 'The researcher at least temporarily subordinates other curiosities so that the stories of those "living the case" will be teased out' (2005, p 445). The assumption here is that the rich and detailed information gained from case research is of value in its own right. It is of such value as to render generalisations from case analysis totally redundant. This also includes the study of policy and administrative issues. According to Gomm et al (2000), analysing a single case in great detail will carry a certain amount of policy weight, providing the case is of sufficient importance both nationally and internationally. Detailed, 'single-site' case studies also have worth, argue Gomm et al, if they are evaluating whether important policy interventions meet their stated objectives.

This intrinsic style of case analysis – its sociologically informed foundations – helped to define the subject matter of early health policy studies; namely, the role of occupational groups within institutional settings and their role in providing health services. One early case study which adopted the intrinsic route towards investigating emergent forms of health provision was Harry Eckstein's historical analysis of the National Health Service (hereafter, NHS) – parochially titled *The English health service* (1958) (see Powell, Chapter Three). Although Bismarck's Germany was the first country to establish a national health system, the British NHS was a highly socialised model, one emulated by other western governments during the second half of the 20th century. The NHS is also regarded as an ideal example of redistributive, social-democratic state intervention. Essentially, Eckstein offers a detailed historical case study, covering, in the main, a 30-year period between 1920 and 1950. Eckstein's book is not the only historical 'case story' of the NHS. One contemporary effort is Rivett's *From cradle to grave* (1998). However, as a compelling, case-based documentation of an emerging health service, Eckstein's study has become something of a classic in its field. But the historical case study was, to an extent, atypical of health research during the early decades of the post-war era.

The aims of Eckstein's historical case study were two-fold. First, there was an attempt to examine how and why 'the Health Service came into being' (1958, p 4). He notes that a universal system of health provision, which covered Scotland and Wales as well as England, was formed, in theory, to address the distributive inequities of the old, privatised medical system that existed before 1946. Towards this, he explored the private medical health system and the nascent public health insurance scheme that were in place during the first decades of the twentieth century. For Eckstein, both were essentially 'philanthropic institutions, and in no subtle sense' (1958, p 18).

There was a second, potentially more significant, rationale underlying Eckstein's historical case study. He sought to conduct an appraisal of what, at the time of his study, was a 'socialised experiment'. Despite its embryonic form, Eckstein maintained that any evaluation of the health service was far from premature – the NHS was 10 years old, after all, by the time *The English health service* was published. Eckstein also justified this evaluation on the grounds that the service was unlikely to change a great deal in the foreseeable future – a forgivable lack of prescience in view of what was to come in the 1980s. Towards this, the third part of Eckstein's book-length case study focuses on the operation of the service, providing a notable before-and-after contrast with the earlier chapters covering the objectives of those who created the NHS. This detailed historical assessment revealed a cleavage between the ideals of the political intelligentsia that created the system and how it worked in practice. The British health service was formed, in the main, to deal with the inequities and distributive problems of the privatised medical care system that existed before universal health provision. The reality was some way removed from the practice: the health service benefited the comfortable middle classes more than the less healthy and socio-economically disadvantaged working classes. The creation of the health service was meant to rationalise and help coordinate medical provision; but the service, for Eckstein, became disjointed, with the Ministry of Health struggling to keep these various elements together (1958, p 241). Eckstein's historical case study also revealed that the policy objectives of the newly formed health service were being undercut by another source: professional practitioners. His findings showed how the NHS benefited the producer interests overseeing service provision, most notably doctors, more than it did the patients, who are there to be helped (1958, p 3). With a modicum of hindsight, he would also have understood how the power and influence of the medical professional would prove a major stumbling block for reformers and policy makers in the future. Such concerns – the unaccountable power of professionals – became increasingly prominent in American public administration research.

Interestingly, the 1960s witnessed a spate of intrinsic case studies of professional bureaucracies by American academics. These cases explored the capability of autonomous professional classes to shape public service institutions as 'professional bureaucracies' in their own image. Sudnow (1965) conducted a case study of the influence exercised by legal professionals in a public defender's office. Weatherly and Lipsky's (1977) case study focused on the Comprehensive Special Law of 1972 in Massachusetts and its effective sabotage at the hands of education professionals. Sociological case studies of health-based professional bureaucracies also appeared. In a sociological study of the medical profession, the American sociologist Anselm Strauss relied on detailed qualitative case analysis of various health professionals; in so doing he furnished research that had implications for health policy. A significant contribution in this respect is Strauss et al's (1964) study of the psychiatric profession – its ideologies and organisation of work. The authors also considered the treatment and fate of patients at the hands of the psychiatric profession. Here, two case studies were developed using team fieldwork, reliant, following the Chicago School tradition, on participant observation. The findings were reported across a mammoth 400-page book, one case study focusing on a private and the other on a state psychiatric hospital, both in the Chicago area. In these settings, policy makers would be interested to note that Strauss et al showed how the social structure of any psychiatric hospital is fashioned by professional practitioners. These cases – detailed and intrinsic in nature – went beneath the surface to understand micro-sociological processes at work. For instance, the researchers demonstrated how occupational ideologies and professional links with external communities, including those made up of expert and lay people, were largely responsible for shaping the objective social structures of the psychiatric hospitals under scrutiny (1964, pp 374–5).

Another notable contribution to the research literature on professional health bureaucracies was overseen by the sociologist Eliot Freidson. Again, his book-length analysis, *Patients' views of medical practice* (1961), centred around three case studies of medical practices in the Bronx. Two of the practices were funded by medical health insurance and the third one was a non-health insurance, solo medical practice. Freidson used the three case studies to explore the relationship between medical professionals and patients, comparing the experiences of patients across diverse organisational entities. The three case studies had a recurring theme:

> since [medical] practice is becoming subject to that external pressure in the course of becoming dependent upon it, it follows that medical culture becomes more and more insulated from patient culture; the amount of control that the patient can exercise over his fate in the consulting-room is being reduced. (Freidson, 1961, pp 226–7)

This story of professional interests trumping those of clients was depressingly familiar. It became a recurring tale for those reading about professional bureaucracies in the public sector. Methodologically, these insights were gained through a combination of semi-structured interviews and participant and non-participant observation. Freidson also employed statistical data generated through questionnaire surveys. The combination of qualitative and quantitative statistical data in this early study provided a foretaste of what in the future became methodological orthodoxy within the fields of public administration and health policy research – the multi-method case study.

The 'scientific' spectre of numbers: the case study and its methodological detractors

The case study's detractors were lurking in the hallowed corridors of academe. As the 1970s progressed, the methodological value of focusing on a specific case was increasingly questioned by social scientists, if not completely dismissed. Donald T. Campbell, the eminent American social scientist and methodologist, was an early, vocal opponent of the case study. His remarks are so cutting as to be worth reproducing here:

> Such studies have such a total absence of control as to be of almost no scientific value ... Any appearance of absolute knowledge, or

intrinsic knowledge about singular isolated objects, is found to be illusory upon analysis. (Campbell and Stanley, 1963, pp 6–7, cited in Flyvbjerg, 2006)

Doubts about the methodological integrity of the case study, in time, also began to surface in political science, a prime example being a 1971 article by Arend Lijphart on the methodological approach of comparative politics. As part of his analysis, Lijphart ranked different methods of political research according to their scientific rigour. How did the case study measure up? The experimental method is described as 'the most nearly ideal method for scientific explanation' (1971, p 683). Although the experimental method can rarely be used in political research, Lijphart listed the statistical method as a scientifically rigorous alternative to the experiment. This was followed by the comparative method, and finally came the case study. Lijphart holds definite reservations about the case method: 'The scientific status of the case study method is somewhat ambiguous, however, because science is a generalizing activity' (1971, p 691). The interpretative and highly descriptive case study that dominated American studies of public administration for much of the 1960s and early 1970s is problematic: 'the direct theoretical value of these case studies is nil, but this does not mean that they are altogether useless' (1971, p 691). He conceded that case studies can furnish the basis for establishing 'general propositions' or form the first step towards 'theory-building' in political science.

Lijphart's attempt to assess the value of the case study in terms of how far it measures up to the standards of scientific inquiry comes as no surprise. He was writing at a time when the academic study of politics was undergoing a professional transformation. The professionalisation of the academy during the course of the 20th century went hand in hand with the growing stature and influence of the scientific methodology. Research activities in the non-science disciplines adopted benchmarks informed by the natural sciences. The research process is less the preserve of the fumbling amateur than of the comprehensively trained professional whose approach is scrupulously methodical. For professionally trained academic political scientists, according to Ricci, 'there are the imperatives of scholarship, which demand that politics be studied scientifically, in accord with certain standards of precision and reliability' (1984, pp 24–5).

The growing stature of scientific methods in political science and cognate disciplines meant one thing: the growing dominance of statistical methods and the decline of narrative-based sociological case studies. The rising importance of quantitative methods is supported by evidence. A notable attempt to conduct a longitudinal survey of the methods employed by political scientists was carried out by Bennett et al (2003). Although the study focuses on American academic practitioners operating in the field of politics, it still proves to be a highly relevant and informative article concerning the fads and fashions of social science methodology. Their research involved coding 2,207 research journal articles obtained from the top seven rated American political science journals across the years 1975, 1985, 1998 and 1999–2000. The results proved informative as far as the reputation of the case study in politics and related research fields is concerned: the qualitative case study is in steep decline across most political science journals.

In the top seven multi-method politics journals, the proportion of research articles using case studies declined dramatically: from 12% in 1975, to 7% in 1985 and to a lowly 1% in 1999–2000 (Bennett et al, 2003, p 373). By the same token, there was a sharp increase in statistical analysis and formal modelling within the American political science community across the same period. A reasonable measure of the growing ascendancy of statistical methodologies concerns the number of such research articles published in journals considered to be disciplinary standard-bearers. For example, between 1965 and 1975, the proportion of articles using statistical methods in the *American Journal of Political Science Review* rose from 40% to 70%. At the same time, the proportion of articles employing case studies fell from 70% to under 10% in the same decade (George and Bennett, 2005, p 3). In fact, by 1998, about 90% of articles in the *American Journal of Political Science Review* were of a statistical nature and around 10% were case studies. Other high-ranking American journals in the politics field also witnessed a similar methodological bias, an asymmetry in the methodical approaches of researchers. In 1998, over 90% of the research articles in the acclaimed *Journal of Politics* employed statistical methods. Around 20% of articles in the same journal for 1998 were case study based (Bennett et al, 2003, p 376).

The methodological makeover of the case study in political and health policy research

The foregoing evidence would suggest that the case study in disciplines related to policy analysis and public administration is an irrelevance – at best. At worst, the case study seems to be a methodological relic that belongs to the past. Bennett et al mourn its waning popularity: 'The dearth of case study articles in *American Politics* ... demands attention as to whether an important approach has been woefully neglected' (2003, p 377). Despite their anxiety, Bennett and his colleagues acknowledge how political and policy scientists have redefined the case study. To paraphrase Mark Twain, it would be premature to start writing the policy case study's obituary. In actual fact, the case methodology in politically informed research did, chameleon-like, adapt to its professional and intellectual habitat. But it did so not under circumstances that many proponents of the case study would have chosen.

Instead of witnessing a progressive and pluralistic era in political research, where methodological integration became the norm, the opposite was true. American political research from the mid-1970s onwards was characterised by methodological fragmentation. Different areas of political interest migrated into distinct methodological communities. Bennett et al (2003) point to the study of comparative politics as an example of how sectarian methodical communities within the same sub-field of political analysis emerged around quantitative and qualitative approaches. Hence, the two leading journals in comparative politics have very distinct methodological profiles. *Comparative Political Studies* is dominated by formal modelling and statistical-based analysis, whereas *Comparative Politics* publishes articles dominated by qualitative approaches. For Bennett and his colleagues, these sectional methodological divisions lead to further insularity: authors, featured in either journal tend to cite previous articles from the very same journal that publishes their work. To an extent, the case method has been embroiled in this methodical *sectarianism*. Within public administration and policy analysis, the sociologically orientated case study, where deep description and ethnographic insights prevailed, has been supplanted. But what emerged in its place?

Case studies of public sector processes and institutions became increasingly sophisticated, the key trend being the way case research in policy-related fields of analysis combined qualitative data with other methods, namely, those that are statistical in nature. In the social sciences during the late 1970s and early 1980s, there was a sense that advocates of the case study were forced into a rapprochement with a quantitative modus operandi in order to deflect growing criticisms of the case study from positivist quarters. Yin, in reply to such criticisms, 'attempted to show that case studies can be conducted systematically' (1981, p 64). This is certainly borne out by evidence in political science. Bennett et al (2003), surveying articles using a multi-method approach, found that there was an increase in published studies combining case analysis with statistical methods: from 33% in 1975 to 50% in 2000.

Scholarly reflection on methodological design within the political and social sciences has made strong claims for the multi-method approach in case analysis. A key contribution is King et al's 1994 book, *Designing social inquiry*. The authors undertook to bring quantitative standards of scientific rigour to qualitative research methods. The authors outline several rules, which for case research involve following a simple formula: researchers should limit the range of variables but increase the number, and diversity, of cases being studied. As George and Bennett (2005) note, King et al's (1994) book was a major contribution to methodological debates within the discipline of political science. Indeed, the book stimulated analysis of the relationship between quantitative and qualitative methods, as well as reassessments of King et al's claims. Prominent among these reassessments is Brady and Collier's (2004) edited collection, *Rethinking social inquiry*. Brady and Collier, and other contributors to the edited collection, criticised *Designing social inquiry* for not adequately addressing the basic shortcomings of quantitative methods. In addition, they claim that King et al (1994) view qualitative methods exclusively through the prism of quantitative methods, failing to acknowledge their distinct strengths. Despite these criticisms, Brady and Collier still praised King et al's (1994) contribution to understanding the relationship between qualitative and quantitative methods. Even these critics did not question King et al's (1994) chief contention: that qualitative and quantitative methods should be combined in case research.

A noteworthy example in the health policy literature of this multi-dimensional, more systematic approach to case research was set out in a study by Alan Meyer (1982). Meyer's analysis was published not in book form but as an academic article, appearing in the most prestigious journal in the field of public administration – *Administrative Science Quarterly (ASQ)*. The research paper written by Meyer examined the way hospitals in the vicinity of San Francisco adapted to a major environmental jolt. The source of this external jolt was an unprecedented strike by doctors, protesting against a substantial increase in malpractice insurance premiums. The strike continued for a month and was supported by most surgeons and referral physicians. It meant that elective surgery declined, as did hospital admissions. The cash flows of various hospitals were affected, leaving them close to bankruptcy. Meyer observes the following about this unique event: 'The doctors' strike afforded a fortuitous natural experiment. By jolting hospitals away from their equilibria, it revealed properties that were not so visible during more tranquil periods' (1982, p 516).

To reveal these properties, Meyer relied on case analysis, but it was a methodological approach that followed King et al's (1994) blueprint for bringing scientific rigour to the case study: a high number of cases combined with a limited number of variables. In terms of cases, Meyer, studied a group of 19 hospitals, making a sample of organisations that were similar and geographically proximate. In these cases, a range of methods were employed, naturalistic observation being combined with quantitative and unobtrusive measures, as well as more in-depth analysis of three hospitals. In terms of causal explanations, the data was used to assess which particular variables were responsible for enabling some hospitals to adapt effectively when the strike action was suddenly instigated. Although adaptations were diverse, Meyer used both qualitative and quantitative data to analyse how four different variables determined effective organisational adaptation. The researchers compared: structures; organisational slack resources, including financial and human responses; antecedent strategies; and ideologies. Meyer found that ideological and strategic variables were better predictors of adaptations to external jolts than were structural variables or measures of organisational slack (1982, p 534). Similar progress towards multi-method forms of case analysis came to the fore in the UK. Indeed, one of the key case studies of the modern UK health system emulated Meyer's study of strategic change, but in the context of policy jolts emanating from central government reforms.

The UK health policy case study, and methodological pluralism

What has been the fate of the health policy study in the UK? In the general field of policy studies and public administration, the spectre of book-length case analyses based on a single episode or a limited range of organisations and groups is a rarity. The approach to case analysis synonymous with Strauss or Freidson is the exception rather than the rule in the British academic firmament. In the policy field, it is now more common for researchers to rely on small-scale, localised and highly episodic case studies. Take, for instance, Maynard's (1975) overview of healthcare in the European Community, made up of nine national case studies from Denmark to Italy. There is a professional rationale at work here. The modern pressure to publish or perish in academia has meant that academics opt for increasing specialisation in their approach to knowledge production. Ricci, in *The tragedy of political science*, makes an interesting observation about specialisation in political science:

> There is ... a propensity constantly to refashion the scope of political science into smaller and smaller realms of expertise, so that some scholars can quickly stand forth as patently competent with regard to subjects that other scholars have somehow overlooked. (Ricci, 1984, pp 221–2)

Ricci's observations apply to any academic discipline. The increased parcelling of knowledge has methodological implications: the multiplication of specialisms is often matched by the proliferation of research techniques. The case study itself has not been immune to this spiralling specialisation. The case study can be used as an 'ontological meat slicer'. It offers a quick and easy way of using empirical data to furnish 'new' and 'novel' research publications.

Despite the pragmatic uses and abuses to which the case study has been subjected, it still retains a certain significance in its own right. Its continued methodological import is evident in ongoing discussions among British social scientists about the reliability and veracity of the case study. The key disagreement centres on the issue of generalisation; or more specifically, on the inability to generalise to a larger population from a single or limited range of cases. Despite notable criticisms, these discussions have also given intellectual and methodological ballast to the case study. In one prominent contribution to the UK debate, Hammersley (1992) outlines how researchers often employ methodological stratagems, and the occasional sleight of hand, to make empirical generalisations from single cases. One such methodological strategy is to claim that the particular microscopic case under investigation is typical of some larger aggregate (Hammersley, 1992, p 86). For Flyvbjerg (2006), writing from a European perspective, those who criticise the use of case studies for lack of rigour, for selling short the hypothetico-deductive model, misunderstand case analysis, overplaying the inability of case analysts to generalise from their findings. Critics also misunderstand the special place of case research in the natural sciences. Major breakthroughs in the natural sciences have relied upon carefully chosen cases for experiments. Flyvbjerg points to the fact that Galileo's bold rejection of Aristotle's dominant ideas on gravity, which had dominated for over two millennia, was not based on large, random samples (2006, p 225). Rather, the alternative theory of gravity offered by Galileo relied on a single experiment – or a case experiment. Other major breakthroughs in physics by the likes of Newton, Einstein and Bohr relied on studies of the specific or the singular.

The case study's methodological staying power and resilience is evident within the academic literature on UK health policy. The trajectory of the health case study in the UK has been shaped, and even given a lease of life, by health service reforms. One prominent example, featured in this collection (see Chapter Twelve, by Hughes), is David Hunter's (1980) *Coping with uncertainty: Policy and politics in the National Health Service*. This is another familiar tale of case research capturing the reform-induced vicissitudes of public health provision. Hunter's book presents a case analysis of resource allocation in two Scottish health boards. The cases were studied during the course of two financial years, from 1975 and 1977, a period that coincided with major central government restructuring and reform of the health service. To explore the politics of health resource allocation, Hunter applied phenomenological spin to mainstream policy theories as a way of understanding administrative decision making. As part of this methodological approach, Hunter's case studies were in-depth and anthropological in their approach, prioritising the voices and views of those practitioners being researched. This methodological modus operandi is reminiscent of the intrinsic case study favoured by American sociologists like Anselm Strauss. The Chicago School tradition, it seems, still had its champions.

Following Hunter's classic case study, there has been no shortage of pressures for change. The NHS, to use Meyer's earlier term, has, during the past 20 years, faced sustained environmental jolts, stemming from central government endeavours to reform the service. 'In the 1980s a new concept of radical shock, where the scale of the repetitive application of a single set of policy objectives, emerged as significant' (Ferlie et al, 1996, p 37). The

Conservative governments of Margaret Thatcher in the 1980s undertook a radical overhaul of the public sector in a bid to roll back the state and render that which was left more efficient and sensitive to consumer pressures. The health service, because of its size, vested professional interests and perceived inefficiencies, became a prime target for a new public management makeover.

Such is the leviathan-like edifice that is the UK health service that the case study became a useful methodological strategy for putting the Conservative reforms of the NHS under the policy microscope. The Nuffield Hospital Trust in the early 1990s supported and published case research of health reforms. One Nuffield-sponsored project was King's (1991) research of the care in the community initiative, a study that focused on the process by which psychiatric patients in Exeter were transferred from institutional settings to community care settings. However, the Nuffield-sponsored case studies of greatest interest were those examining the impact of new public management reforms on the health service. Paton and Bach's (1990) Nuffield-published book, containing six separate case studies, captured a health system in transition. According to Paton and Bach, the Thatcher-led Conservative governments, fuelled by a New Right ideology, with its valorisation of the market, adopted two strategies in reforming the health service during the 1980s (1990, pp 4–8). First, emphasis was placed on local hospital managers, borrowing from private sector techniques and personnel, to act as harbingers of efficiency and transparency. This was the objective of the Griffiths Inquiry Report of 1983 (see Macfarlane et al, Chapter Nine). Second, the Conservative governments used successive legislative interventions to prescribe market-led changes within the health service. Paton and Bach used case examples of specific locations and areas of health policy to understand the extent to which these Conservative health reforms reshaped medical services. Choosing a topic for case analysis was also guided by specific criteria: cases had to be relevant to management personnel over time and not just examples of in-vogue innovations; topics were chosen on the basis of whether they had resulted in significant change, including both constructive or disruptive changes; topics were also chosen to highlight the great diversity of policy making within the health sector over time.

The authors used largely thick, narrative description. This was the type of research approach to case study work associated with the intrinsic, sociological tradition. As noted, the case studies were conducted across different locations and policy areas – the authors did not stick to the single case or site, which was popular among policy researchers in the 1960s. Indeed, Paton and Bach embraced two types of research strategy when it came to developing their health policy case studies (Paton and Bach, 1990, pp 10–11). First, they devised organisational and behavioural case studies to trace the fate of a local or national policy initiative over time. The purpose behind this case approach is clear: to identify the key actors and decision-making processes behind policy initiatives, as well as the main interest affected by policies. For instance, the 'Northville' case study examined the planning of new acute services, while the Greenbelt case study was used to trace the origins and development of competitive tendering in the NHS. The second approach used by Paton and Bach was the analytical case study. Analytical cases emphasised micro-management problems, especially those concerning resources, and the solutions devised at a local level to deal with such issues. For instance, the Riverside case examined how local health authority managers responded to the demands of hospital closures and restructuring. My own case analysis of the Tomlinson reorganisation of London's health services, though not sponsored by the Nuffield Trust, was a companion piece to the Riverside case study (see Marinetto, 1999).

Clearly, there now exists something of a body of literature on case research tracing the public management health policy experiments since the 1980s. The case studies, though, have been small in scale and have been highly localised. Paton and Bach's book typifies the dominant approach to health policy research. Their book is made up of a diverse range of self-contained, 'within case studies', set in various locations – a conscious strategy by the authors in order to highlight the variety of health policies that had mushroomed over the course of the 1980s. However, there was one prominent exception to the self-contained, micro-case study rule. And this was Pettigrew et al's (1992) *Shaping strategic change*, central to which are 11 case studies (Pettigrew et al, 1992, p 301) (see Locock and Dopson, Chapter Thirteen). Each of the 11 cases threw a spotlight on different types of health service provision and policy change, the underlying research aim being to understand why there is substantial variability in the way general management can bring about constrictive change in particular circumstances but not in others. Unlike the within case approach of Paton and Bach, these studies were longitudinal in scope, allowing the authors to make cross-case comparisons:

> A case study methodology has been used, although one which is more longitudinal, processual and comparative in nature than conventional single case work. (Pettigrew et al, 1992, p 4)

The case approach in Pettigrew et al's study has a greater affinity with Meyer's multi-dimensional and more systematic case methodology than Paton and Bach's self-contained narrative style. The 11 cases were constructed around 400 interviews, observations, archival sources and secondary statistics. The authors comment on the rationale for drawing upon a diverse range of sources:

The design choice in this study has been to conduct intensive analyses of relatively few cases, rather than a more superficial analysis of a larger number. Such are the complexities of … strategic change issues … that such superficial analyses would be in danger of missing key components of the explanation. (Pettigrew et al, 1992, p 301)

Conclusion: the extended case study and methodological pluralism

What should be the way forward for case research, particularly in the field of health policy? The way Paton and Bach and Pettigrew respectively handled case methodology is valid and has a place in case-led research of health policy. This conclusion is not a gross example of intellectual fence sitting. Far from it. Rather, here I am echoing George and Bennett's (2005) ideas concerning the future of the case study in the social sciences. In their contribution to the ongoing methodological debate about the case study, they maintain that the progress, and continued vitality, of case research can be achieved only through methodological pluralism. They emphasise the complementarity between quantitative and qualitative research and indicate how researchers can draw on the strengths of both, rather than subsuming case analysis under quantitative style methods. It is interesting that Pettigrew et al's case studies contain little in the way of number crunching. But the depth of empirical material opened up the research to generalisations and theory development. There should be room for such an in-depth, longitudinal form of case research, which ultimately gives priority to a variety of qualitative data. There should certainly be a place in the health policy field for what Burawoy (2009) terms extended case analysis. The question is whether professional demands and resource constraints would allow such extended methodological pluralism. Or whether there will be a retreat to type: to the small, localised and self-contained health case study. It would be worth finishing this introduction with a quote from one of the contributing authors to this collection. Hughes (in Chapter Twelve) makes a telling observation about the status of David Hunter's 1970s' research as compared to the ongoing *progress* of case research: 'As one of the few studies of NHS management work that utilises in-depth case studies, involving ongoing engagement with subjects over a substantial time period, Hunter's study provides an attractive alternative model to the small-scale case studies often completed today.'

References

Allison, G.T. (1971) *Essence of decision: Explaining the Cuban missile crisis*, New York: Harper Collins.

Barnes, L.B., Hansen, A.J. and Christensen, C.R. (1994) *Teaching and the case method*, Boston, MA: Harvard Business School Press.

Bennett, A., Barth, A. and Rutherford, K.R. (2003) 'Do we preach what we practice? A survey of methods in political science journals and curricula', *PS: Political Science and Politics*, vol 36, no 3, pp 373–78.

Brady, H.E. and Collier, D. (2004) *Rethinking social inquiry: Diverse tools, shared standard*, Lanham, MD: Rowman & Littlefield.

Burawoy, M. (2009) *The extended case method: Four countries, four decades, four great transformations, and one theoretical tradition*, Berkeley, CA and London: University of California Press.

Campbell, D.T. and Stanley, J.C. (1963) *Experimental and quasi-experimental designs for research*, Chicago, IL: Rand McNally.

Derthick, M. (1972), *New towns in-town: Why a federal programme failed*, Washington, DC: Urban Institute.

Eckstein, H. (1958) *The English health service: Its origins, structure, and achievements*, Cambridge, MA: Harvard University Press.

Ferlie, E., Ashburner, L., Fitzgerald, L. and Pettigrew, A. (1996) *The new public management in action*, Oxford: Oxford University Press.

Flyvbjerg, B. (2006) 'Five misunderstandings about case-study research', *Qualitative Inquiry*, vol 12, no 2, pp 219–45.

Freidson, E. (1961) *Patients' views of medical practice: A study of subscribers to a prepaid medical plan in the Bronx*, New York: Russell Sage Foundation.

George, A.L. and Bennett, A. (2005) *Case studies and theory development in the social sciences*, London: MIT Press.

Gerring, J. (2004) 'What is a case study and what is it good for?', *American Political Science Review*, vol 98, no 2, pp 341–54.

Gerring, J. (2007) *Case study research: Principles and practices*, Cambridge: Cambridge University Press.

Gomm, R., Hammersley, M. and Foster, P. (2000) 'Case study and generalization', in R. Gomm, M. Hammersley and P. Foster (eds), *Case study method: Key issues, key texts*, London: SAGE.

Hammersley, M. (1992) *What's wrong with ethnography? Methodological explorations*, London and New York: Routledge.

Heclo, H. and Wildavsky, A. (1974) *The private government of public money: Community and policy inside British politics*, London: Macmillan.

Herring, P. (1940) *Presidential leadership: The political relations of Congress and the chief executive*, New York: Farrar and Rhinehart.

Hunter, D. (1980) *Coping with uncertainty: Policy and politics in the National Health Service*, Letchworth: Research Studies Press.

King, D. (1991) *Moving on from hospitals to community care: A case study of change in Exeter*, London: Nuffield Provincial Hospitals Trust.

King, G., Keohane, R.O. and Verba, S. (1994) *Designing social inquiry: Scientific inference in qualitative research*, Princeton, NJ: Princeton University Press.

Lijphart, A. (1971) 'Comparative politics and the comparative method', *American Political Science Review*, vol 65, no 3, pp 682–93.

Marinetto, M. (1999) *Studies of the policy process: A case analysis*, London: Prentice Hall.

Maynard, A. (1975) *Health care in the European Community*, London: Croom Helm.

Meyer, A.D. (1982) 'Adapting to environmental jolts', *Administrative Science Quarterly*, vol 27, no 4, pp 515–37.

Mogey, J.M. (1955) 'The contribution of Frédéric Le Play to family research', *Marriage and Family Living*, vol 17, no 4, pp 310–15.

Neustadt, R.E. and Fineberg, H.E. (1978) *The swine flu affair: Decision-making on a slippery disease*, Washington, DC: Government Printing Office.

Paton, C. and Bach, S. (1990) *Case studies in health policy and management*, London: Nuffield Provincial Hospitals Trust.

Pettigrew, A.M., Ferlie, E. and McKee, L. (1992) *Shaping strategic change: Making change in large organizations: The case of the National Health Service*, London: Sage.

Pressman, J.L. and Wildavsky, A.B. (1973) *Implementation*, Berkeley, CA: University of California Press.

Putnam, R.D. (1993) *Making democracy work: Civic traditions in modern Italy*, Princeton, NJ: Princeton University Press.

Ricci, D.M. (1984) *The tragedy of political science: Politics, scholarship, and democracy*, New Haven, CT: Yale University Press.

Rivett, G. (1998) *From cradle to grave: Fifty years of the NHS*, London: King's Fund.

Schattschneider, E.E. (1935) *Politics, pressures and the tariff: A study of free private enterprise in pressure politics, as shown in the 1929–1930 revision of the tariff*, New York: Prentice-Hall.

Stake, R.E. (2005) 'Qualitative case studies', in N.K. Denzin and Y.S. Lincoln (eds), *The Sage handbook of qualitative research*, 3rd edn, Thousand Oaks, CA: Sage, pp 443–66.

Stein, H. (1952) *Public administration and policy developments: A case book*, New York: Harcourt, Brace and Company.

Strauss, A., Schatzman, L., Bucher, R., Ehrlich, D. and Sabshin, M. (1964) *Psychiatric ideologies and institutions*, London: Collier-Macmillan/Free Press.

Sudnow, D. (1965) 'Normal crimes: sociological features of the penal code in a public defender's office', *Social Problems*, vol 12, no 3, pp 255–76.

van Wynsberghe, R. and Khan, S. (2007) 'Redefining case study', *International Journal of Qualitative Methods*, vol 6, no 2, pp 80–93.

Weatherly, R. and Lipsky, M. (1977), 'Street-level bureaucrats and institutional innovation: implementing special education reform', *Harvard Educational Review*, vol 47, no 2, pp 171–97.

Yanow, D., Schwartz-Shea, P. and Freitas, M.J. (2010) 'Case study in political science', in A.J. Mills, G. Duperos and E. Wiebe (eds) *Encyclopaedia of case study research*, Thousand Oaks, CA: Sage Publications.

Yin, R.K. (1981) 'The case study crisis: some answers', *Administrative Science Quarterly*, vol 26, no 1, pp 58–65.

Part Two

Creation, consolidation and disillusion (1948–1980s)

The first foray into our case studies covers the period from the inception of the NHS in 1948 until the 1980s. The starting point is, naturally, the creation of the NHS. We do not consider the political or organisational antecedents of the NHS; we take these for granted in our analysis. (For analysis of pre-NHS healthcare, see Powell, 1997, chs 2–3.) However, the end-point is less clear cut. The 1980s reflected the erosion of the post-war welfare state consensus and the emergence of 'new public management'. A specific date is somewhat arbitrary, though the 1979 general election (bringing Margaret Thatcher into power) is perhaps the most obvious point.

This period is marked by relative stability; for example, the first major reorganisation was 26 years after the NHS's inception, in 1974. Certainly, the initial periods of optimism gave way to disillusion as the challenges that were to beset the NHS ever since became noticeably manifest. The pattern described in Klein's (2010) analogy of the NHS 'opera' – actors shift around the stage as thematic melodies recur – became apparent.

The six chapters in this section address the whole of the period covered by the section. Martin Powell (Chapter Three) charts the creation of the NHS in terms of some of the leading commentaries on it, noting their different interpretations. The chapters by John Mohan (Chapter Four) and Ian Greener (Chapter Five) explore two iconic policies of the 1960s and 1970s – the Hospital Plan and NHS 'pay beds' respectively. They address these issues from different perspectives – from commentaries on the Plan and from Klein's (1979) analysis – but both illustrate the persistent challenges of the health policy process.

The following two chapters, by Joan Higgins (Chapter Six) and Justin Keen (Chapter Seven), can be read together in the sense that they address the origins of the patient safety movement. Higgins draws on John Martin's (1984) study of 'Hospitals in trouble', which examined the scandals of the long-stay institutions from the 1960s onwards. Keen takes Perrow's (1999) study of the nuclear plant at Three Mile Island in the US to examine the ways his ideas filtered into the healthcare sector, showing their enduring influence upon the development of patient safety.

Finally, Peckham and Willmott (Chapter Eight) examine Alford's (1975) classic study of healthcare interest groups. Though he wrote about New York healthcare in the 1970s, Alford's analysis has been applied to the NHS. Indeed, Peckham and Willmott consider it especially relevant nearly 40 years later.

References

Alford, R. (1975) *Health care politics: Ideological and interest group barriers to reform*, London: University of Chicago Press.

Klein, R. (1979) 'Ideology, class and the National Health Service', *Journal of Health Politics, Policy and Law*, vol 4, no 3, pp 464–90.

Klein, R. (2010) *The new politics of the NHS: From creation to re-invention*, 6th edn, Oxford: Radcliffe Publishing.

Martin, J.P. (1984) *Hospitals in trouble*, Oxford: Basil Blackwell.

Perrow, C. (1999) *Normal accidents: Living with high risk technologies*, Princeton, NJ: Princeton University Press.

Powell, M. (1997) *Evaluating the National Health Service*, Buckingham: Open University Press.

three

NHS birthing pains

Martin Powell

Introduction

This chapter focuses on the creation of the NHS. It examines contributions from different times, perspectives, academic disciplines and approaches that yield some different conclusions. However, the extent to which all these contributions are 'case studies' is not fully clear. The definition of a case study is far from certain, and case studies come in all shapes and sizes (Yin, 2009, see also Chapters One and Two). Yin (2009, pp 8–14) sets out three conditions of the case study method: the type of research questions used, the extent of control that an investigator has over actual behavioural events, and the degree of focus on contemporary as opposed to historical events. The case study is the preferred method when a 'how' or 'why' question is being asked about a contemporary set of events over which the investigator has little or no control (Yin, 2009, p 13). Although Yin argues that there are not sharp boundaries between different methods and that there are large overlaps among them (p 8), he insists that the case study differs from history in that it focuses on contemporary events (p 11). Taken to extremes, Yin's argument that case studies cannot be historical is bizarre, given that all case studies are historical because, the moment after an event occurs, it becomes 'historical'. However, he argues that the case study relies on many of the same techniques as a history but adds two sources of evidence not usually included in the historian's repertoire: direct observation of events being studied and interviews of the persons involved in the events. Although case studies and histories can overlap, the case study's unique strength is its ability to deal with a full variety of evidence – documents, artefacts, interviews and observations – beyond what might be available in a conventional historical study (Yin, 2009, p 11).

Yin (2009, pp 185–90) sets out the criteria of an 'exemplary case study': it must be significant, complete, consider alternative perspectives, display sufficient evidence and be composed in an engaging manner. The creation of the National Health Service (NHS) appears to satisfy most of these criteria. Most would agree that the creation of the NHS was 'significant' (p 185). Completeness can be characterised in at least three ways. First, the complete case is one in which the boundaries of the case are given explicit attention. Time intervals and spatial boundaries are considered, with (as we shall see below) some writers arguing that the NHS has longer or shorter historical roots, but most writers focus on the English NHS, pointing out that Scotland had different legislation. Second, the investigator should expend exhaustive effort in collecting the relevant evidence, with critical pieces (for example, those representing rival propositions) receiving 'complete' attention. While some historians do not explicitly consider rival propositions, the vast majority are keen to include all sources and 'fillet' the archives, with extensive footnotes being seen as a badge of honour. Third, studies should not be ended prematurely on account of resource constraints. This is more difficult to establish, although my impression is that few historians are likely to 'cut corners' in this way. Historians do not tend to explicitly consider rival theoretical propositions, although the narrative generally considers differing perspectives. Similarly, most historical studies tend to display sufficient evidence. Finally, the issue of whether the case study was composed in an 'engaging manner' is surely in the eye of the reader.

The 'case' might be one author's study (meaning that we have many cases) or the creation of the NHS (meaning that we have one case). Marinetto (Chapter Two) regards Eckstein (1958) as a detailed historical case study. Willcocks (1967) regards his study of the creation of the NHS as a 'case study'. The one major issue of whether historical policy studies can be case studies concerns the question of complete evidence. Studies can and do use interviews (for example, Berridge, 1996) and witness seminars (for example, Evans and Knight, 2006). However, contemporary history studies that conduct interviews generally cannot access official documents under the '30 year rule', although this is changing under the influence of freedom of information legislation. For example, Berridge (1996, pp 2–3) did not have access to official documents. In other words, no individual policy history can be 'complete' because accounts focusing on older issues cannot draw on interviews (the participants are no longer able to be interviewed) and accounts focusing on more recent issues cannot draw on full official documentation. However, while individual 'cases' cannot be complete, the cumulative 'case' of the creation of the NHS can draw on older studies with interviews and on more recent studies that draw on The National Archives. As we will see below, as the sources on the creation of the NHS change, there are some shifts in interpretations and conclusions. Second, it is not clear whether the 'creation' of the NHS focuses on philosophy, principles or aims of the service, or on the initial structure, or on the institutional bricks and mortar that imperfectly captured those aims. There is a tendency to focus on decisions that were taken, and the 'Bevan template' is often examined: Nye would or would not approve of this new policy (cf Berridge, 2008, 2010). However, it is important to examine decisions that were not made, or roads that were not taken (cf Powell, 1997).

The remainder of the chapter provides a brief review of the major book studies of the creation of the NHS in chronological order, before discussing different general approaches, themes (implicit and explicit) theories and conclusions.

Review of studies

This section briefly introduces the selected studies, books that either focus on the creation of the NHS or cover it in some detail as part of their wider content. It then critically examines the accounts, comparing sources, conclusions and explanations (cf Gorsky, 2008).

The studies are varied in a number of ways (Table 3.1). First, they cover a wide time-scale, from the first study by Ross (1952), which appeared within five years of the 'Appointed Day', to Rintala's study (2003), which was published after the NHS's 50th birthday. Second, the writers include American visitors (such as the early studies by Eckstein, Gemmill and Lindsey) as well as many UK authors. Some writers (such as Honigsbaum, Webster and Rintala) are historians. Others are political scientists (Eckstein), social policy academics (Abel-Smith, Willcocks, Klein) and biographers (Foot, Campbell). Rivett (1998) is a former GP and Deputy Chief Medical Officer. Pater (1981) was a Principal at the Ministry of Health at the time of the creation of the NHS. However, he notes that 'the account is not based on reminisence' (p xi), and stresses that his book was the first to be based on Public Record Office archives (but see Honigsbaum, 1989). Navarro (1978) and Doyal (1979) set out to provide Marxist accounts of health policy.

Sources

One of the first disagreements concerns 'standard' sources. According to Klein (2006, p 21, note), in many ways the best account remains Eckstein's (1958). At the time of its writing, government documents were not accessible and the book is perhaps biased by the sources that were available: Eckstein's exclusive emphasis on the central role of the medical profession reflects the fact that the main sources available were the published accounts of negotiations in the medical press. However, Campbell (1994, p 153) claims that Pater's is the most authoritative history of the creation of the NHS, while Stewart (1999) writes that 'the standard and best account of the creation of the NHS is Webster's' (p 205, note). On the other hand, some accounts, such as Gemmill's (1960) and Grimes' (1991), are rarely cited, and there has been limited use of sources such as Dunn (1952) on the emergency medical services (EMS).

There is a major division between the later accounts, which were able to incorporate the records in the Public Records Office (PRO)/The National

Table 3.1: Studies of the creation of the NHS

	Primary sources	Main secondary sources	Conclusions	Explanations
Ross (1952)	Limited: *Hansard*, medical press and newspapers		Consensus, evolution	
Eckstein (1958)	*BMJ*, *Hansard*, newspapers	Titmuss (1950)	EMS medical profession, non-ideological	Path dependency
Gemmill (1960)	Limited: *BMJ*, *Lancet*	Titmuss (1950), Ross (1952)	Progression, consensus	Path dependency
Lindsey (1962)	*BMJ*, *Lancet*, newspapers, *Hansard*	Ross (1952), Eckstein (1958)	Evolution, consensus, medical reports, war, EMS	
Abel-Smith (1964)	Many: *BMJ*, *Lancet*, hospital, *Hansard*	Titmuss (1950), Eckstein (1958), Lindsey (1962)		
Stevens (1966)	*BMJ*, *Lancet*, interviews	Eckstein (1958), Eckstein (1960), Lindsey (1962), Abel-Smith (1964)		Medical profession; little on conflict
Willcocks (1967)	*BMJ*	Titmuss (1950), Ross (1952), Eckstein (1958), Eckstein (1960), Lindsey (1962), Abel-Smith (1964)	EMS, Beveridge Report, medical profession, minimises Bevan	Pressure groups
Forsyth (1973 [1966])	Limited	Eckstein (1958)	Conflict	Pressure groups
Foot (1975)	*BMJ*, *Lancet*, *Hansard*, interviews, newspapers	Eckstein (1958), Eckstein (1960), Lindsey (1962)	Bevan's battle with doctors	'Great men': Bevan
Navarro (1978)	Limited	Eckstein (1958), Abel-Smith (1964), Stevens (1966), Willcocks (1967), Forsyth (1973)	Doctors as capitalist class, war, minimises Bevan, and Beveridge	Class conflict/ Marxism
Honigsbaum (1979)	Public Record Office: Cabinet, Ministry of Health, *BMJ*	Titmuss (1950), Ross (1952), Eckstein (1958), Lindsey (1962), Abel-Smith (1964), Stevens (1966), Willcocks (1967)		
Campbell (1994 [1987])	Public Record Office: Cabinet, *Hansard*, newspapers, *BMJ*, Attlee Papers	Eckstein (1958), Eckstein (1960), Abel-Smith (1964), Foot (1975), Pater (1981), Klein (2006 [1983])		
Pater (1981)	Public Record Office: Cabinet, Ministry of Health, medical archives, *Hansard*, *BMJ*, *Lancet*, newspapers	Limited: Eckstein (1958), Eckstein (1960), Foot (1975)		

(continued)

Table 3.1 (continued)

	Primary sources	Main secondary sources	Conclusions	Explanations
Klein (2006 [1983])	Public Record Office: Cabinet, Ministry of Health, *Hansard*, interviews	Eckstein (1958), Abel-Smith (1964), Willcocks (1967), Foot (1975), Godber (1975), Honigsbaum (1979), Pater (1981)		
Webster (1988)	Extensive National Archives research, medical and nursing journals	Extensive	The decisive impact of Bevan	Impact of Second World War, Bevan, political conflict, medical pressure
Rivett (1998)	Herbert (1939), hospital surveys, medical and nursing journals, Taylor (1981), Godber (1988)			
Webster (2002)	PEP (1937), hospital surveys, command papers, National Archives: Cabinet	Titmuss (1950), Pater (1981)	The decisive impact of Bevan	Impact of Second World War, Bevan, political conflict, medical pressure
Rintala (2003)	Attlee, Bevan, Horder, Moran, Hill, Macnalty, Morrison material, Royal College of Physicians (RCP), medical books and journals, no National Archives research	Abel-Smith (1964), Eckstein (1960), Foot (1975), Campbell (1987), Forsyth (1973 [1966]), Fox (1986), Gemmill (1960), Goodman (1970), Grimes (1991), Hollingsworth (1986), Honigsbaum (1979, 1989), Klein (1983), Lindsey (1962), Pater (1981), Rivett (1986)	Politicians prescribe, doctors differ, disciples decide. Little on civil service. Alliance between Lord Moran and Bevan	Examines interpretations of national consensus, Labour Party and Bevan

Archives (TNA), and the early accounts, which relied heavily on the medical press. Pater (1981) writes that his book was the first to be based on PRO records, but Honigsbaum (1989) notes that the PRO has changed since Pater. For the first time, it is possible to obtain a fairly complete picture of what went on within the portals of government. Moreover, medical files were largely available. Within the world of consultants, only the internal debates that took place in the Royal College of Surgeons remain obscure (Honigsbaum, p xi).

Some studies included interviews (Lindsey, Stevens, Foot, Klein). Few accounts are comprehensive, tending to devote little attention to sources such as *Hansard* (but see, for example, Pater, 1981). The House of Commons debates are 'especially disappointing', the debates in the House of Lords between Horder and Moran being 'much livelier' (Rintala, 2003, p 133). Reports tend to focus on well-defined issues, such as contrasting Bevan's performance with that of Conservative spokespersons (for example, Webster, 1988, 2002), but few focus on criticism of Bevan's proposals from his own side, from Fred Messer (see Powell, 1997). Few accounts cover the Standing Committee on the NHS Bill (but see Pater, 1981, Powell, 1997). Even after the PRO/TNA sources become available, they are mined selectively, with a focus on the retreat from early radical Coalition proposals. The Labour Cabinet discussion tends to receive little attention. Webster (2002, p 15) argues that Cabinet deliberations were little more than cursory, except on the sole issue of hospital nationalisation. According to Honigsbaum (1989, p 217), Bevan's method was to hold conferences and solicit views: if civil servants wanted to influence him, they had to do so openly. This explains why there are so few position papers in the PRO for the period after July 1945.

Significance

One of the first points of disagreement is on the significance of the NHS, the issue of evolution or revolution and the 'implementation gap' between original and final plans. Navarro (1978, pp 45–7) writes that the importance of the Beveridge Report and Bevan has been exaggerated. Bevan missed the opportunity to regionalise and to integrate the entire hospital sector. Regarding the creation of the NHS as a revolutionary step is a 'hyperbole': the NHS represented an extension of National Health Insurance (NHI) to the entire population – not a minor step, but hardly a revolutionary one. Honigsbaum (1989, pp 217–18) writes that Bevan had the good fortune to spearhead a movement that already had force. Willcocks (1967, p 28) writes that Bevan introduced little that was new, the only major point being the nationalisation of the hospitals, which is a little like saying that Orson Welles appears for only a few minutes as Harry Lime in *The Third Man*. Klein (2006, p 13) argues that after the election of the 1945 Labour government, Bevan's scheme 'represented one dramatic break with the immediate past – to the extent that it represented a return to MacNalty's 1939 proposal'. According to Willcocks (1967, p 104), Bevan was less of an innovator than he is often credited with being: his plan came at the end, albeit the important and conclusive end, of a series of earlier plans. He 'created' the NHS 'but his debts to what went before were enormous'. Similarly, Campbell (1994, p 165) states that too much can be claimed for Bevan. Viewing the NHS as his personal creation is a 'distortion of the long and cumulative process by which the Service came into existence in 1948'. Klein (2006, p 17) states that, in many ways, Bevan's scheme was less radical for general practice than the 1944 White Paper. For example, GPs would remain independent contractors rather than salaried employees, but the buying and selling of practices would cease – 'the only point on which Bevan was more radical than the 1944 White Paper'. Similarly, Campbell (1994, p 177) writes that Bevan nationalised the hospitals while leaving the GP service essentially undisturbed.

It has been claimed that the significance of the NHS was reduced by concessions, but commentators stress different concessions. Webster (2002, p 11) points to the concessions of the Coalition government, with the 'dilution' of the 1944 White Paper representing a 'major retreat'. However, other commentators point to Bevan's concessions. Klein (2006, pp 15–16) points out that concessions were given to the medical profession, such as merit awards, private practice and special status for Teaching Hospitals. Campbell (1994, p 174) writes that, during the 18 months to the 'Appointed Day', Bevan was obliged to make concession after concession to the doctors. Honigsbaum (1989, p 96) states that Bevan's concessions were quick to come. Rivett (1998, pp 28, 31) writes that in the final round of negotiation Bevan accepted key demands from the doctors. Although Bevan might have considered the NHS as pure socialism, it was closer to impure liberalism, in that doctors and local administrations enjoyed considerable freedom.

Explanation

A number of explanations of the NHS have been advanced in terms of who and how.

Who?

Early accounts tend to stress the importance of the doctors. According to Eckstein (1958, pp 2–4), the legislation of 1946 culminated a long preparatory process that had lasted almost three decades and in which socialists did not in any sense play the leading part. The NHS Act was a 'doctor's measure' much more than a 'patient's measure', with the leading role played by members of the medical profession rather than by doctrinaire politicians of the left. Of all the people and organisations articulately concerned with medical reform before the war, the socialists were the last and, in some ways, the most half hearted in the field (Eckstein, 1958, p x). Lindsey (1962) claims that a series of important reports between the wars on the coordination and improvement of medical facilities contain most of the basic ideas that were to shape the framework of the NHS. The medical profession played the most enlightened role of all in many of its proposals. The British Medical Association (BMA) reports of 1938 and 1942 were 'classic examples of impartiality, constituting the high-water mark of progressive thought for that organisation' (pp 25–6). 'Very little found its way into the NHS Act of 1946 that had not been recommended or discussed by the earlier reports and studies' (Lindsey, 1962, p 31). Similarly, Rintala (2003, pp 48–9) writes that health policy was not a high priority for Labour in the inter-war period. The 1943 document 'National Service for Health' was by far the most impressive Labour Party statement about health policy before 1945, but it 'appears to have been virtually ignored by all of its possible audiences, including the Labour Party' (but see Stewart, 1999). Honigsbaum (1989, pp 217–18) writes that the NHS was the result of a complex of forces. The civil service played no small part in the development of the NHS, but in the end no one within the civil service could match the influence of those outside. The doctors – led by Hill and Moran – all but imposed their will on the department. Willcocks (1967, pp 102–3) writes that there is no doubt whatever that the *Lancet* was right when it said in 1946 that the Act derived 'more from the long discussion between the profession and the Ministry of Health than it does from any doctrinaire idea of the Minister's party'. Rivett (1998, p 29) cites a *BMJ* editorial in 1960, on Bevan's death, that claimed that the medical profession rather than Bevan was the principal architect of the NHS. Eckstein (1958, p 136) writes that it is generally supposed that credit for the NHS belongs to all the major parties in equal measure. 'This is substantially, but not quite, correct' (Eckstein, 1958).

There is some debate about whether the doctors' contribution was positive (in suggesting plans) or negative (in vetoing unacceptable government plans). Eckstein (1958, p 118) discusses the importance of medical reports, notably *Lancet*, Medical Planning Commission (MPC) and Medical Planning Research (MPR) reports, with the latter seen as the 'most remarkable plan for self-reform in the history of the British [medical] profession', with 'immense' effects on government planning. 'It is certainly a curious fact that the leaders of the profession, during the war, produced precisely the sort of grandiose plan they were so desperately to oppose afterward.'

More recent commentators point to a difference between the Coalition and Labour governments. Webster (2002, p 14) writes that Bevan 'immediately re-established the minister's supremacy in policy making, acting with remarkably little reference to outside interests, Whitehall departments, or even his own senior officials or ministerial colleagues'. According to Honigsbaum (1989, p 217), unlike earlier ministers, Bevan was not led by his civil servants. Klein (2006, p 7) argues that in the earlier period civil servants took the initiative in generating policy options, unprompted, as far as can be judged from the records, by the politicians. Indeed, politicians entered the game late. 'For most of the time in the period covered, politicians play the role of Fortinbras [in Shakespeare's *Hamlet*]: when he comes on stage in the last scene, the trumpets may sound – but all the protagonists of the action are dead. Only occasionally, and exceptionally, do the politicians play a central role in the drama.' He contrasts the politics of compromise under the Coalition government, during which politicians are fringe figures, and the politics of innovation under the Labour government, when politicians take the centre stage.

'Great men' thesis

Turning to individuals, some commentators point to influential individuals, whether politicians, civil servants or doctors (cf Berridge, 2008). Honigsbaum (1989, p 23) writes that Sir John Maude became Permanent Secretary at the Ministry of Health in February 1941 and 'dominated policymaking within the department until 1945', when he retired at the age of 62 upon Labour's assumption of office. Abel-Smith (1964, pp 475, 501–2) stresses the importance of Bevan, and his Chief Medical Officer, Sir William Jameson. Honigsbaum (1989, pp 217–18), writes that Maude, Rucker, Jameson and Hawton – in that order – all exerted influence.

According to Pater (1981), credit for the NHS must be 'widely shared' – from Lord Dawson, with contributions from Beveridge as an impetus to its creation, Moran, ministers such as Brown, Willink and Bevan, civil servants such as Sir John Maude (Permanent Secretary), Sir John Wrigley (Deputy Secretary), Sir Arthur Rucker (Deputy Secretary 1942–47) and Sir John Charles (Deputy Chief Medical Officer, 1944–50). However, there is no doubt that the main credit must rest with two other officers of the Ministry – Sir William Jameson (CMO 1940–50) and Sir John Hawton (Deputy Secretary 1947–51, later Permanent Secretary to 1960).

Rintala (2003) outlines the interpretations that the NHS was created by national consensus, the Labour Party and Bevan, but tends to dismiss these, arguing that the part played by individuals is often overlooked (p 70). He stresses the importance of the 'Medical Lords' Moran and Horder: the 'battle of medical giants' (p 72). Moran described a future British NHS in a BBC broadcast in 1942 which was 'remarkably similar' to that outlined in the NHS Bill of 1946. Moran's maiden speech in the House of Lords in 1943 repeated most of the prescription of his broadcast (p 108). Moran became Bevan's closest as well as his most important ally in creating the NHS (p 111). In creating the NHS, Bevan 'prematurely closed his ears to all other voices except one' (p 140). Klein (2006, pp 15–16) considers that, in particular, one of the key actors in Bevan's manoeuvres was the President of the Royal College of Physicians, Lord Moran.

How: consensus versus conflict

Early accounts tended to stress consensus. Gemmill (1960) argues that the NHS was the logical outcome of a project that had been launched 35 years earlier, shaped by all political parties (p 15). He cites *The Times* on the 10th anniversary of the service stating that it was conceived by a Liberal [Beveridge], nurtured by a Coalition government under a Conservative [Churchill] and brought to life by a Labour government [headed by Attlee] (pp 15–16). He outlines the 'brief and consensual route' to the White Paper of 1944 (pp 18–20), but claims, in a mastery of understatement, that the doctors were less enthusiastic than Parliament about the White Paper (p 20). Bevan's plan differed considerably from the one that had been proposed by the Coalition government, though its ultimate objective was the same (p 20). Lindsey (1962) claims that the scheme was the result of more than two decades of planning and thinking, was evolutionary rather than revolutionary, with support coming from all political parties (p 23).

Some writers have presented a 'conflict within consensus' thesis. Fox (1986, p 111) claims that, by the end of the war, disputes about health policy were about means rather than ends. Gemmill (1960, p 20) argues that Bevan's plan differed considerably from the one that had been proposed by the Coalition government, though its ultimate objective was the same. Klein (2006, p 5) writes that various proposals put forward during the inter-war period had all come up with somewhat different schemes. If everyone was agreed about the end of policy in a general sort of way, there was little by way of consensus about means. He continues that the Coalition's White Paper was based on two principles that were to remain the foundation of the NHS as it eventually emerged in 1946: namely, comprehensive, and free at the point of use. However, although the proclaimed ends of the 1944 White Paper were the same as those of the 1946 Act, the institutional means were different (p 8).

Although Abel-Smith (1964) was one of the first writers to stress conflict rather than consensus, Webster (1988, 2002, see also 1990) presents the most developed critique of consensus (see Gorsky, 2008). Webster (1988, pp 390–1) writes that once the NHS was established as a national institution there was a tendency to read back consensus into earlier history. However, he gives only 'moderate' support to that interpretation. Webster (1988, p 24) notes that schemes were 'rival and incompatible'. The themes of the 1944 White Paper – free and comprehensive –were both subject to significant reservations (p 55). Webster (2002, p 3) argues that the path to the NHS was by no means an inevitable and logical progression. There was no smooth process over evolutionary change and a noticeable absence of consensus over the most basic aspects of healthcare policy.

Long versus short roots

There is also disagreement between accounts of the 'starting point' of the evolution of the NHS. 'Short' accounts are given in Stevens (1966), while

Willcocks (1967) begins his account with the creation of the EMS. On the other hand, Ross (1952) starts his account in 1850. Lindsey (1962) claims that the roots of the NHS reach back to the first decade of the 20th century and even earlier. Honigsbaum (1989) begins with the NHI Act of 1911. Pater (1981, p 2) gives the most relevant starting point in the Royal Commission on the Poor Laws (RCPL) of 1909. Webster (1988, p 16) argues that it is arbitrary to identify a starting point for initiation of planning for the NHS. Conventionally, the wartime crisis and the EMS are regarded as crucial, but the inter-war crisis also played its part. He traces the origins from RCPL.

Factors

Even accounts that stress a long evolutionary process argue that more recent factors 'speeded up' the path to the NHS. The importance of the Second World War is stressed by Navarro (1978) and Doyal (1979). According to Lindsey (1962, pp 23–4), the ordeal of the war, with its levelling effect, certainly helped to create the proper climate for parliamentary action, with war regarded as a 'powerful catalyst'. Webster (2002, p 6) writes that it took a second world war to shatter the inertia of the established regime. Anticipation of bombing led to EMS. He cites Political and Economic Planning (PEP) (1941, p 3) that 'the bombing plane ... has forced on us a transformation of our medical services', adding that the Luftwaffe achieved in months what had defeated politicians and planners for at least two decades.

Willcocks (1967, p x) argues that the events of the EMS and the Beveridge Report precipitated the decision to create an NHS. However, Webster (2002, p 17) writes that the Emergency Hospital Scheme (later Emergency Medical Scheme) (EHS) as a springboard for the nationalisation of hospitals had occasionally been canvassed during the Second World War, but this idea had been rejected in all the major planning documents, adding that 'there is virtually no direct evidence about the course of Bevan's thinking'. Eckstein (1958, p 134) claims that the wartime government's medical planning was derived from three main sources: the EMS, the MPR, and the Beveridge Report. The latter is 'generally assigned the most important place among the factors leading to the NHS'. However, this emphasis is 'probably misplaced'. Announcements of reform predated Beveridge. 'So as far as its detailed recommendations are concerned the Beveridge Report is one of the least important steps leading to the NHS.'

Theory

Few accounts tend to use theory in an explicit way. Eckstein (1958, pp 5–6) hints at the importance of path dependency: the new system had to be adjusted to the old. It is no exaggeration to say that at least some of the things for which we are likely to blame the administrative judgements of today's ministers and civil servants ought more properly to be attributed to the Poor Law Amendment Act of 1834. However, it is disappointing that an author of a book on pressure group politics (Eckstein, 1960) devotes so little attention to this theme. With an implicit nod to path dependency, Lindsey (1962, p ix) argues that 'had the new service been built from scratch, a more integrated system would surely have been conceived'. Rivett (1998, p 1) writes that the designers of the NHS did not start with a clean sheet of paper. Campbell (1994, p 177) touches on path dependency and on interest groups, stressing the 'art of the possible': 'the fact is that the local authority option was not a practical possibility in 1945'. Webster (2002) argues that the interest groups responded to Beveridge by retreating to their entrenched positions. The polarisation of attitudes experienced at this time cast a long shadow over the future NHS. Honigsbaum (1989, pp 213–14) hints at rational versus incremental decision making and at interest groups: civil servants failed to understand medical politics, stressing a tidy, rational 'paper' solution. Forsyth (1973, pp 1–2) discusses 'influential pressure groups', arguing that the effect of pressure groups is to take decision making out of the public eye. Despite the book's subtitle, Willcocks (1967, p 102) argues that we may have overstated the importance and power of the pressure groups and may have undervalued, thereby, other important factors such as public opinion, ad hoc groups and so on.

Some writers have suggested counterfactuals. Honigsbaum (1989, p 217) suggests that there might have been a very different outcome if Horder had become Royal College of Physicians President rather than Moran. The onset of war probably made some kind of health service inevitable. For Campbell (1994), the historian's problem is to identify and try to evaluate Bevan's distinctive contribution to the NHS. In what precise ways might it have been different had the Tories won the 1945 general election? Or if another Labour minister had been responsible for introducing it? How much of the overall shape, and how many of the structural or conceptual flaws, can be specifically attributed to him? There can be no doubt that some form of NHS would have come into being after 1945, whoever had won the general election. In addition to the limited use of theory, there is also limited use of an evaluative template (but see Powell, 1997).

Conclusion

This section revisits Yin's (2009) criteria for case studies. The case studies of the creation of the NHS satisfy many of Yin's criteria (2009): significant, 'complete', considering alternative perspectives, displaying sufficient evidence, composed in an engaging manner. They use multiple sources of evidence and consider rival explanations or plausible rival hypotheses (Yin, 2009).

It is difficult to dispute that the creation of the NHS is significant. It is less clear whether the accounts are complete. The early accounts do not display sufficient evidence and are incomplete because they lacked access to the archives. Willcocks (1967, p 11) writes that without access to the minister's and his advisers' papers, one can rarely be sure which was the true answer. Few accounts feature interviews. Some sources, such as *Hansard* and Cabinet minutes, tend to be dismissed. The accounts tend to present a 'narrative' view, with little explicit theory, and do not explicitly consider rival explanations.

Although there is significant agreement on some issues, such as the skilful 'divide and rule' tactics used by Bevan, and that more concessions were given to specialists as compared to GPs, disputes and unanswered questions remain. To some extent, some different conclusions are explained by the fuller range of sources available to later writers. 'Turning points' and 'decisive' contributory factors are elusive. Forsyth (1973, p 2) writes that how the NHS acquired some of its characteristics still remains a mystery. Willcocks (1967, p 1) gloomily concludes that case studies never 'prove' anything (Eckstein, 1960). Like Stevens' (2000) verdict on studies of the wider NHS, studies on its creation exhibit 'mixed messages, diverse interpretations', illustrating the 'contested interpretation of historical interpretation' (Berridge, 2010, p 799)

However, the definition of the 'case' remains unclear. Yin (2009, p 29) writes that the case can include decisions, programmes, the implementation process and organisational change, making the creation of the NHS the case. However, he adds that definition of the unit of analysis or case is related to the way that you have defined your initial research questions (Yin, 2009, p 30), so that if one issue relates to the interpretations given by different accounts, then the case might be the individual book. Moreover, it is not clear when the case ends. This could be taken as the NHS Act of 1946 or the 'Appointed Day' in 1948. It could be argued that the early years of the NHS should be included, so as to check for 'snagging' problems. Finally, it could be claimed that 'creation' has not ended, in the sense that the initial features of the service still cast a long shadow over the service today and that we are still on the 'path' laid down in the 1940s. However, whatever interpretation is taken of the definition of the case or the features of the case study, the creation of the NHS shows that 'history matters' (Berridge, 2008) and that 'thinking in time' (Neustadt and May, 1986; Berridge, 2010; see also www.historyandpolicy.org) remains important.

References

Abel-Smith, B. (1964) *The hospitals, 1800–1948*, London: Heinemann.

Berridge, V. (1996) *AIDS in the UK: The making of policy, 1981–1994*, Oxford: Oxford University Press.

Berridge, V. (2008) 'History matters? History's role in health policy making', *Medical History*, vol 52, no 3, pp 311–26.

Berridge, V. (2010) 'Thinking in time: does health policy need history as evidence?', *Lancet*, vol 375, no 9717, pp 798–9.

Campbell, J. (1994) *Nye Bevan. A biography*, London: Richard Cohen Books (first published as *Nye Bevan and the mirage of British socialism*, London: Weidenfeld & Nicolson, 1987).

Doyal, L. (1979) *The political economy of health*, London: Pluto Press.

Dunn, C. (1952) *The emergency medical services*, 2 vols, London: HMSO.

Eckstein, H. (1958) *The English health service*, Cambridge, MA: Harvard University Press.

Eckstein, H. (1960) *Pressure group politics. The case of the British Medical Association*, London: Allen and Unwin.

Evans, D. and Knight, T. (eds) (2006) *'There was no plan!' The origins and development of multi-disciplinary public health in the UK*, Report of witness seminar held at University of the West of England, Monday, 7 November 2005, Bristol: University of the West of England.

Foot, M. (1975) *Aneurin Bevan, A Biography, vol 2: 1945–1960*, St Albans: Paladin.

Forsyth, G. (1973) *Doctors and state medicine*, 2nd edn, London: Pitman Medical (first published 1966).

Fox, D. (1986) *Health policies, health politics. The British and American experience, 1911–1965*, Princeton, NJ: Princeton University Press.

Gemmill, P. (1960) *Britain's search for health*, Pennsylvania, PA: University of Pennsylvania Press.

Godber, Sir G.E. (1975) *The Health Service: Past, present, and future*, London: Athlone Press, 1975.

Godber, Sir G.E. (1988) 'Forty years of the NHS', *British Medical Journal*, 297, pp 37–43.

Goodman, N.M. (1970) *Wilson Jameson: Architect of national health*, London: George Allen and Unwin.

Gorsky, M. (2008) 'The British National Health Service 1948–2008: a review of the historiography', *Social History of Medicine*, vol 21, no 3, pp 437–60.

Grimes, S. (1991) *The British National Health Service: State intervention in the medical marketplace, 1911–1948*, New York: Garland.

Herbert, S.M. (1939) *Britain's Health*, Harmondsworth: Penguin.

Hollingsworth, J.R. (1986) *A political economy of medicine: Great Britain and the United States*, Baltimore: Johns Hopkins University Press.

Honigsbaum, F. (1979) *The division in British medicine*, London: Kogan Page.

Honigsbaum, F. (1989) *Health, happiness and security. The creation of the National Health Service*, London: Routledge.

Klein, R. (2006) *The new politics of the NHS*, 5th edn, Abingdon: Radcliffe Publishing (first published 1983).

Lindsey, A. (1962) *Socialized medicine in England and Wales. The NHS, 1948–1961*, Chapel Hill: University of North Carolina Press.

Navarro, V. (1978) *Class struggle, the state and medicine. An historical and contemporary analysis of the medical sector in Great Britain*, Oxford: Martin Robertson.

Neustadt, R. and May, E. (1986) *Thinking in time. The uses of history for decision makers*, New York: The Free Press.

Pater, J. (1981) *The making of the National Health Service*, London: King's Fund.

Political and Economic Planning (PEP) (1937) *Report on the British Health Service*, London: PEP.

PEP (1941) *Planning 177*, London: PEP.

Powell, M. (1997) *Evaluating the National Health Service*, Buckingham: Open University Press.

Rintala, M. (2003) *Creating the National Health Service. Aneurin Bevan and the Medical Lords*, London: Frank Cass.

Rivett, G. (1998) *From the cradle to grave. Fifty years of the NHS*, London: King's Fund.

Ross, J.S. (1952) *The National Health Service in Great Britain. An historical and descriptive study*, London: Oxford University Press.

Stevens, R. (1966) *Medical practice in modern England. The impact of specialization and state medicine*, New Haven, CT: Yale University Press.

Stevens, R. (2000) 'Fifty years of the British National Health Service: mixed messages, diverse interpretations', *Bulletin of the History of Medicine*, vol 74, pp 806–11.

Stewart, J. (1999) *The battle for health*, Aldershot: Ashgate.

Taylor, S. (Lord) (1981) 'How the NHS was born', *British Medical Journal*, 223, pp 1446-8.

Titmuss, R.M. (1950) *Problems of social policy*, London: HMSO.

Webster, C. (1988) *The health services since the war. Volume I. Problems of health care. The National Health Service before 1957*, London: HMSO.

Webster, C. (1990) 'Conflict and consensus: explaining the British health service', *Twentieth Century British History*, vol 1, no 2, pp 115–51.

Webster, C. (2002) *The National Health Service. A political history*, 2nd edn, Oxford: Oxford University Press.

Willcocks, A. (1967) *The creation of the National Health Service. A study of pressure groups and a major social policy decision*, London: Routledge and Kegan Paul.

Yin, R.K. (2009) *Case study research: Design and methods*, 4th edn, London: Sage.

four

Hospital policy in England and Wales: of what is the 1962 Hospital Plan a case?

John Mohan

Introduction

> Researchers probably will not know what their cases are until the
> research, including the task of writing up the results, is virtually
> completed. What *it* is a *case of* will coalesce gradually, sometimes
> catalytically, and the final realization of the case's nature may be the
> most important part of the interaction between ideas and evidence.
> (Ragin, 1992, p 6; italics in original)

In 1962 the Conservative Minister of Health, Enoch Powell, launched what
he characterised as an exercise in planning not previously attempted this
side of the Iron Curtain. This was the Hospital Plan for England and Wales
(Ministry of Health, 1962) – a 10-year programme of hospital construction
and reconstruction involving 90 new and 134 substantially remodelled
hospitals. It was simultaneously an attempt to modernise hospital stock,
to save capital expenditure by imposing a degree of standardisation on
hospital construction, to reduce revenue expenditure by cutting running
costs and to redistribute resources on the basis of need. The intention was
to produce a national network of District General Hospitals (DGHs) –
hospitals of 600–800 beds, serving populations of 100,000–150,000, with
specialist services being organised on a regional basis in teaching hospitals.
The implicit organisation led Daniel Fox (1986) to characterise the Hospital
Plan as 'hierarchical regionalism', an ideal-typical form of organisation
which he regards as having been widely adopted during the 20th century. It
marked, arguably, the zenith of such efforts, at least in terms of its published
aspirations. And if we think of a further theme that has dominated health
policy over the last century, that of central–local relationships, the Plan was
highly centralist in character and raised questions about how (and indeed
whether) the laudable aims of the NHS towards delivering an egalitarian,
genuinely *national*, service could be realised.

Nearly half a century on, how should we view the Hospital Plan? It has generally had a good press in both academic and non-academic texts – Timmins (1995), for example, describes it as 'Enoch Powell's great Hospital Plan' – while it received positive verdicts from prominent health policy analysts such as Klein (1983) and Ham (1992). The latter draw on the principal academic study of the Plan itself, by David Allen (1979). Given the time at which he was writing, Allen did not have access to archival sources – national papers on policy making being subject to the 30-year rule – so he drew on interviews, parliamentary and press sources, as well as medical and professional journals. He produced a chronology of the decision-making process which he then 'tested' against idealised models (political, process, rational and bureaucratic) of rationality in decision making.

Although Allen's book was welcomed in some standard texts on health policy, there were critical voices. Gwyn Bevan (1981) pointed out that Allen's approach is problematic: it assumes that an objective, stable and coherent narrative account could be produced, and that different models could be brought to bear on that reality. There are numerous other points which may be made about Allen's work. It's not very critical; even at the time of the Plan's launch there were extensive public criticisms of the limitations of the evidence base for the Plan, but these received relatively little attention in Allen's book. In addition, the temporal focus is limited to consideration of a single event, but this means that there is nothing about the Plan as a process rather than an event, no consideration of implementation issues, and no discussion of whether and to what extent the Plan's objectives had been attained. All of these would have meant a lengthier book, but historical distance might have lent a bit of critical perspective. Forsyth's (1981) review was more positive, arguing that some of these models have a ring of truth in explaining certain aspects of the decision-making process. However, Allen's overall conclusion seems somewhat lame: 'so what occurred was affected by history, the social process producing consensus, economic conditions, the organisational structure of government and the NHS, values of the organisations, the personalities of those in critical positions and their personal motivations' (Allen, 1979, p 180). This doesn't leave much out, but nor does it really give us guidance as to the relative importance of these factors.

What might be gained from revisiting the Plan and, more specifically, what role can case study research play in policy analysis? Before conducting a case study, we need to answer a prior question, which is the one hinted at in the epigraph at the head of this chapter. Of what, exactly, is the Hospital Plan a case? Sociological definitions would suggest that a 'case study is a detailed study of a single social unit', that the units have clear boundaries which make them easy to identify (school, factory, street gang) and, furthermore, that the social unit selected should be a single example of the many cases that make up the type of unit in question. None of these seems to fit the

Hospital Plan, for several reasons. It was an event (the launch of a public commitment on the part of government to raise capital investment in hospital services), rather than a social unit. Second, that event was only one point in a process – in this case, the process of top-down planning. The boundaries of the Plan are difficult to draw both chronologically (when did it begin and end?) and in terms of substantive content (to what extent is it valid to speak of an era of central planning in hospital provision?). Thus, we might focus on the development of the Plan itself, which would give us an obvious end-point in 1962. In effect, Allen sees the Plan as a singular event (a decision), but Gwyn Bevan saw the Plan as being a proposal and only part of a much wider process. An alternative would be to carry the study forward into the implementation of the Plan, in which case we would have problems deciding when it was over. A revision in 1966 dropped references to the 'Plan' – it was titled the 'Hospital Building Programme' (Ministry of Health, 1966). Alternatives might include key dates at which challenges to the concept of a DGH were debated and rejected (for example, 1969: the Bonham-Carter Report [Central Health Services Council, 1969]) or promulgated (such as 1980: the Conservatives' 'Future pattern of hospital provision' [DHSS, 1980]); or 1973, at which point capital expenditure was cut in real terms for the first time. This poses the question of when a case study should end, but it also challenges us to think about the stability of our analyses over time.

Third it is not clear what other comparable cases there might be. The Plan was, arguably, unique in a British context, although one might draw some comparisons with the rapid expansion of capital investment under the Labour government after 1997. As for other parallels, we might find these in other areas of state intervention – for example, investment in the educational or housing infrastructure, though in neither case are the individual building projects as complex as those associated with hospital development. Alternatively, we might find them in the health systems of other countries but, given the characteristics of the public-private mix for healthcare in comparable nation-states, one tends not to find the same degree of top-down planning.

These comments point towards the uniqueness of the Plan, and they highlight what John Walton (1992) describes as a 'fundamental duality' in the various uses of terms like 'case' and 'case study'. The term implies particularity – cases are 'situationally-grounded, limited views of social life' – but it also implies a sense of generality – that is, the particular is a case of something else. Consequently, we should consider the Plan as an exemplar of wider social processes or phenomena, and this entails attention to its symbolic content as well as its substantive content.

There are several general phenomena of which the Hospital Plan might be seen as a case. We can see the Plan as a rhetorical device designed to convince the electorate of Conservative commitment to welfare, an example of rational central planning, an illustration of 'state failure', a case study of the role of key individuals in a decision, a symbolic exercise in modernisation and/or an illustration of modernist principles. All of these offer some insights, and the Plan might be all of them simultaneously. As Diane Vaughan (1992) argues, in developing case studies we are elaborating a theory of interest to specify more carefully circumstances in which it does or does not apply, rather than attempting, in a positivistic fashion, to reject a formal hypothesis. Harry Eckstein (1958, p 15), in a widely quoted phrase, argued that 'case studies never "prove" anything; their purpose is to illustrate generalisations which are established otherwise, or to direct attention to such generalisations'.

I argue that revisiting case studies of historical events can help us in at least three respects. Most obviously, the emergence of new sources might lead us to change the emphases we give, for example to the underlying rationality of the Plan. We have policy papers which weren't available to previous authors (though they have been used for example, by Webster, 1994) as well as some private correspondence from individuals. So there is a case for looking at these; we are not, in Webster's (1998) phrase, poring over the remains of the same 'paltry entrails' long scrutinised by generations of researchers at The National Archives, which would be the case if we were attempting to extract a revised version of the origins of the NHS, for example. Second, there are advantages in being able to place analyses in a longer-term perspective. As Wievorka (1992, p 169) puts it, this enables us to assess the stability over time of our analyses and to enquire into the appropriateness of a different time-scale for understanding; so, for example, what was once a case study of a single decision becomes contextualised as part of an examination of different methods of regulation and distribution of healthcare resources. Third, we can look through new intellectual lenses – for example, revisiting the Plan in the light of debates about modernity and modernisation, or about 'state failure'. I argue that it is possible to generate a more multi-dimensional and richer view of the Plan and a reinterpretation of its role: albeit with the benefit of hindsight, we can see the Plan was a flawed but partially successful attempt to redistribute resources and improve the infrastructure in the NHS. In contrast to the era of sporadic and uneven construction that preceded the NHS, this was a considerable achievement. Bearing these comments in mind, I concentrate on three key themes: the Plan as an exercise in rational, bureaucratic planning; the Plan as an exercise in modernisation and in the use of modernist rhetoric for largely symbolic purposes; and the Plan as an illustration of 'state failure'.

'A durable asset politically': rationality and planning, or an exercise in spin?

How successful was this as an exercise in planning? The prior question here is how we might define planning. Presumably, looking through early 21st-century lenses, we would expect it to be based on evidence, and the evidence base was pretty thin. The Plan proposed bed norms for the guidance of planners, but these were based on a small number of studies of the use of hospitals in small urban centres with rural hinterlands and few, if any, competing hospitals. These were not representative and their limitations were acknowledged. Nevertheless, bed ratios were viewed as a 'useful tool … rather like giving a blind man a stick – it may help him even though it won't improve his sight',[1] though decisions were thought to incorporate an element of 'art as well as science' and would inevitably include a large element of 'by guess and by God'.[2] The bed norm finally chosen – 3.3 acute beds/1,000 population – was later criticised for its arbitrary and inflexible nature; the norms were used as maxima, and hospital boards which assumed that they could plan beyond that level were given 'firm orders' to reduce excesses.[3] Thus the norms became a vehicle whereby conformity could be imposed. So this was apparently scientific, but also politically convenient, as it provided a way of capping the ambitions of some Regional Hospital Boards (RHBs). The internal discussions about bed norms were echoed publicly at the time, notably by one MP who complained in the parliamentary debate on the Plan that the Minister had simply stuck his finger in the list of possible norms and pulled out a politically convenient figure.

The bed norms were combined with the concept of the DGH, which emphasised economies of scale in service provision and comprehensiveness of service (Godber, 1958, 1959; Abel and Lewin, 1959; Farrer-Brown, 1959). Concepts such as that of the 'area hospital' (Abel and Lewin, 1959, p 111) were proposed; such facilities were to serve every 'natural area' of population. The implicit assumption was that the DGH would provide better-quality care at reduced unit costs. The scope of the DGH followed from the need to provide all the services thought to be required locally; the scale was defined in terms of an appropriate medical staffing structure (Harrison and Prentice, 1998, pp 14–32). However, the concept of a DGH had been arrived at by 'rather imprecise socio-medical studies' (Taylor, 1960) and was 'inevitably ill-defined' because the Ministry of Health had 'nothing empirical to go on'.[4] The Deputy Secretary in the Ministry, Enid Russell-Smith, was privately more critical: 'we are really making up a policy as we go along … I really do not think we have been very well-served by the medicos'.[5]

The Plan ostensibly aimed to facilitate integration of hospital and community health services; improved complementary community services were to facilitate the discharge of patients as soon as they no longer required hospital treatment. However, only vague statements were made about this. In the preparation the Plan, the intention was to include a 'general picture of local authority developments' in the field of community care. These, in their turn, 'would involve certain assumptions about the amount that could be left to voluntary effort'.[6] This was prescient – few of the RHBs, the primary planning organisations, had taken account of local authority service provision in formulating their proposals, despite ministerial assertions to the contrary.[7] The same general observation could apply to the links between hospitals and other parts of the health service. Ministry of Health officials considered that 'the only part [of the Plan] that can be clearly seen is the list of hospital projects'.[8]

The notion that the Plan represented a comprehensive and national blueprint – something that wasn't being attempted outside Eastern Europe – is also suspect. Being based on the submissions of individual Boards, which had varying technical abilities and capacities, variation in quality was inevitable. The Deputy Secretary of the Ministry commented that the building programmes, 'instead of being founded on calculation, reason, logic and mathematical projection … rest on no ascertained facts whatever'.[9] The lack of evidence of any clear philosophy and strategy is evident in the characterisation of one regional draft as 'a study of individual hospitals with little view of a wider field'. This is not strong evidence to support the claims made by Powell about the virtues of central planning and it does not inspire confidence in the view of the Plan as a child of rational, bureaucratic policy.

The obvious counterfactual question, though, is whether the Ministry could have done any better and, perhaps more to the point, whether it needed to do so. Given the lukewarm commitment of the Conservative government to the NHS (Webster, 1994), further quibbling from officials, MPs or professionals might have delayed action even further. Consequently, the Plan's assumptions were shaky at best, heroic at worst, and the result was an increase in capital investment without clear foundations. Nevertheless, there is little sign in the Ministry of Health papers that officials attempted to dissuade Powell: it was very clear that he was going to drive this through in some form to maximise credit for the government. This raises the question of the Plan as a case of something else: a symbolic political gesture. The Plan was launched with hyperbolic references to key political developments of the 20th century. We have already noted Powell's 'Iron Curtain' reference, while the Permanent Secretary of the Ministry, Bruce Fraser, raised expectations by speaking of a 'new deal' for hospitals.[10] Considerable political capital was invested in the Plan: unusually, although it merely involved expanding an established programme, it was launched with a White Paper. It was a large-scale, highly visible and discrete programme which assumed totemic significance. It therefore became a lodestone of commitment to the welfare state – which also rendered it a hostage to fortune. This raises the question of whether it was purely a symbolic gesture or whether there was real substance to the Plan and the promises it gave.

First, financial commitments were far less generous than the publicity would lead us to believe. The Guillebaud Committee's (1956) criticisms of underinvestment are sometimes viewed as having paved the way, but the Treasury was firmly focused on undermining the case made by Guillebaud.[11] The parameters of policy were set by the Government's 1959 election pledge to increase the rate of hospital building, but there were arguments about the minimum that could be committed; this led to a target of £50m a year, reached via incremental growth of £5m a year,[12] even though it was clear that this would leave the NHS some way short of being a 'service whose problems are only those of replacement'. Powell felt that the Plan was 'the least we could justify', but even so he financed it through concessions to the right of the Conservative Party, by increasing NHS charges, and in fact revenue from the charges imposed in 1960 amounted to more than the annual average rate of investment envisaged by the Plan. Thus, the Plan did not mark a dramatic departure or a shift in public expenditure priorities; the burden of financing it fell on the users of the service (Webster, 1994; Timmins, 1995).

Second, the assumptions on which the Plan was based were, at best, shaky. Powell had yielded to Treasury demands to constrain NHS revenue growth, but even allowing for savings from projected hospital closures, ministry officials acknowledged that there would be insufficient revenue to fund new developments; the assumptions of the Plan were described as 'guff'. Heffer, Powell's biographer, glosses over the weaknesses, arguing that 'it was inevitable that some current costs would be sacrificed' (1998, p 27), but this is disingenuous: the underlying weaknesses were well known. Furthermore, complementary community care provision was essential if higher hospital throughput was to be achieved, yet the considerable variations in the provision of community services by local authorities were simply ignored. Two key developments were required if the Plan was to achieve its aims: a vigorous programme of hospital closures, and considerable investment in complementary community care. These both implied political commitments, but ministers were reluctant to engage with the former, and local authorities could not be relied upon to deliver the latter. This contributes to a revised assessment of the Plan's coherence. It was subject to heavy political spin, with strong emphasis being placed on new investment, but, as medical commentators were quick to point out, not unlike subsequent Conservative and Labour efforts, most of the projects announced were in the pipeline anyway and the Plan merely brought some of them forward (Mohan, 2002, p 134).

The extent of the weaknesses in existing knowledge becomes clear only with the passage of time and the release of policy papers. And given the low level of investment in the hospital stock, change could not have been delayed indefinitely. Even so, Allen (1979) offers fairly limited criticisms, preferring to focus on the incomplete knowledge available rather than on deficiencies in that knowledge, and tending to neglect the criticisms that were publicly aired at the time. Revisiting the policy making underlying the Plan shows convincingly its limitations as an exercise in planning. But the Plan had further, unanticipated consequences. First, it became a lodestone of commitment to welfare. This meant that hospitals continued to attract a disproportionate share of resources. In effect, the Plan defined the nature of healthcare – centralised, remote, professionalised – and precluded alternatives (Manson, 1979, p 42). Second, perhaps because of the underlying weaknesses and unresolved issues, as well as its long-term nature, it was a candidate for cuts and postponements: its frustration potential was enormous.

It may appear unfair to impose – even if implicitly – a utopian and *post hoc* definition of rationality on the whole exercise, and perhaps those involved did the best they could. But if that is the case, it could equally be argued that less grandiose claims ought to have been made for the Plan. It might better be viewed as an exercise in spin – the weaknesses were well known to those responsible for the Plan, but they also knew that careful presentation would be, as Macmillan recognised in a congratulatory note to Powell, a 'durable asset politically'. Furthermore, to the extent that it is possible to regard the plan as a milestone, we could also see it as a millstone (compare Lowe, 1997, p 199, on the Plowden Committee's contemporaneous proposals): it effectively constrained debate about health policy because the scale of the building programme became a political virility symbol. The mantra of 'schools and hospitals' – so characteristic of recent policy squabbles – has, arguably, had a negative influence on health policy. For comparisons, we might look no further than developments under the Private Finance Initiative (PFI). An electorally driven policy to increase the level of capital investment in and replacement of the hospital stock has produced political dividends, but, as in the Hospital Plan before it, heroic assumptions have been made about throughput targets and the availability of the supporting community services.

'Ruthlessly breaking with habit and tradition': modernisation and modernity

To what extent can the 1962 Plan be seen as part of a modernisation strategy? Jessop (1992) notes the various connotations of modernisation: 'corporate planning, economies of scale, mass production, investment in science and technology, pursuit of standardisation and centralised control, active state sponsorship of Fordist economic growth and a general belief that big was beautiful' (p 23). In the context of the welfare state Murray (1991) and

Mulgan (1991) have noted similar parallels: 'hospitals of the Fordist era were like factories in the Green Belt' (Murray, 1991, p 22). This may be over-simplistic: most hospitals in green belt areas were long-stay institutions that could not be characterised as Fordist insofar as they could be characterised as having assembly-line treatment methods. Nevertheless, economies of scale and mass production were implicit in the Plan's emphasis on centralisation and revenue-saving capital investment (criticised by Manson, 1979 as an attempt to introduce 'capitalist rationality' into the NHS). Proposals for even larger-scale developments were advanced in the 1960s with the Bonham-Carter Report, though Richard Crossman, as Secretary of State for Social Services, had described some such proposals as 'a case of elephantiasis' (quoted in Mohan, 2002, p 149).

Standardisation and industrialised building were seen as one way of reducing pressure of demand on the construction industry in a context of labour scarcity, and as a way of cutting costs, and this was endorsed in discussions: Henry Brooke (the Home Secretary) stated that the Plan meant 'standard provision at standard cost'. However, the record in hospital policy is mixed.[13] Moves towards standardisation had not advanced far by 1962, and made unsteady progress thereafter through central guidance about the content, design and administration of building schemes (Vann-Wye, 1992, p 171). These initiatives logically pointed towards standardisation of the design and construction of whole hospitals and the use of industrialised construction methods. However, these developments did not gain much purchase: some relied (as did the Plan itself) on strong assumptions about the availability of appropriate support from complementary services, and another reason was 'undue deference' to the wishes of hospital consultants (House of Commons, 1970). Following a process of experimentation with various standard designs, the restrictive public expenditure climate of the 1970s finally persuaded health authorities to accept standardisation in the form of the 'Nucleus' design (Vann-Wye, 1992; Mohan, 2002, ch 8). It cannot be said, then, that the aim of 'standard provision at standard cost' had even begun to be achieved in the 1960s. The adoption of standardisation was a somewhat reluctant process, driven by economic necessity.

An alternative view is to see the Plan as an exercise in modernity – that is, the sweeping-away of a problematic past. Eckstein (1958, pp 262–3) argued that a key aim of the NHS was to 'make subject to calculation what had previously been left to chance ... [and] replace spontaneous adjustment with deliberate control'. The modernist rhetoric is immediately apparent. The Plan's claims to modernity include a desire to create an integrated and hierarchical regional organisation, and a concomitant willingness to override community opposition to hospital closures, in order to produce a more rational distribution of services.

Of course, idealistic blueprints were not new and the wartime Ministry of Health papers and the Hospital Surveys contain forward-looking visions. However, forward planning in the early years of the NHS was regarded by officials as a largely hypothetical exercise. As the resource straitjacket was loosened in the mid-1950s there is more evidence of a long-term vision, encapsulated in the realisation that 'haphazard development [was] even more wasteful than ribbon development and urban sprawl'.[14] The case was gradually accepted, but there was further implication of the process of rationalisation. The aspirations of the Plan to modernity were most severely tested when it had to be acknowledged that, if the aims of increasing efficiency were to be achieved, many hospitals would have to be sacrificed. Civil servants could advocate closure of hospitals dating from the 'horse-and-buggy age, in which modern treatment cannot be given', but this was not something that a Conservative government could easily acknowledge publicly. Misgivings were expressed about closing many institutions which had been founded on legacies, maintained by donations until 1948, and which continued to attract substantial voluntary commitment.[15]

Powell sought to soften the blow by consultation about the continued role of voluntary effort in the NHS, but he nevertheless emphasised the importance of 'ruthlessly breaking with habit and tradition where they conflict with reason and common sense';[16] he went so far as to propose that he could even 'close hospitals ceremonially' to demonstrate commitment to modernisation. Since no such events took place before he left office, we may infer that he was dissuaded from this course of action![17] Criticism of hospital closures emanated not just from those distressed at the prospect of losing cherished hospitals, but also from opposition to any variant of 'planning': 'the ideological centralization proposed in the Hospital Plan is about as realistic as would be a plan to scrap all the ships in the fleet except the aircraft carriers, and about as moral as would be a plan to close all the parish churches on the grounds that the work done in them could be more efficiently organised in cathedrals'.[18]

The Plan was therefore an uneasy compromise between modernity and tradition. Of course, that is arguably true of many policies, but it is difficult to think of another public initiative which proposed closing so many cherished institutions in the name of a scientific vision of progress. Indeed, when the experience of the hospital system had been one of 'incessant construction' (Webster's [1988] phrase) the idea that large numbers of hospitals should be removed, for the greater good, was bound to pose problems. And so it proved, as critics pointed to traditional, if not anti-modern, virtues of localism and voluntarism. Resolving these tensions was not helped by the underlying weaknesses of the Plan. When the promised results seemed unlikely to be achieved, ministers soon adopted a softer line on closure policy rather than insisting on carrying the Plan through to the letter (Mohan, 2002). So, as has been argued by Daunton and Rieger (2001, pp 7-11) and other historians of modernity, this exemplifies the selective and compromised adoption of modernist rhetoric.

The Plan and 'state failure'

A distinctive feature of policy under the Blair and Brown governments was a quite deliberate and systematic attempt to distance New Labour from the era of central planning in which the state demonstrated unequivocally its inability to deliver. The Hospital Plan is not mentioned explicitly, but it hovers in the background. While in office, Labour spokesmen repeatedly referred to the 1960s and 1970s as an era of inadequate cost control and endless bureaucratic delays. The implication was plainly that central planning – if not state intervention itself – had failed, and such arguments were used to lever into position the controversial proposals for the PFI and, later, Foundation Hospitals. The reality was that the Plan was launched into what soon became very difficult economic circumstances, and relied for its implementation on a construction industry that was clearly not up to the task (as again was recognised by the Ministry of Health in advance of the Plan's launch). So in what sense can we characterise the era of planning as an exemplar of state failure?

Two external influences need to be given more weight in order to counter this charge. Most obviously, there was the changing economic environment. The Plan was launched in relatively unpropitious economic circumstances, which soon became worse. Throughout the 1960s and 1970s there was a succession of crises in public expenditure planning which were dealt with by cutting back on anticipated capital expenditure for reasons of political expediency, often on an ad hoc basis, in response to external pressures such as the demands of the International Monetary Fund or oil price hikes. As a consequence, the Plan was swiftly relabelled as a 'building programme', but this was not enough to stem criticism. The anodyne versions of Cabinet discussions in this period should be complemented by a reading of the diaries of Crossman (1976) and Castle (1980) to get a sense of the political difficulties these circumstances posed. Crossman refers to 'demented' discussions designed to squeeze small sums out of the building programme while prominent medical politicians deplored continued 'astronomical' spending on defence commitments; Castle argues that any sense of rationality had gone out of the window in the face of Treasury demands for cuts: 'pleading sudden crisis or necessity ... how could I get my health authorities to plan the NHS properly?' (1980, pp 359-60).

The second external factor was the state of the construction industry. First, there was the problem of cost control. Because of capacity constraints in the economy in the early 1960s, the real-terms cost of hospital building soon began to rise steadily; it was acknowledged to be a 'relatively "easy" climate from the point of view of the contractor'.[19] The construction industry was also characterised by large numbers of small firms, many of which were not capable of the large-scale work required. Contractor bankruptcies could cause major disruption. RHB witnesses to the 1970 inquiry by the House of Commons Select Committee on Estimates suggested that the construction industry was not known for its 'highly organised management factor' and RHBs therefore had to make allowances for the 'generally inefficient' way of doing things.[20]

It was therefore believed that, without substantial gains in productivity, 'the [construction] industry would not be able to meet the country's building needs'.[21] But little could be done to reorganise the industry; the indicative planning of the 1960s 'had little effect' on construction (Smyth, 1985, p 172). To the extent that the state could do anything about this, it was via reorganising the demands placed on the construction industry, via attempts at standardisation and at streamlining the processes involved in commissioning construction, but none of these came to very much.

This era has been characterised disparagingly as one in which a 'command-and-control' bureaucracy moved with sloth-like speed to produce a set of half-built, cumbersome and inflexible hospitals which the nation could not afford. Norms-based planning is the villain of the piece here (see, for example, Mallender, 2000). Alan Milburn, for example, argued that top-down planning had stifled innovation.[22] However, given the scale of the task faced by the NHS and the need to prioritise, given limited resources, it must be acknowledged that, despite its inflexibilities, the Plan was at least a starting point; bed norms, however arbitrary, gave a basis for determination of priorities. It was also the case during this period that attempts were made more systematically to steer revenue and capital resources towards areas of greater need.[23]

Such a view also represents RHBs as automata, yet the evidence from this period also shows flexible responses to changing needs. Thus, reviews of the capital programme took account of differential and selective population change as well as attempting to make allowances for the needs of new towns and for rural areas. There may be an argument that there could have been more flexibility, but consider the counterfactual case: what would have happened if RHBs had arbitrarily interfered with their declared order of priorities? Hospital boards were implementing a set of development proposals within a constrained budget; the size of individual projects meant that shuffling the order of schemes, once they were under way, was almost impossible. This may have given an appearance of inflexibility, but the problems arose from the need constantly to refer development proposals up to the Ministry of Health and the Treasury. RHBs had little scope to depart from agreed plans without authorisation, and this caused much frustration among senior RHB officers.[24] In short, flawed though the Plan was, what we see in this region at least is an attempt to maximise the resources available to the region and ensure that (allowing for the inevitable 'lumpiness' of large investments) efforts were made to respond to changing circumstances.

For all the criticisms of the era of planning in the welfare state, consideration of historical evidence would lead us to bring in a more balanced verdict. It's unlikely that ministers are familiar with the historical evidence surrounding hospital policy. It's more likely, as Hay and Watson (2003) argued, that, rather than contemporary policy being shaped by interpretation of the evidence, instead the interpretation of evidence is shaped by a pre-selected policy trajectory. In this regard, initial indications from the Coalition government show considerable continuity, with new Secretary of State for Health Andrew Lansley echoing many previous top-down stereotypes in his announcement of a policy designed to remove such restrictions on competition in the NHS as had been left in place by Labour.

Concluding comments

I will conclude with two reflections. The first is from Lewis Carroll's allegorical poem 'The Hunting of the Snark'. This is a description of an expedition, by boat, to capture a mythical marine animal, the Snark. It becomes clear that the crew and the Captain don't really know what they are looking for, despite the Captain's apparent certainty. The 'map' on which the crew rely to find it is a flight of cartographic fancy, the 'unmistakeable marks' by which one might recognise a Snark prove to melt away into the fog surrounding the creature when it materialises and, just as they think they have caught up with it, it vanishes altogether. I am not the first to recognise the parallels for social science, and Allen (1979) himself acknowledged them: '"the decision" became like a mirage I tried to chase and every time I reached it, it disappeared, until one asks whether there is such a thing as "A" decision'. One might respond, though, with the argument that it is unrealistic to expect to be able to put clear boundaries around a major political and policy event and in that way to freeze and capture it. In this chapter I have shown – albeit with hindsight – how several other accounts of the Plan are possible which would lead us, at the very least, to mount multiple Snark-hunting expeditions in several different directions.

The second reflection is the comment of Umberto Eco's monk, at the end of *The Name of the Rose*: at the end of a novel containing multiple layers of meaning, the narrator, by now an aged monk, writes that: 'it is cold in the scriptorium; my thumb aches. I leave this manuscript. I know not for whom; I no longer know what it is about: *stat rosa pristina nomine, nomina nuda tenemus.*' An approximate translation of this is 'what is left of the rose is only its name, the bare name which we hold'.[25] The Hospital Plan exists – and existed – in name only, but there are multiple interpretations of what it symbolised; it is far more than a case of decision making. Some interpretations lead, using new evidence, to a revised verdict on the Plan's coherence and on the arguments advanced in previous case studies. New lenses will enable us to look at events in different ways and with the benefit of longer-term perspectives – as in the discussion of the Plan as an exemplar of modernity and modernisation. Finally, some re-examinations of historical case studies will be selective and, arguably, predetermine their conclusions, as in the Labour government's characterisation of the apparent failures of previous eras of planning.

Should we be concerned about this? There are clearly multiple narratives, and the answer to the question in this chapter's title is probably that the Plan is many things to many people. In this postmodern age academics probably don't have to worry too much about how (if at all) we should decide between the competing cases. The point at which we might be concerned is when lessons are being drawn for policy. In this regard policy makers would be well advised not to rely on case studies which approach their object from only one angle or, even worse, to prejudge case studies by seeking what they want to find. Future generations of policy makers may well discover that the era of central planning in the NHS actually had a number of virtues after all.

Acknowledgements

This chapter draws extensively on Mohan (2002) and paraphrases material presented there in more detail – particularly in chapters 5–7. Footnote references are to material held in The National Archives (Cabinet [CAB], Ministry of Health [MH] and Treasury [T] papers), Churchill College, Cambridge (Russell-Smith [RUSM] and Clarke [CLRK] papers) and Tyne-Wear Archive Service, Newcastle upon Tyne [TWAS]. I am grateful to staff in those archives for their assistance.

Notes

[1] MH 123/278, Proceedings of joint conference on Hospital Planning, 30 June 1960, paper by Dr N. Goodman.

[2] *Ibid.*

[3] MH 88/325, 'Bed norms', 16 June 1961.

[4] MH 123/242, Robinson-Douglas, 16 November 1960.

[5] RUSM 1/21, 13 November 1961.

[6] T227/1311, Russell-Smith-Robertson, 27 January 1961.

[7] Maclay, HC Debates, vol 661, cols 35–6, 4 June 1962; also Ministry comments on RHB draft plans in MH 88 file series.

[8] T227/1311, Douglas-Robertson, 30 December 1960.

[9] RUSM 1/21, 15 June 1961, 20 June 1961, 28 August 1961.

[10] CLRK 1/3/1/1, Clarke-Robertson, 29 June 1960.

[11] MH 137/41, Fraser-Clarke, 17 November 1960.

[12] *Ibid.*

[13] *British Hospital and Social Services Journal*, 28 February 1964, 12 June 1964.

[14] MH 88/27, Tatton-Brown-Davies, 3 March 1960.

[15] CAB 134/1984, Home Affairs Committee, 19 December 1961.

[16] MH 156/72, 4 August 1961.

[17] MH 90/83, Meeting between Powell and RHB Chairmen, 20 December 1960.

[18] Dr M. Emrys-Roberts, letter to *The Times*, 26 September 1962.

[19] T227/1313, Church-Douglas, 10 April 1962.

[20] House of Commons Select Committee on Estimates (1970), *Evidence*, Q.459–533, 2245–2254, 3371–3383.

[21] Geoffrey Rippon, Minister of Public Building and Works, speaking in 1966 – quoted in Smyth, 1985, p 171.

[22] www.publications.parliament.uk/pa/cm200203/cmhansrd/vo030108/debtext/30108-08.htm.

[23] MH 166/586, Yellowlees Paper.

[24] TWAS, HA/NR/19/221–5 for files dealing with management of the capital programme.

[25] For Eco's own version of this see: http://cs.fit.edu/~ryan/rose.html.

References

Abel, A.L. and Lewin, W. (1959) 'Report on hospital building', *British Medical Journal*, (Supplement), pp 109–14.

Allen, D. (1979) *Hospital planning. The 1962 Hospital Plan for England and Wales. A case study in decision-making*, London: Pitman Medical.

Bevan, G. (1981) 'Review of *Hospital Planning* by David Allen', *Journal of Management Studies*, vol 18, pp 242–5.

Castle, B. (1980) *The Castle Diaries, 1974–76*, London: Weidenfield and Nicolson.

Central Health Services Council (1969) *The functions of the District General Hospital*, London: HMSO.

Crossman, R. (1976) *The diaries of a cabinet minister*, 3 vols, London: Hamish Hamilton and Jonathan Cape.

Daunton, M. and Rieger, B. (eds) (2001) *Meanings of modernity: Britain from the late-Victorian era to World War II*, Oxford: Berg.

DHSS (Department of Health and Social Security) (1980) *The future pattern of hospital services in England and Wales*, London: DHSS.

Eckstein, H. (1958) *The English NHS: Its origins, structure and achievements*, Cambridge, MA: Harvard University Press.

Farrer-Brown, L. (1959) 'Hospitals for today and tomorrow', *British Medical Journal*, (Supplement), pp 118–22.

Forsyth, G. (1981) 'Review of Hospital Planning by David Allen' *Public Administration*, vol 57, pp 489–91.

Fox, D. (1986) *Health policies, health politics*, Princeton, NJ: Princeton University Press.

Godber, G.E. (1958) 'Health services, past, present and future', *Lancet*, vol 272, issue 7036, pp 1–6.

Godber, G.E. (1959) 'The physician's part in hospital planning', *British Medical Journal*, (Supplement), pp 115–18.

Guillebaud Committee (1956) *Report of the Committee of Enquiry into the Cost of the National Health Service*, Cmnd 9663, London: HMSO.

Ham, C. (1992) *Health policy in Britain*, 3rd edn, London: MacMillan.

Harrison, A. and Prentice, S. (1998) *Acute futures*, London: King's Fund.

Hay, C. and Watson, M. (2003) 'The discourse of globalisation and the logic of no alternative: rendering the contingent necessary in the political economy of New Labour', *Policy and Politics*, vol 31, pp 289–305.

Heffer, S. (1998) *Like the Roman: The life of Enoch Powell*, London: Harper Collins.

House of Commons (1970) *Hospital building in Great Britain: Evidence submitted to Sub-Committee B of the Select Committee on Estimates*, London: HMSO.

Jessop, B. (1992) 'From social democracy to Thatcherism; twenty-five years of British politics', in N. Abercrombie and A. Warde (eds) *Social change in contemporary Britain*, Cambridge: Polity, pp 14–39.

Klein, R. (1983) *The politics of the NHS*, Harlow: Longmans.

Lowe, R. (1997) 'Milestone or millstone? The 1959–61 Plowden Committee and its impact on British welfare policy', *Historical Journal*, vol 40, pp 463–91.

Mallender, J. (2000) 'The National Beds Inquiry: where next?', *Health Care UK*, Autumn, pp 7–10.

Manson, T. (1979) 'Health policy and the cuts', *Capital and Class*, vol 7, pp 35–45.

Ministry of Health (1962) *A hospital plan for England and Wales*, Cmnd 1604, London: HMSO.

Ministry of Health (1966) *The hospital building programme*, Cmnd 3000, London: HMSO.

Mohan, J. (2002) *Planning, markets and hospitals*, London: Routledge.

Mulgan, G. (1991) 'Power to the public', *Marxism Today*, May, pp 14–19.

Murray, R. (1991) 'The state after Henry', *Marxism Today*, May, pp 22–7.

Ragin, C. (1992) 'Introduction: cases of "What is a case"', in C. Ragin and H. Becker (eds) *What is a case? Exploring the foundations of sociology*, Cambridge: Cambridge University Press, pp 1-18.

Smyth, H. (1985) *Property companies and the construction industry in Britain*, Cambridge: Cambridge University Press.

Taylor, S. (1960) 'Hospitals of the future', *British Medical Journal*, ii(5201), p 753.

Timmins, N. (1995) *The five giants: A biography of the welfare state*, London: Harper Collins.

Vann-Wye, G. (1992) 'Hospitals in the UK: a history of design innovation', in R. Loveridge and K. Starkey (eds) *Continuity and crisis in the NHS*, Milton Keynes: Open University Press, pp 157–78.

Vaughan, D. (1992) 'Theory elaboration: the heuristics of case analysis', in C. Ragin and H. Becker (eds) *What is a case? Exploring the foundations of sociology*, Cambridge: Cambridge University Press, pp 173–200.

Walton, J. (1992) 'Making the theoretical case', in C. Ragin and H. Becker (eds) *What is a case? Exploring the foundations of sociology*, Cambridge: Cambridge University Press, pp 121–38.

Webster, C. (1988) *The health services since the war, Vol I*, London: HMSO.

Webster, C. (1994) 'Conservatives and consensus: the politics of the NHS, 1951–64', in A. Oakley and S. Williams (eds) *The politics of the welfare state*, London: UCL Press, pp 54–74.

Webster, C. (1998) 'Birth of the dream: Bevan and the architecture of the NHS', in G. Goodman (ed) *The state of the nation: The political legacy of Aneurin Bevan*, London: Gollancz, pp 106–29.

Wievorka, M. (1992) 'Case studies: history or sociology?', in C. Ragin and H. Becker (eds) *What is a case? Exploring the foundations of sociology*, Cambridge: Cambridge University Press, pp 159–72.

five

The case study as history: 'Ideology, class and the National Health Service' by Rudolf Klein

Ian Greener

Introduction

This chapter argues that by exploring case studies from the NHS's past, we can gain insights into the dynamics of its organisation and policy in the present. To this end, a classic paper examining conflict in the 1970s, Rudolf Klein's 'Ideology, class and the National Health Service', will be explored in terms both of what it tells us about the NHS in the 1970s and also of what it can tell us about the dynamics of health organisation today. First, we will explore Klein's original case study in depth, bringing out its key messages and themes. We will then explore how these themes can illuminate NHS policy and organisation in the 2010s, before going on to a conclusion.

Background to the case study

Klein published 'Ideology, class and the National Health Service' at the end of the 1970s in a leading US journal (Klein, 1979). The paper (see also Klein, 2006, ch 4) covers conflict within the Labour government, and between the Labour government and the medical profession, from 1974 and 1976 over the issue of beds set aside in NHS hospitals for the treatment of private patients (pay beds). Klein does not explicitly describe his work as a case study, although he does refer to it as the 'case of the pay beds issue' (p 487). It is a case study in that it is an exemplar of the relationship between policy makers and vested interests in the 1970s, based on empirical data and provides analysis that is generalisable beyond the scope of its particular example. It is therefore attempting to make an argument that by studying case studies from the history of the NHS we are better able to understand the present. This chapter invites (as well as presenting) a comparison of the events of the 1970s with those of the present, in order to better understand both.

Klein presents the pay beds case as being important for a number of reasons. First, he argues, because it questions 'the basic concordat on which the NHS was built' (Klein, 1979, p 465). The 'concordat' he refers to is based upon work of his that suggests that the creation of the NHS represented a tacit deal between the state and the medical profession, with the state, on the one hand, agreeing to allow the NHS the autonomy to run the service, while the medical profession, more or less facing a monopoly purchaser of its services in the state, agreed to work within the budget that was set for it (see, for example, Klein, 1990). This created a dynamic in which there was 'conflict within consensus' (Klein, 1979, p 464), where there was plenty of scope for the state and the medical profession to fall out, but definite limits about the criticisms each could make of the other because of their mutual dependence.

Second, Klein argues that the conflict brought into opposition the Labour Party and the trade unions, on the one hand, and the Conservative Party and the medical profession, on the other, creating a conflict about a health issue that had the capacity to reflect a clash of class interests. This is another important claim. For much of the history of the NHS it has been regarded, because of its principles of offering (mostly) free and (mostly) comprehensive care on the criteria of need rather than ability to pay, as a remarkably progressive example of social engineering (Greener, 2008). These tensions again raise important questions about health reform which are worth exploring both in terms of the 1970s and for today.

'Ideology, class and the National Health Service'

Klein structured his paper by first presenting some facts about private medical practice in the UK, following this by a brief account of the events surrounding the pay beds dispute between 1974 and 1976. He then went on to consider the conceptual difficulties of analysing the case, the role of the Labour Party, trade unions and medical profession in the dispute, and to present his conclusion, which discussed the implications of the paper for the study of the politics of health.

Private practice in the 1970s

Pay beds can be regarded as one of the oddities in the organisational structure of the NHS. Allowing private practice in NHS hospitals was not the result of deliberate design, but instead one of the compromises offered by Bevan to the consultants during the period leading up to the creation of the NHS. Bevan's strategy in setting up the NHS was effectively to split the medical profession (Honigsbaum, 1989), first getting the consultants on board through offering concessions such as allowing the use of pay beds, and thus for NHS consultants to practise private medicine in NHS hospitals, and then entering into a protracted negotiation with the general practitioners, having first secured the hospitals doctors' commitment to joining the NHS when it came into operation in 1948 (Rintala, 2003).

Klein begins by exploring the structure of private medical practice in the UK. He makes a number of points: that private practice takes a number of forms; that the scale of private practice is difficult to determine; that information about the incomes doctors receive from private practice is scarce; and that pay beds are only a tiny proportion of all NHS resources. What this amounts to in Klein's argument is the suggestion that not only was private practice 'marginal to the NHS' both in terms of its 'scale of operations and finance' and 'administratively and politically' but also there was a 'paucity of information' (Klein, 1979, p 467) about it. This lack of information signified the lack of political salience of pay beds in health politics in the years before 1974, making the rather explosive dispute that emerged between 1974 and 1976 even more remarkable.

The political battle between 1974 and 1976

This section presents a summary of Klein's research on the pay beds dispute between 1974 and 1976.

After four years of Conservative government, Labour was returned to power in 1974, winning not an emphatic majority, but on a minority vote. Klein presents a pledge contained in the Labour manifesto, in by no means a prominent place, that 'A Labour Government will revise and expand the National Health Service; abolish prescription charge; introduce free family planning; phase out private practice from the hospital service and transform the area health authorities in democratic bodies.' Labour called a second general election in 1974 in an attempt to achieve a majority, pledging this second time that the Labour government had already 'started its attack on queue-jumping by increasing the charge for private pay beds in National Health Service hospitals and is now working out a scheme for phasing private beds out of these hospitals'.

Between the two elections, Labour found its policy towards pay beds being forced by trade unions. The National Union of Public Employees (NUPE) took industrial action against pay beds at Charing Cross Hospital, with its members refusing to serve meals to or to help in the care of private patients. Members of the Confederation of Health Service Employees (COHSE) joined the strike, spreading it to other hospitals and catapulting the issue onto the front pages of newspapers and into television bulletins. In response, the British Medical Association's (BMA) Central Committee for Hospital Medical Services, the body that represented the consultants, threatened to adopt a work-to-rule for its members unless the Secretary of State, Barbara

Castle, took action to restore normal working and to rescind the union ban on pay bed admissions.

Barbara Castle was forced in these circumstances to make a decision about the future of pay beds. She met with representatives of the medical profession and unions and worked out an agreement in which the unions agreed to call off their industrial action and the consultants withdrew their work-to-rule threat. In return, a decision over pay beds was effectively postponed, being referred to an already-appointed working party that was negotiating a new contract for hospital consultants. Castle did, however, make the statement that she felt NHS facilities should not be made available on the basis of the ability to pay rather than need, those two different ideas being 'incompatible in the NHS'. Castle went further, on a subsequent occasion, using the metaphor of a church to describe the NHS and asking the question 'What would we say of a person who argued that he could only serve God properly if he had pay pews in his church?' The battle lines were clearly becoming drawn, with the trade unions flexing their muscles and Labour politicians either agreeing with the case they were making or acknowledging the power of the unions in the formulation of Labour policy at that time. Klein seems to argue more in favour of the former explanation, suggesting that the issue of pay beds was becoming framed in 'terms which made it central to the Labour Party's vision of itself as a crusader for social justice' (Klein, 1979, p 468).

In August 1975 the government outlined proposals for the separation of private practice from NHS hospitals. Labour would first legislate to revoke the authorisation of pay bed facilities in the NHS and then establish a licensing system for the private sector in order to freeze its size as at March 1974. Labour, then, wanted not only to remove pay beds from the NHS but also to prevent any further growth in private medicine. Things were not helped at the Labour Party conference in 1975, when NUPE put forward a resolution for the eventual abolition of all private practice and all private insurance schemes. The stakes, for both government and medical profession, were growing higher.

The new proposals reached the medical profession at a time when negotiations over the new consultant contract were already stalling. The Council of the BMA responded by recommending that senior hospital doctors limit their work to caring for emergencies and existing patients only, and began to collect undated resignations (a strategy that the BMA had also used in the 1960s to campaign for reforms in GP pay). Junior hospital doctors, in the meantime, were already embroiled in a pay dispute and had already introduced an emergencies-only rule, making it seem that hospitals, the vanguard of high-profile, high-technology medicine, were grinding to a halt.

NUPE responded in turn by threatening to blockade pay beds in retaliation for any consultant who followed the BMA call. Crisis meetings were held between the government and the medical profession, with Lord Goodman being brought in by the prime minister to mediate, and which led to a compromise formula that was to form the basis of subsequent legislation and become the basis of a new agreement on private practice. If we judge policy success by the ability of interested parties to reach a compromise, then this was a success.

The Goodman compromise was based on two principles: that private beds should be separated from the NHS, and that the government should allow private practice to be maintained in Britain, with doctors being entitled to work both privately and for the NHS. Around a quarter of pay beds (about 1,000 at that time) were to be phased out immediately, and decisions about the rest were to be taken by an independent board made up of representatives from the medical profession and appointees nominated in consultation with trade unions, and with an independent chair who had a casting vote, if necessary. No limits were set on the future size of the private sector and no date was set for completion of the phasing out of pay beds. The Conservative Party opposed the eventual legislation that put the compromise in place, putting forward (with the support of the BMA) 400 amendments and a number of new clauses during its passage through parliament. At one point it seemed that the Conservatives might succeed in bringing the Bill down by its exceeding available parliamentary time; but Labour, under threats of further industrial action from the trade unions, pushed the measure through by cutting short parliamentary discussion.

Analysing the case

After his outline of the case (which is longer than that presented above, which can be considered a summary of his summary), Klein goes on to paint some additional context that allows him to begin to present his analysis.

First, he suggests that Labour's position in the negotiations over pay beds was shaped by the common view that 'Labour Ministers tended to take it for granted that opposition to private practice within the NHS had always been an article of faith for the party' (Klein, 1979, p 472). This was because the allowance of pay beds was the result of a compromise that Bevan felt he had to make during the creation of the NHS rather than being a deliberate choice. Labour ministers' actions therefore 'represented the delayed implementation of what had always been the Labour Party's aims. Immanent policy had simply become explicit action' (p 472).

However, under Klein's scrutiny, this claim is shown not to make a great deal of sense. If pay beds were such an affront to Labour, and it had always intended to remove pay beds, why had it not removed them (or even made them much of issue) during the 1960s Wilson administration? Wilson's government had been far more concerned with abolishing prescription charges, the introduction of which had been one of the stated reasons for Bevan's resignation from the first post-war Labour government in 1951 (Campbell, 1987). Prescription charges were a much more live issue for Labour because they represented an affront to the idea that the NHS should be provided free of charge. However, by the 1970s they also represented a humiliating memory: Labour had abolished prescription charges to great fanfare in 1964, only to have to reinstate them two years later in the face of a budgetary crisis. As we saw earlier, the first Labour manifesto of 1974 made a commitment to abolish both prescription charges and pay beds, but it was pay beds that were carried forward to legislation. Why was this?

Klein suggests (p 473) that the problem was not that private practice had grown much during the 1970s, forcing itself onto Labour's policy agenda. Growth was incremental and marginal. Instead, he suggests that there was some evidence that although private medicine had not increased in size, it had increased in impact, with the 1971/72 House of Commons Employment and Social Services Sub-Committee carrying out an inquiry into NHS facilities for private patients and the Labour majority on the Committee using the opportunity to highlight what it saw as the abuses of private practice within the NHS. These findings were subsequently removed by the Conservative majority on the main Public Expenditure Committee, but they provided a forum and a means to gain impetus for raising an overtly ideological issue within government.

For Labour members of the Sub-Committee, private practice represented 'queue-jumping for non-medical reasons', which was unfair both on the public as a whole and on the clinicians who had to treat them. It led to dual standards of service and encouraged the most highly skilled consultants to become concentrated in areas of the country that held the greatest scope for private practice rather than medical need. This can be regarded as a consultant version of the inverse care law, whereby general practitioners tend to gravitate away from the areas where medical need is greatest because those areas also tend to offer a lower standard of living (Tudor-Hart, 1971).

Klein suggests that the Sub-Committee found little or no evidence of queue jumping or other abuses by private patients, but that this lack of evidence and the subsequent overruling of its report by the Conservative-dominated Public Expenditure Committee did not prevent the report from gaining wide currency. Indeed, on reading Klein's account now, a reader can't help wondering if the overruling of the report might have given it greater cachet among Labour politicians, who frequently invoked it between 1974 and 1976.

Klein, however, suggests that the main reason for the issue of pay beds becoming so live was a combination of the new Labour government's needing to do something to satisfy its activist left-wing and the difficult economic situation it inherited in 1974, with inflation, unemployment and the balance of payments deficit all rising. Labour ministers therefore had limited room for manoeuvre in terms of improving the NHS. Unions were being asked to accept wage restraint to reduce inflation through the 'Social Contract', but any additional budgetary settlement for health services was still going to be largely absorbed in pay settlements. In these circumstances, ministers had to make a political impact – keeping the unions, in particular, on board – but with little money to spend in achieving it. In addition to this (but absent in Klein's account), Labour had inherited the first major reform of the NHS, planned by both Labour and Conservative governments (Ministry of Health, 1968; DHSS, 1970, 1971; Secretary of State for Health and Social Services, 1972) but falling to Labour to implement, and so had to focus a great deal of time and energy on making the new reforms work.

The decision to focus on pay beds rather than on abolishing prescription charges makes a great deal of sense in this situation. Abolishing prescription charges would have been expensive, but removing pay beds was largely cost free (in economic terms, at least). Both policies would have helped to satisfy calls from trade unions for the government to show its commitment to the political left, but the latter also met the economic criterion of being affordable. It also allowed the government to challenge the consultants to offer a full-time commitment to providing NHS services, and so to bring them under greater managerial control and allow a more rational planning of healthcare manpower.

In the present era, when the Labour Party has been openly critical of union strike action, we also need an explanation as to why the government of the 1970s was so keen to act in concert with the trade unions. Klein suggests a number of reasons. A first issue is about context: the first general election of 1974 was called by Prime Minister Heath on the issue of who governed the country (Ling, 1998) – the government or the trade unions. The early 1970s, in the wake of the breaking economic crisis of the period, was characterised by antagonistic relationships between powerful trade unions and a government attempting to put into place industrial relations strategies. This had culminated a national strike by the coal miners and Heath's attempt to assert governmental authority in order to challenge union power. The election gamble failed, and resulted in the return of first, the minority and then, the majority Labour governments, which instead attempted to put in place a more corporatist approach to government in which the unions were increasingly incorporated into decision-making processes. This was partly ideological, but also the result of necessity: reducing inflation in a time of strong unions and collective bargaining arrangements required either significant union reform or an increase in union cooperation in order to make pay bargains stick.

In the NHS, professional organisations such as the BMA were growing in power and influence, and the number of unionised workers was increasing, the proportion being estimated at three-fifths of all NHS workers in 1974. There were significant rises in membership of COHSE and NUPE. This rise in membership offered far greater scope for industrial action to be a powerful negotiating tool, especially over pay.

In the early 1970s greater militancy appeared to be paying dividends, with rates of pay for NHS workers rising, and it culminated in 1973 with strikes by ancillary workers against the government's incomes policy. It also led to increased competition between COHSE and NUPE, and also had the potential to create competition between these groups and bodies such as the Royal College of Nursing, leading to the unions' effectively advertising their ability to strike better deals for members and potential members as a result of their militancy.

In 1973 the national conference of the National and Local Government Officers' Association (NALGO) called for the abolition of private pay beds, the first time the issue had been given prominence at a trade union conference. Subsequently, the removal of private practice became official Trade Union Congress policy, but this was hardly the result of a groundswell of activism at the local level. This claim is backed up by a survey commissioned in 1976, albeit by the body representing independent hospitals, which found 42% of trade unionists were in favour of keeping pay beds and only 25% were in favour of their removal. Klein suggests that industrial action was centred in London, because this is where the provision of pay beds was most politically visible, and that the political visibility might, in turn, have resulted from activists' perceptions of unfairness, rather than a general sense of discontent from other staff. This sense of unfairness arose from consultants' being able to increase their incomes at the expense of support staff, who had to support the private patients in NHS hospitals but received no extra reward for doing so.

However, it seems that consultants' income from private practice may also have been rather marginal. By 1973 the percentage of consultants with part-time contracts allowing them to undertake private practice had fallen below 50%, and although a small minority made large incomes from their private work, for most of the profession the amounts earned were relatively small. So why was the issue such an important one for the medical profession?

First, inflation and the fall in economic growth of early 1970s had resulted in the medical profession's perceiving a threat to its standard of living. Pay settlements in the 1970s saw doctors slipping down the earnings hierarchies, and living standards for general practitioners and consultants fell by a reported 20% between 1975 and 1977. The argument over pay beds has to be seen in the light of negotiations over a new consultant contract that began in 1974, the aim of which was to link reward more closely to effort. Labour also wanted to add incentives in favour of full-time consultants (for both ideological and planning reasons) and to encourage consultants to move into shortage specialities and deprived parts of the country. These new payments would the replace the distinction awards presently offered to specialists, and which were decided within the profession.

The contract negotiations dragged on for over a year before being abandoned, with the consultants coming to believe that the government's pay beds policy was the beginning of a process to remove opportunities for private practice entirely. This was fuelled by trade union activism, and also by the proposals to reward full-time commitment to the NHS and create a state monopoly over healthcare.

This suspicion was further fuelled by rivalry between the BMA and the Regional Hospital Consultants and Specialists Association, both of which claimed to represent the NHS consultants. In this environment, for most of the consultants, private practice increased in importance because of identification of the doctor as 'an independent entrepreneur, rather than a salaried civil servant' even if most earned a small amount of money from it.

However, the real extent of opposition from the consultants was revealed in BMA surveys of consultants in 1976. Although 73% were opposed to the separation of private practice from the NHS, only a minority were prepared to fight for this principle by resigning from the NHS, while 63% were prepared to accept the Goodman compromise. Only 54% of those eligible took part in the ballot, suggesting the issue was not as salient for most doctors as the rhetoric of their leaders might have suggested.

The politics of health

From the earlier analysis of the Labour government, the trade unions and the medical profession, Klein makes a number of points.

First, that the pay beds dispute was the result not of an emerging, independent and pressing problem in its own right, but of the importance of politics in deciding what issues come to the fore in healthcare.

Second, that the ideological position of the Labour government was not a deciding factor in the dispute. Rather, it was a 'predisposing factor' (p 484) that was activated because the Labour government of 1974 became dependent upon support from the trade unions and there had been a shift in the balance of power towards organised labour.

Third, that the shift in power towards organised labour allowed the trade unions to exert political pressure on the Secretary of State, and action on pay beds was the price that had to be paid for collective trade union support on national pay issues. Policy on pay beds appeared to be an (economically) inexpensive way of obtaining union support. Civil servants, however, saw the issue differently, taking into account the potential effects on relations with the medical profession, and so they were not in support of the changes.

Fourth, that the NHS requires the cooperation of a large variety of organised groups because it is dependent upon a 'complicated mix of specialized skills' (p 485). The NHS needing the co-operation of a wider range of organised groups meant that the medical profession were unable to prevent the issue of pay beds coming to the fore in health politics. But in order for the government to push through its programme of change, it still needed the support of the doctors to make the changes work.

Fifth, that the pay beds dispute represented the emergence of a new set of actors in the policy arena of the NHS: the trade unions. This change, Klein suggests, did not lead to the radicalisation of health politics, but did create a situation where more pluralistic bargaining was necessary, with the problem for policy analysts being how to account for the interaction of a whole set of organised interests. This leads to a paradox: the structure of health policy interests shapes and provides the language of pluralistic bargaining, but it is the interactions between these interests that determine the outcomes of any particular policy dispute.

'Ideology, class and the National Health Service' in retrospect

Klein's analysis of the 1970s is important in its own terms. It provides a snapshot of the politics of health at that time which shows how an issue that seems, in the larger scheme of the NHS, to be relatively unimportant came close to bringing the health service to a standstill. When we consider that this was in an era before 24-hour news and continual television coverage of industrial disputes, this is all the more remarkable. It is sobering and alarming to imagine how such a high-profile dispute would be conducted today.

An initial reflection on the case is the sense of how very different the policy environment was in the 1970s. The Office of National Statistics now reports national union membership density at about 28%, half of what it was in the 1970s. It is hard to obtain figures for the unionisation rate in the NHS, but it seems fair to claim that union power has been dramatically reduced. This is the result of a number of factors.

First, the contracting out of ancillary services under the Conservative government of the 1980s led to the destruction of the ability of those workers to engage in collective bargaining and markedly reduced their ability, except at a local level, to engage in any industrial action. Even that ability was minimal, because of the power that the private firms who now employed workers such as cleaners held to replace such workers. There is little prospect of the health service's being brought to a halt by ancillary workers now.

If ancillary workers are unable to affect the NHS through industrial action, what about the clinicians? In terms of the doctors, a key turning-point was at the end of the 1980s. The Thatcher-led government's health review effectively excluded the doctors from consultation, and then put in place legislation directly against the wishes of the medical profession. In the 1970s, the doctors, as we saw earlier, effectively held a veto over policy that they did not like because their cooperation was regarded by politicians as being necessary for any kind successful implementation. By the end of the 1980s things were rather different. One reason for this was the introduction of general managers into health services during the 1980s, and faith in management as providing the solution to the health service's ills.

In the 1970s, doctors effectively ran health services, but by the end of the 1980s this was no longer true. The Conservative government, buoyed by a large parliamentary majority even if its leader was becoming increasing weak, put in place an internal market for care, despite a concerted BMA campaign against it. The government legislated what were, at the time, the most radical reforms the NHS had seen, directly in the face of medical opposition, and, over time, watched the doctors' campaign against the reforms gradually wind down and evaporate. Politicians learned a valuable lesson from this: that it was possible to put in place radical health policy changes in the face of medical opposition. The subsequent rather incremental adoption of the internal market suggested, however, that legislating radical reform and implementing it were two separate things, and that the doctors were still needed to make change happen. However, medical influence over government decision making had been comprehensively challenged and found to be an optional rather than a compulsory part of policy making. The terms of negotiation for NHS reform were to be rather different in the 2000s.

Another factor explaining the reduced influence of the medical profession in the 1990s and 2000s has its roots in another element of Klein's account of the 1970s – the heterogeneity of the doctors. The traditional split in British medicine is between the interests of general practitioners and those of consultants, with the BMA attempting to represent both but often struggling to balance the interests of the two groups. What Klein's account showed was that the leaders of the consultants, having to take account of rival representative bodies and possibly taking a London-centric view, were found to be a good deal more radical than many of the members.

The gap between the representative bodies of the medical profession and the rank-and-file doctors has increased as doctors themselves have become more diverse. One difference is in the matter of gender: as more women entered the medical profession in the 1980s and 1990s they increasingly found that their interests were not taken into account by the male-dominated leaders of their profession and that their voice was not represented by them. Second, as the number of doctors has risen, they have become a more socially diverse grouping, coming from a wider variety of medical schools, and so having less in common. This, again, leads to a divergence of interests and makes it more difficult to create common ground for any medical leadership to speak for the profession as a whole. Third, as consultants have increasingly taken on managerial as well as clinical roles this has created another division, where more recently qualified doctors often have very different expectations of their roles, which may be based on non-clinical as well as clinical principles, and so are more sympathetic to attempts to improve the efficiency of health services than are their older peers.

If doctors have become less radical over time in their opposition to health reform (Greener, 2006), what about nurses? There is a history, particularly in the 1970s, of nurse activism (Hart, 1994), but it is striking that, for the most part, rather than being a part of a pluralistic approach to health policy making, nursing has instead found itself on the sidelines. Despite nurses being the largest group of health service workers, the most prestigious nursing representative body, the Royal College of Nursing, has for most of its history had an explicit policy of being anti-strike, thus removing a key negotiating tool from its armoury, and is generally regarded by governments as being the professional group in the NHS that is most compliant to reform (Traynor et al, 2007). Indeed, surveys of health workers' attitudes to reform issues find that the most supportive group of all is made up of nurses who have taken on managerial roles (Degeling et al, 2003) – a group that seems able to support most efforts to reorganise health services in a more managerial way. Given this, and the lack of a recent history of nursing industrial action, it seems that it would require a very significant change for nurses to become an integral part of analyses of the politics of health.

As such, the politics of health has changed dramatically since the time of Klein's article. Health policy formulation has become an increasingly closed shop, with politicians able to construct White Papers more or less as they wish and with negotiation over the content of policy taking place behind closed doors, often involving a substantial role for private sector lobby groups and policy advisers. Whether this is any more pluralistic, as Klein envisaged would be the case, is open to question. On the one hand, lobby groups and advisers may provide new and different perspectives that the corporatism of the 1970s often did not take into account, but on the other hand, this wider involvement of groups has not led to greater transparency because the consultations often take place outside of public forums. As I wrote this, the Conservative-Liberal Democrat Coalition government published a White Paper that was probably the most radical in NHS history (Secretary of State for Health, 2010) within 100 days of entering office and with barely any consultation with any health service group (or anyone else for that matter), and only provoked widespread protests from doctors after it had been passed in the Commons, even if recent surveys suggest there is very little public or professional support for the reforms. This makes a remarkable contrast with the policy area of the 1970s. Understanding how the politics of health has become so neutered since the 1970s is important, not least because, although it would not make sense to argue in favour of a return to the way politics was conducted then, introducing a countervailing force to untrammelled government policy making would surely be a positive move.

It is interesting to consider why, in direct contrast to the 1970s, it is possible for the government today to put in place a radical reform agenda that is opposed by the majority of those working in the NHS. One reason is the greater heterogeneity of the medical profession, already noted above. In the 1970s medical leaders were regarded as being more legitimately representative of doctors at all levels than they are today. Equally, the bruising encounter between the BMA and the Conservative government in the late 1980s showed that it was possible for the government to legislate directly against the wishes of the doctors – the most articulate and, at that time, most politically active group within the NHS (Klein, 1995) – and appears to have led to the doctors' becoming far more circumspect about again attempting to launch a national campaign against health reform.

Klein's study, for all its positive points, is not without its weaknesses. Klein did not foresee the remarkable changes that the NHS was to undergo in the 1980s and 1990s as general management and then the first internal market were introduced (Macfarlane et al, Chapter Nine; Wainwright and Calnan, Chapter Eleven; Allen, Chapter Eighteen), along with the concerted challenge to the medical profession and trade unions that this policy making represented. This is a rather unfair criticism, however, as it would have required him to foresee Thatcherism, which would have been an impossibility at the time of writing his article. Klein could not have foreseen, in particular, how the Conservative government would be prepared to take on the doctors directly over the introduction of the internal market (see earlier), even if was, by that time, an extension of the government's approach of attempting to tackle what it regarded as the 'vested interests' that were blocking attempts to reform Britain (Thatcher, 1993).

What is perhaps a more rounded criticism is that Klein appears to have been suggesting, by the end of his paper, that policy making in the 1980s was set to become more pluralistic. This is entirely understandable, given the end point of his case, with both the doctors and trade unions having exerted considerable influence over the pay beds dispute. However, it was possible to read the 1970s as a period in which corporatist policy had reached its zenith, and was therefore almost inevitably going to collapse through its own contradictions in the 1980s. Even Labour, with 'In Place of Strife' in the early 1970s, had acknowledged that trade union reform was necessary, even if the government at that time simply did not have the will to face up to its logic. Even as Klein published his article, the country tipped into the 'winter of discontent', when unions flexed their muscles and the Conservatives began to plan for a very different approach to industrial and economic policy making. Again, to predict the very different path of the 1980s is asking rather a lot of Klein, but, given his later prescience in picking up potentially radical change (Klein, 1998), it is also a measure of how much we expect from him.

What of private medical practice?

The main point of Klein's paper was not to explore private beds per se, but instead to explore the politics of health through that lens. But what happened to private practice afterwards?

The increase in private medicine during the 1980s, encouraged by government, is well documented (Richmond, 1996). Its growth stalled towards the end of the decade in the face of economic hard times, but instead of being frozen or abolished, has grown in importance because of the increasing blurring of boundaries between NHS and private medicine. During the 1980s, initiatives to reduce NHS waiting lists made use of private facilities, often staffed by the same doctors who would have provided the care had it taken place in NHS facilities. The internal market of the 1990s did not allow competition between public and private providers, but in the 2000s the 'mixed economy of care' created an environment where not-for-profit and private providers of care entered into contracts to provide NHS care on an unprecedented scale. The aim of these reforms was to increase competition and drive up quality. It is still far from clear whether it achieved these goals, but it may have increased the capacity of the NHS by offering additional beds, and so have contributed to a reduction in waiting times. But the most important factor is that private medical practice has gone from being an anathema to the NHS and its workers, to being a direct competitor for NHS funds.

At the same time, however, private practice has also been represented by policy makers as having a dark side. During the New Labour government, in particular, private practice became regarded as a symptom of a local 'closed shop' in which waiting lists were often locally manufactured by consultants so that they could preserve their private work while continuing to receive the benefits of working for the NHS. It is no coincidence that, as well as making greater use of the private sector as a means of increasing NHS capacity, reforms have focused on bringing new private and not-for-profit entrants into healthcare, in an attempt to foster competition, as well as on increasingly specifying in the terms of their contracts the hours and times that consultants are obliged to offer the NHS.

Equally, the present Coalition government has proposed to abolish the cap on the proportion of income that NHS hospitals can earn from private income, a change that will lead to their having to consider carefully the balance between public and private income that they want to earn. Pay beds, rather than withering on the vine as a result of the compromise of the 1970s, never went away. They have been a mainstay of television dramas about hospital care such as *Casualty* and *Bodies*, in which greedy consultants are portrayed, in line with the parliamentary Sub-Committee report of the 1970s, as allowing queue-jumping for their own private enrichment. Even in the 2000s, claims and counter-claims have abounded of hospitals allowing 'rich' patients to 'queue-jump' using NHS facilities (Browne, 2002). The pay beds issue has become less prominent at a national level, but has never really gone away.

What is new is that the government now appears to be actively encouraging NHS facilities to chase increasing amounts of private practice by removing the private income cap. In a similar way that universities have been encouraged to pursue increasing numbers of overseas students, who pay higher fees despite receiving effectively the same service, NHS hospitals can now decide for themselves the balance of fee income that will suit them best. Again, the lack of co-ordinate response from doctor, nurse or trade unions bodies in opposition to the changes until they had already become law is a sign of the rather anaemic level of political debate that now prevails in UK healthcare.

Conclusion

Klein's paper is, in my view, a hugely valuable study from the 1970s that provides key insights into the very different way that the politics of healthcare in the NHS work today. This contrast is not just about nostalgia; it reminds us that the rather sterile, non-confrontational relationship between the doctors and the state today wasn't always so, and of the strong reactions that private medicine, until very recently, raised for many people working within the NHS.

Klein's paper is not as widely cited as I would have hoped (just 20 citations on Google Scholar, although of course this does not pick up contemporary books that cite it). Studies that have cited it tend to use it as an example of how the relationships among vested interests changed in the 1970s, or to use its theoretical ideas around more pluralistic policy making to inform an understanding of veto-points, or as a basis for a comparison between the UK and the US. Here, however, it has formed the basis of a comparison between the politics of health in the 1970s and in the 2010s.

The confrontational and highly politicised health-policy arena of the 1970s is in marked contrast to that of today. The influence of the trade unions over health policy was to prove relatively short lived because of the Conservative government's confrontation with trade unions more generally in the 1980s and its specific policy of contracting out ancillary services in the NHS. Medical influence declined after the profession's unsuccessful attempts to campaign against the internal market reforms later in that decade, and also as a result of its increasing heterogeneity and the inability of the leaders of the medical profession to campaign on behalf of the majority of their members. Nursing has never managed to have the influence over health policy that its centrality to the NHS would suggest.

As such, the plurality that Klein suggested might become the norm in health politics (at least conceptualised as representing public debate between interested parties) never really surfaced. However, another of his conclusions, that of the NHS's dependence upon a diverse group of workers arranged in complex patterns of organisation, remains true. It remains within the power of doctors and nurses, in particular, to campaign, mobilise and, should they wish, to bring the NHS to a standstill. We are now facing the most radical (and potentially damaging) proposals for health reorganisation in the history of the NHS – but whether clinicians will mobilise against them seems unlikely. Until clinicians re-establish their role as leaders of opinion for health reform, and become prepared again to use their industrial muscle, it seems as if policy will be led by politicians, their advisers and the lobby groups that are most able to make their presence felt.

References

Browne, A. (2002) 'Scandal of NHS beds auction', *Guardian*, 6 January.

Campbell, J. (1987) *Nye Bevan and the mirage of British socialism*, London: Weidenfeld and Nicolson.

Degeling, P., Maxwell, S., Kennedy, J. and Coyle, B. (2003) 'Medicine, management, and modernisation: a "danse macabre"?', *British Medical Journal*, vol 326, no 7390, pp 649–52.

DHSS (Department of Health and Social Security) (1970) *National Health Service: The future structure of the National Health Service*, London: HMSO.

DHSS (1971) *National Health Service reorganisation: Consultative document*, London: HMSO.

Greener, I. (2006) 'Where are the medical voices raised in protest?', *British Medical Journal*, vol 330, p 660.

Greener, I. (2009) *Healthcare in the UK: Understanding continuity and change*, Bristol: Policy Press.

Hart, C. (1994) *Behind the mask: Nurses, their unions and nursing policy*, London: Bailliere Tindall.

Honigsbaum, F. (1989) *Health, happiness and security: The creation of the National Health Service*, London: Routledge.

Klein, R. (1979) 'Ideology, class and the National Health Service', *Journal of Health Politics, Policy and Law*, vol 4, no 3, pp 464–90.

Klein, R. (1990) 'The state and the profession: the politics of the double-bed', *British Medical Journal*, vol 301, pp 700–2.

Klein, R. (1995) 'Big bang health care reform – does it work? The case of Britain's 1991 National Health Service reforms', *Milbank Quarterly*, 73, pp 299–307.

Klein, R. (1998) 'Why Britain is reorganizing its National Health Service – yet again', *Health Affairs*, vol 17, pp 111–25.

Klein, R. (2006) *The new politics of the NHS: From creation to reinvention*, Abingdon: Radcliffe Publishing.

Ling, T. (1998) *The British state since 1945: An introduction*, Cambridge: Polity.

Ministry of Health (1968) *National Health Service: The administrative structure of the medical and related services in England and Wales*, London: HMSO.

Richmond, C. (1996) 'NHS waiting lists have been a boon for private medicine in the UK', *Canadian Medical Association Journal*, vol 154, pp 378–81.

Rintala, M. (2003) *Creating the National Health Service: Bevan and the medical lords*, London: Frank Cass Publishers.

Secretary of State for Health (2010) *Equity and excellence: Liberating the NHS*, London: The Stationery Office Limited.

Secretary of State for Health and Social Services (1972) *The National Health Service reorganisation: England*, London: HMSO.

Thatcher, M. (1993) *The Downing Street years*, London: Harper Collins.

Traynor, M., Drennan, V., Goodman, C., Mark, A., Davis, K. et al (2007) '"Nurse entrepreneurs" a case of government rhetoric?', *Journal of Health Services Research and Policy*, vol 13, pp 13–18.

Tudor-Hart, J. (1971) 'The inverse care law', *Lancet*, vol 1, pp 405–1.

six

Hospitals in trouble

Joan Higgins

Introduction

The notion that hospitals can do harm as well as good was not a new one when John Martin published *Hospitals in trouble* in 1984. Contemporary accounts of conditions in 18th-century hospitals talked of the high mortality and infection rates, the unhygienic conditions and the fact that they frequently 'killed' rather than 'cured'. Later, in 1863, Florence Nightingale, in her *Notes on hospitals*, declared that 'it may seem a strange principle to enunciate, as the very first requirement in a hospital, that it should do the sick no harm' (p iii). She went on to explain that people who were admitted to hospital were actually at higher risk of infection, or even death, than sick people with the same illness outside hospitals. These two books – a century apart – had in mind different kinds of 'harm' and identified different causes. Both, however, made the point that institutions which were designed to care for and treat sick people sometimes damaged or, occasionally, killed them. It is a paradox that remains today in every health system, and is the reason why this case study is of continuing importance.

Description of the case study

- The main research question is 'How is it that institutions established to protect vulnerable people sometimes do them harm?'.
- The first inquiry report into failing hospitals was published in 1969.
- There are nine key elements of failure, common in all inquiries

Martin's book began with the central question: 'How is it that institutions established to care for the sick and helpless can have allowed them to be neglected, treated with callousness and even deliberate cruelty?' The book was the first systematic analysis of failures of care in long-stay NHS hospitals and it covers the period 1965–83. The hospitals were primarily caring for people with mental health problems and learning disabilities, neglected groups who were, in every sense, 'out of sight and out of mind'. The hospitals had been built, quite deliberately, in isolated areas and their patients had often lived there, beyond the gaze of mainstream society, for many years. The plight of these people came to public attention in November 1965 when *The Times* published a letter from a number of peers, academics and social workers which deplored what they described as the shocking treatment of older people in 'mental hospitals'. They complained that the Ministry of Health had ignored their concerns and called for a national investigation. The letter was followed up, in 1967, by a book, *Sans everything: A case to answer*, edited by Barbara Robb, one of the signatories to the letter. This set out in some detail the appalling conditions in a number of hospitals, and shortly afterwards the Minister of Health commissioned the first in a series of inquiries into failures of care in the NHS.

The purpose of Martin's book was to learn lessons from the inquiry reports that were published after 1969 (see also Keen, Chapter Seven; Exworthy and Oliver, Chapter Nineteen). It also described how the NHS responded to these reports, and drew out the implications for the management of the NHS and for NHS staff in particular.

Lessons from the inquiries

The analysis of the inquiry reports threw up a remarkable number of common themes, even though the hospitals concerned were in different parts of the country and of different types and sizes. The main factors involved in the failures of care were:

- isolation
- lack of support
- the 'corruption of care'
- failures of leadership
- poor administration and lay management
- lack of resources
- power of trade unions
- inadequacies of training
- personal failings.

It is worth examining these themes in turn because of their relevance to health services today and as a way of demonstrating the significance of the case study in health policy analysis.

Isolation of and *in* the failing hospitals took many forms. The hospitals were usually geographically isolated; they had been built away from towns and cities and often had their own extensive facilities and grounds (including farms for growing their own produce). They had few visitors and were beyond the normal scrutiny which occurs when family, friends and others come and go. Abuse took place behind closed (often locked) doors where no one could see what occurred. There was isolation *within* the hospitals too. Different wards had different regimes, with some of them described as 'little fiefdoms' (p 81). Staff were vulnerable and afraid to complain. Medical staff rarely visited the wards; their workloads were heavy, ward rounds were infrequent and many were out of touch with the day-to-day treatment of patients. Staff in these hospitals were intellectually isolated: they did not attend courses and were not up to date with the latest thinking in their disciplines. As Martin points out, 'they were cut off from their professions as much as from the world outside the hospital' (p 81). Many years later, in the Bristol Hospital Inquiry, the very same observation was made. Although Bristol Royal Infirmary was a leading teaching hospital in the centre of a large city, the junior staff described some of their senior colleagues as being in a 'backwater', left behind by recent developments in their disciplines.

Lack of support for vulnerable patients was a common theme in the inquiries. These people had often been abandoned by family and friends and many had been 'put away' for life. They risked becoming scapegoats when things went wrong and were the butt of 'practical jokes' and cruel humour. Inspection regimes tended not to identify these issues and professional supervision did not address them adequately. Staff had become adept at resisting external scrutiny. As one nurse put it: 'As a charge nurse I am head of a household, therefore a person resistant to outside peering and prying eyes' (p 83).

The 'corruption of care' was evident throughout the accounts of these hospitals. The primary aim of caring for vulnerable people had become secondary to the maintenance of the regime and 'the preservation of order, quiet and cleanliness' (p 87). Staff had lost touch with why they were there and the routines had become ends in themselves. People who had been attracted to a caring profession had lost their values and sense of purpose.

Failures of leadership ran through all the hospitals where care was poor. Senior staff did not establish, or display, appropriate standards of behaviour and showed little interest in the job satisfaction of their colleagues. There was victimisation of staff who stepped out of line and who drew shortcomings in care to the attention of management. There was little willingness to acknowledge or respond positively to criticism. Doctors were often invisible. In most cases they showed no leadership and were resented by nursing staff, who worked long hours for much lower rates of pay. In some hospitals doctors were known for over-prescribing and over-treating, but there was no means of challenging their clinical practice and protecting patients from these excesses. In these hospitals, doctors could be overbearing and autocratic, with few restraints on their powers.

Poor administration and lay management were a feature of many, if not most, of the hospitals that were criticised. The inquiries spanned a period when there was considerable organisational and management change in the NHS. In the beginning, Hospital Management Committees were at the apex of the organisational tree; by the end, it was District Health Authorities. All of these different bodies had lay membership, and it is upon this that Martin focuses in looking at the weaknesses of the regimes. He describes how many of these 'inadequate local worthies' (p 90) were simply not up to the task of management. They had a very loose job description and concentrated on issues that were inappropriate to their lay role. They tended to fall back on commenting upon obvious physical defects of the buildings rather than on standards of care, so that Martin says their reports read as if they had been produced by a 'trainee Clerk of Works' (p 90) rather than a lay manager. He says that they also displayed 'the very English weakness of parochialism' (p 91) and that there was a failure to understand, or take account of, innovations and developments elsewhere in the NHS. They had no comparators, so did not appreciate that their hospitals had fallen out of step with what was normally regarded as good practice. They were sometimes too empathetic to staff and were ill equipped to challenge or question them. In some cases, staff deliberately kept them in the dark so they had no opportunity to comment or to put things right.

Lack of resources contributed significantly to poor care. The hospitals were often chronically understaffed, and even when staffing improved, from 1969 onwards, they still did badly, compared with other hospitals. Whittingham Hospital, for example, in 1969 had one doctor to 714 patients. Lack of staff was often said to be the single most important explanation for the low standards in these long-stay hospitals. However, other factors, such as the attitude and values of the staff, were important too. Many had lost touch with the expectations of their professional bodies. Their *raison d'être* was to get through a series of tasks, and the 'good patients' were those who conformed uncomplainingly to the institutional regimes (p 219).

The power of trade unions was very evident in some of the failing hospitals and it was often a malign influence that set the interests of staff against those of vulnerable patients and 'management'. Some of them sought power for its own sake and in order to exercise control within these isolated institutions. 'Whistleblowers' who complained about the treatment of patients and the behaviour of their colleagues were marginalised and, in the worst cases, seriously victimised.

Many of the inquiry reports point to *inadequacies of training*, poor recruitment practices and a lack of supervision. Staff received very little support in what could be alarming and threatening situations and some were promoted well beyond their capabilities. They had responsibilities for which they had no training or talent and the reports were critical of the senior managers who had allowed this situation to persist. Colleagues turned a blind eye to practices which they knew to be wrong, because they had to continue to work on that ward next day and next week – possibly for the rest of their working life.

Finally, Martin attributes failures of care to the *personal failings* of staff who provided and managed that care. Some were simply weak and did not challenge the behaviour of colleagues when they knew it to be wrong. Others failed to demonstrate leadership and to set appropriate standards of behaviour. They sometimes felt inadequate and threatened themselves; this showed itself in intimidation and bullying of more junior staff. Attempts at humour were misplaced, and jokes at the expense of patients reinforced the already obvious power differentials. Martin talks of 'permissive sub-cultures' (p 96) in which cruelty and harshness were tolerated and where outright brutality and criminality could occasionally be found.

Although the inquiry reports described some of the very worst conditions in hospitals in the UK in the 1970s and 1980s, these same characteristics of failure can still be found in the NHS today. Some, such as the negative power of trade unions, may have less prominence, but the factors listed by Martin would still be recognisable by any analyst of health policy a quarter of a century after his book was published.

Methods and analysis

- A mix of contemporary history, administration and sociology
- Inquiry reports used as a valuable source of data, rich in detail
- Inquiries can serve many purposes, not just fact finding.
- Despite their strengths, inquiry reports are variable in quality and an imperfect vehicle for gathering data and understanding failure.
- Case studies can provide good contemporaneous knowledge and context and a sense of historical perspective.

Three particular aspects of a discussion of methodology are relevant in this case study. First, we discuss the methodology that Martin used to study hospital failure. Second, we can use his work to examine the 'inquiry' itself as a method of fact finding and lesson learning in British social policy. The 'inquiry' has become an extremely popular tool over the last 40 years, not just in hospitals but in social care (especially in services for children) and in mental health services. The first major childcare inquiry (into the death of Maria Colwell) was published in 1974 and it was followed by other high-profile inquiries into the ill-treatment of children, such as, in recent years, Victoria Climbié and 'Baby P'. As this section will demonstrate, inquiries can serve a variety of purposes apart from the obvious aim of gathering information and establishing what went wrong. Third, we can reflect on the values of a case study approach in analysing a 'classic text' such as *Hospitals in trouble*.

The methods used in Hospitals in trouble

Martin described his book as 'a mixture of contemporary history, administration and sociology, with a bias towards the practical rather than theoretical, but conceived at the level of principle rather than the details of administration' (p xiii). The methods he used were both familiar and simple. His book is based upon a detailed textual analysis of 21 inquiry reports and other relevant documents. The key themes from these reports are identified and analysed in depth. Before, during and after the process of identifying the most important issues which were emerging, Martin interviewed staff in the hospitals concerned, senior officials and policy makers in the Department of Health and Social Services (DHSS), the Health Service Commissioner, senior members of professional bodies such as the General Nursing Council and other academics working in similar areas. The interviews were an opportunity to gather more data and also to test out the robustness of the conclusions that were emerging from the analysis of the inquiry reports. The first half of Martin's book describes the different aspects of 'the problem' that was identified through this analysis, while the second half identifies a number of 'remedies' to address the problem.

Inquiry reports in social policy

Over the last 40 years inquiry reports have proved to be a rich source of data for policy analysts. They capture not just legislative intent and implementation at particular periods but also the 'mood of the time'. They describe practices that may have been commonplace when the reports were published, but that seem callous and insensitive in retrospect.

Martin's book shows how inquiries themselves changed over the years. The Ely Hospital Inquiry, which was the first of its type, took just 15 days to hear the evidence and completed its work within a year. Nevertheless, it ran to 83,000 words and was comprehensive in its coverage. Before long, however, the public inquiry had become a major undertaking. As Martin points out, the Farleigh Inquiry heard 56 witnesses, Whittingham 85 and South Ockendon 116. Inquiries started to employ their own solicitors, and sometimes barristers as well, and the costs rose accordingly (p 73). The major inquiries of more recent years, such as the Royal Liverpool Children's Hospital Inquiry, the Bristol Royal Infirmary Inquiry and the Shipman Inquiry each lasted several years and resulted in many volumes of evidence and analysis. They have been the subject of great public and professional interest and have had an increasing impact upon policy. An analysis undertaken in 2002 shows that public inquiries are increasing in number (Walshe and Higgins, 2002). There were two in the 1970s, five in the 1980s and 52 from 1990 to 2002. In 1994, the Department of Health issued a circular (HSG(94)27) which required that an inquiry be held into every case in which a person receiving treatment for mental health problems committed homicide. The overall number of inquiries subsequently increased very markedly.

Walshe and Higgins' analysis suggests that inquiries may serve at least six purposes, which are not, of course, mutually exclusive:

* establishing the facts
* learning from events
* providing an opportunity for reconciliation and resolution
* reassurance and rebuilding of public confidence
* establishing accountability and identifying culpability
* providing a political response, showing that action was taken.

It is probably obvious that the main purpose of an inquiry is to discover 'what went wrong', and perhaps who or what was to blame. Increasingly, public bodies have also made an explicit commitment to learning from inquiries and responding formally to their recommendations. What may have been less obvious is the way in which inquiries can provide catharsis for patients, families and communities. People have an opportunity to tell their story, a chance to reflect on the impact of the events for all concerned and to grieve openly. This was probably at its most stark in Liverpool when the Royal Liverpool (Alder Hey) Inquiry was taking place, in Stafford during the Mid Staffordshire Inquiry and in Hyde, Greater Manchester, during the Shipman Inquiry. Many families, and whole communities, were affected. In Bristol, during the Bristol Royal Infirmary Inquiry, there was a clear determination that 'this must never happen again'. Professional bodies and politicians sought to reassure the public that the Inquiry would leave no stone unturned, that vested interests would be exposed and that measures would be introduced to ensure fundamental changes in policy and practice. Thus, the public inquiry can serve a number of purposes, some explicit and others more subtle.

Since Royal Commissions became unfashionable there have been few methodologies, apart from inquiries such as these, that examine an aspect of social policy in such forensic depth. They are enormously valuable for understanding organisational norms, individual behaviour and how gaps between policy making and implementation can arise.

Nevertheless, they have their critics. The Department of Health has itself said that 'there is an impression of variable focus, different levels of rigour, differences in methodology and in the way that recommendations are framed and adopted' (DH, 2000, p 65). An editorial in the *British Medical Journal* was equally harsh (Smith, 2000). It argued that there were growing suspicions that some inquiries were set up not simply to get at the facts but 'to divert the heat from politicians' (p 715). It concluded that there was a growing urgency to clarify what inquiries were for, how they should be run, what criteria should govern the launch of an inquiry and what processes would be used for appointing inquiry members. It suggested that, unless these processes became more transparent, inquiries and their conclusions would lack credibility and be suspected of 'bias, corruption or incompetence' (p 715).

These reservations about inquiries are well founded but they do not challenge the conclusion that, taken together, inquiries into failures of care over 40 years have thrown up consistent and clear messages about what goes wrong in organisations that were designed to protect vulnerable people.

The value of a case study approach in analysing a 'classic text'

Perhaps the greatest value of analysing 'classic texts' arises from the fact that they are very much 'creatures of their time'. In the policy world, they tend to reflect the preoccupations of the moment. Although policy themes recur, they adopt a different shape and emphasis at different points in time. Texts like this help us to understand the historical context of social policy and they enable us to identify patterns and issues that seem to be part of the fabric of our social institutions, as well as of professional practice.

The benefit of hindsight helps us to understand policy problems that may look glaringly obvious from a distance but that are complex and impenetrable at the time. Anyone trying to analyse contemporary social policy is trammelled by extraneous factors that may or may not be relevant to the debate. It is difficult to tell, when one is deep in the middle of it. A book such as John Martin's brings clarity to the task. It does not claim to contribute to grand theory but it uses an intelligible, systematic structure for finding an answer to an important research question.

The contemporary relevance of the case study

- We are now beginning to quantify 'adverse incidents' and failures in the NHS.
- Governments are more active in promoting learning from failure, in a coherent manner.
- Many changes in policy and practice derive from the recommendations of inquiry reports.
- Martin's work emphasises the importance of understanding failure in its broader context.
- 'Human error' is rarely the sole cause of failure. Systemic problems are usually at the heart of what goes wrong.

Quantifying failure

The modern NHS is beset by complaints about failures in hospitals that result in harm to, or the death of, patients in its care. In 2000 the government published a report entitled *An Organisation with a Memory*. It was the outcome of an expert group that had been established to learn from 'adverse events'. The report explained that, although the great majority of NHS care was of a very high standard, serious failures nevertheless occurred. What is more, the same type of failure was happening repeatedly, 'displaying strong similarities to incidents which have occurred before and in some cases almost exactly replicating them' (DH, 2000, p vii). Following the publication of the report, the government introduced a series of measures to identify and quantify the things that went wrong and to respond to them robustly. One outcome was the creation of the National Patient Safety Authority (NPSA) in 2001 and the introduction of a mandatory system for recording and reporting 'adverse events'. For the first time, there was a national system for gathering and analysing data and a determination to learn from things that go wrong. Between October 2003, when the NPSA first started to collect data, and November 2009 there were 3,875,241 recorded incidents in the NHS, most of them in acute hospitals. In recent years the number has reached 1 million incidents per annum and this is increasing steadily. By far the largest category of incidents is 'patient accidents' – often referred to euphemistically as 'slips, trips and falls'. This accounts for around 32% of all incidents each year. The next biggest categories are 'treatment/procedure' (13%); 'medication' (10%); 'infrastructure', for example staffing/facilities (7%); 'documentation', for example patient records (7%) and clinical assessment, for example diagnosis/scans (3%–6%). These figures show that it is not the well-publicised hospital-acquired infections (such as MRSA or *C. difficile*), medication errors or inappropriate clinical interventions that are the biggest problems in the NHS, but often quite simple failures of care, such as ensuring that patients do not fall out of bed or slip in the bathroom (NPSA, 2009). Most of these incidents are not serious and very few result in claims for compensation; however, around 10,000 each year do result in 'severe harm or death' (NPSA, 2009).

What the NPSA has been able to do, unlike the inquiry reports of previous years, has been to gather data systematically over a period of years. Although it can quantify only 'reported incidents', there is evidence that the collection of data, and its accuracy, is improving each year. While the inquiry reports produced evidence in considerable depth, often in vivid detail, they could not give any indication of the size of the problem.

Learning from failure: better regulation

The obvious question to arise from Martin's study is how to prevent failure from occurring in the future. Before the publication of Martin's book in 1984, there were no systematic attempts to draw together the threads of the different inquiries or to respond to them in a coherent manner. In 2000, *An Organisation with a Memory* said that 'The time is right for a fundamental re-thinking of the way the NHS approaches the challenge of learning from adverse health-care events. The NHS often fails to learn the lessons when things go wrong, and has an old fashioned approach in this area compared with other sectors' (p xi).

Since then there have been significant improvements. The government now responds formally to the major reports and spells out how it intends to deal with their recommendations. There are many explicit examples of policy change arising directly from the reports. More generally, 'regulators' such as the Care Quality Commission (CQC) and the NHS Litigation Authority (NHSLA) have been given the specific responsibility to develop measures that reflect learning from failure. The NHSLA, for example, indemnifies healthcare providers against claims for clinical (and other) negligence. It has created a set of standards, based upon claims experience and knowledge of high-risk activities, against which its members are assessed on a regular basis and there are financial incentives for members to improve their practice. The Bristol, Alder Hey, Shipman and Climbié inquiries, among others, all led to major policy changes across a wide range of activities, including death registration, revalidation of doctors, improved consent practice and data sharing between different agencies. This does not mean, of course, that tragedies will not occur in future. However, there is now a more intelligent and consistent approach to learning from, and dealing with, failure than those that prevailed in earlier decades.

Putting things in perspective

Any individual inquiry into a failure of health and social care systems, whether it is about hospital patients, child protection or homicides by people with mental health problems, can seem to identify a singular and unique set of events. Individual doctors may be blamed, individual social workers may be called to account, failing hospitals may be identified.

However, what Martin's book and others like it have shown is that there are deeply ingrained patterns of failure in some of our social institutions. These are never 'one off' events and there are clear and identifiable organisational risk factors in each set of circumstances. There are, of course, rogue individuals who indulge in acts of omission, cruelty or even criminality, but they usually go undetected because of long-established systemic weakness. Our ability to predict failure, based on past experience, is remarkably strong.

There is a mass of evidence from other sectors (for example the Audit Commission's findings in 2002 on the causes of the Oldham riots, and reports on airline and shipping disasters), and from other countries, that demonstrates that the messages are consistent. What may seem to be isolated incidents, when disasters occur, can be shown to be part of the well-established fabric of failure. The tendency to blame 'human error' or particular individuals is distracting and rarely gets to the heart of the problem. Martin's book emphasises the complexity of failure and cautions against rushing to judge the individuals at the centre of the crisis.

Resisting 'moral panic'

It is not unusual for governments and the media, when faced with public concern about failures of care in the NHS, to over-react to the problems and to focus upon the wrong issues. One current example would be the present government's response to healthcare acquired infections (HCAIs) such as MRSA and *C. difficile*. There is no doubt that such infections are traumatic for patients who acquire them and that they can result in death. It is also an indictment of modern hospitals that hygiene and cleanliness have not had higher priorities and that national intervention has been necessary to correct the problem. However, as the NPSA data demonstrates, the proportion of 'reported incidents' involving HCAIs is very small and it pales into insignificance when compared with the harm caused by 'patient accidents' (HCAIs accounting for 2% of incidents, compared with 33% for patient accidents, in 2008). HCAIs frequently feature as front-page news in the national press and the coverage has fuelled patients' anxieties about whether hospitals are safe places for sick people. The response to this concern – better hand washing – has been, in part, symbolic. Although more effective hand washing can certainly reduce some infections, it has no impact on others and it is not a panacea.

Having an understanding of the wider issues that the inquiry reports and Martin's book touch upon, as well as a sense of history, can enable policy analysts to evaluate the latest 'health scare' in a balanced way. For over 40 years the press has demonised individuals, hospitals and particular clinical practices. As Martin observed, coverage of the inquiry reports was 'sensationalized' and members of staff were 'reviled and ostracized' (p 183). At the same time, the press and investigative journalists played a valuable role in highlighting and exposing failure when traditional routes had not done so. It is important to understand this context and to sift carefully the data produced by the press and other media. Some of it may be an exaggeration, but other information might be hugely valuable. It can detract from the key issues or it can spotlight them starkly. Any desire to address social problems must be based upon a sound analysis of what went wrong. Martin's book demonstrates the need for a balanced and informed approach, and not one based upon selective and partial media concerns.

Summary

The purpose of this chapter has been to demonstrate the value of using a case study in health policy analysis. In this case it was a single study about why hospitals fail, but it covered a period of nearly 20 years. The study shows that the roots of failure go very deep and can rarely be attributed to the actions of one or two rogue professionals. Things that go wrong have to be seen in the context of systemic failure, deriving from problems of organisational culture, poor leadership and other complex factors. The main data source for the case study was the official inquiry reports into hospital failure, published from 1969 onwards. These provide a rich vein of information and are valuable contemporary documents. They help us to understand policy, practice and values in health policy at particular points in time. One of the benefits of a case study such as Martin's is the depth of analysis that is possible when a single question is analysed using data spanning nearly two decades. However, the inquiry reports do not paint a comprehensive picture and are gradually being supplemented with more systematic data collection and analysis, which provides a greater breadth of understanding. The single most important contribution of a case study of this kind in health policy is that it lends perspective. Looking back, it is possible to discern trends and patterns that are difficult to see in the heat of the moment, when things go wrong. The sometimes natural inclination to blame individuals is diluted with the benefit of hindsight, when the full complexity of systemic problems can be understood more easily. This case study, like many others, helps us to stand back, reflect and bring a sociological analysis to bear on some of the most challenging problems of our time.

References

DH (Department of Health) (2000) *An organisation with a memory: Report of an expert group on learning from adverse events in the NHS*, London: The Stationery Office.

Martin, J.P. (1984) *Hospitals in trouble*, Oxford: Basil Blackwell.

NPSA (National Patient Safety Agency) (2009) *Patient safety incident reports in the NHS: Reporting and learning system quarterly data summary; Issue 14, November 2009*, England.

Nightingale, F. (1863) *Notes on hospitals*, 3rd edn, London: Longman, Green, Longman, Roberts and Green.

Robb, B. (1967) *Sans everything: A case to answer*, London: Nelson.

Smith, R. (2000) Editorial: 'Inquiring into inquiries', *British Medical Journal*, vol 321, pp 715–16.

Walshe, K. and Higgins, J. (2002) 'The use and impact of inquiries in the NHS', *British Medical Journal*, vol 325, pp 895–900.

seven

Normal accidents: learning how to learn about safety

Justin Keen

Introduction

Healthcare delivery is inherently complex, and we know that people make mistakes in every health service every day. Mistakes can and do harm patients, and we should be concerned to learn from them in order to ensure safer care in the future. There is a large and rapidly growing literature on errors and their prevention and no shortage of practical guidance, suggesting that there is indeed a desire to learn (see Higgins, Chapter Six). But closer inspection reveals a puzzle. Most research and guidance focuses on the avoidance of errors made by individual clinicians, and on the need to identify immediate causes when mistakes are made. Yet high-profile reports (Institute of Medicine, 1999) and inquiries into tragedies in health and social care (Kennedy, 2001; Laming, 2003) have concluded that failures should be attributed to poorly designed and performing systems of care. We therefore have two very different types of explanation of errors, one focusing on individuals and the other on the organisation of care. Which one is right?

This chapter argues that systemic explanations of safety and failure are honoured in the breach in health services and in health services research, and that as a result research and guidance are misdirected. Charles Perrow's *Normal accidents*, first published in 1984 and updated in 1999, is used to highlight the nature of this misdirection, and one way of getting back on track. Perrow was invited to study the near-meltdown of the Three Mile Island nuclear power plant in the US in 1979 and used his research there as the basis for a wide-ranging review of complex technological systems and the ways in which they can fail. There are obvious and important differences between nuclear power plants and healthcare, but *Normal accidents* can still help us to reflect on the merits of current assumptions about safety in healthcare, and ways in which we can study it. Perrow's use of evidence and argument is described in the next section. The rest of the chapter draws on his book to identify lessons for the conduct of case study research into safety in healthcare settings, case study design and the challenges of learning from past events.

Normal accidents

Perrow starts his book with a description of an accident at the Three Mile Island nuclear power plant in Harrisburg, Pennsylvania in 1979. The accident started in the plant's cooling system. The cooling system has two related functions, to keep the reactor core from overheating and to use the heat generated in the core to produce steam, under pressure, which drives turbines that generate electric power. After the event, it became clear that a small amount of water – perhaps a cupful – had leaked into a system that drove a number of instruments in the plant's control room. Moisture in the instrument system triggered two valves to close, even though nothing was wrong with the reactor itself. This led to the cooling pumps stopping, and hence the cooling water supply to the generator being turned off.

The reactor core was still hot, and the heat had to be removed. At Three Mile Island there was, as one might expect, an emergency cooling system, but, as it happened, its pipes were blocked. The emergency pumps came on but the operators did not know that they were pumping water into a closed pipe and that the reactor was not being cooled. A sequence of events followed that were a mix of the automatic (valves opening or closing) and operators in the control room acting on the basis of the information from the various dials and alarms in front of them. The upshot was a situation in which the reactor core was uncovered and there was a genuine risk of nuclear material escaping into the environment. Fortunately, disaster was averted, in significant part because, some two hours after the initial failure, an operator in the control room made a correct decision to shut a particular valve. He later testified that his decision was a matter of luck, as he had not understood the status of the reactor at the time: he just happened to make the right decision.

Perrow relied mainly on a review of documents, including the report and background papers from the official inquiry set up after the accident (the Kemeny Commission), supplemented by site visits. The view after the accident was that the operators had made a series of errors and that the accident was their fault. But, if one placed oneself in the control room at the time, then, the paperwork showed, it would not have been possible to work out what was happening. There were a number of reasons for this. The sequence of events that led to the accident had not been anticipated, and so was not in the minds of the operators when things began to go wrong. Some of the emergency processes in the reactor were not well understood: they turned out not to produce the expected results. At one point there were three audible alarms and many of the 1,600 or so lights in the control room were on or blinking, a straightforward case of information overload. And some of the instruments were either broken or faulty, providing misleading information.

Perrow asked himself whether the Commission and other commentators had produced accounts which fitted the known facts. He concluded that the official inquiry had fallen into the trap of making judgements with the benefit of hindsight. The operators' mistakes looked stupid, and hence worthy of blame, only afterwards. Perrow believed that many of the individual decisions could be defended on the basis that they were reasonable in the context of the available information. He arrived, instead, at the view that the accident resulted principally from poor design and regulation. More precisely, he accepted that individuals can make mistakes but argued that some of those mistakes occurred because the environment they were working in made mistakes more likely.

Perrow's next step was to ask a policy question: Are we at risk of more accidents? He addressed the question by developing a conceptual framework that was designed to capture the reasons why complex technologies can fail and why major failures are mercifully rare. He coined the term 'normal accidents' to emphasise the point that accidents are not phenomena from Greek mythology, attributable to Fate. They are the product of events that occur during routine operations. A normal accident is characterised by (i) multiple failures in a complex system that do not unfold in a linear sequence and (ii) the irreducible incomprehensibility of the system. The second point was particularly important in understanding the accident at Three Mile Island: viewing things from the control room, the team had to act on incomplete, unreliable and conflicting information.

He further argued that complex technologies can usefully be characterised along two dimensions. The first focuses on the ways in which the various components of any large system interact with one another. In the majority of cases, even in large and complex systems, the interactions are linear: a change in one component will trigger a predictable change in the next one, in a sequence. On the other hand, there are complex interactions where components can turn out to be related in ways that the designers and operators did not foresee. As a result, those interactions can produce unfamiliar or unexpected effects which are either not visible or not immediately comprehensible to those responsible for a system.

The second dimension distinguishes between tightly and loosely coupled components. Tight coupling captures the idea that a change in one component is likely to lead to a change in another. A production line is a good example, where the stages of the production process are intimately linked to one another. Where components are loosely coupled, their operations are relatively independent of one another. In the Three Mile Island accident, Perrow argued, parts of the plant that were assumed to be independent from one another turned out to be more tightly coupled than anyone realised and generated complex interactions that nobody in the control room could have understood as events unfolded.

This line of analysis suggested why major accidents were rare. They occurred as a result of specific sequences of events, but where the conditions for the sequence occurred only rarely. (In Three Mile Island, for example, the initial water spill and the pipe blockage were likely to occur at the same time.) Major accidents were generally avoided, in part because the dangerous sequence of events was arrested part way through, either because of automatic safety procedures working or because operators discovered and rectified problems before they escalated. One interesting implication of this line of thinking was the possibility that relatively minor, localised problems occurred all the time but were generally identified in the normal course of events and either solved or tolerated. Thus, major accidents were rare, but usefully understood in the context of continuous monitoring and repair (Edgerton, 2006).

The final step in Perrow's methodology was to survey a number of other technology-intensive industries. In doing so, he was seeking to explore the nature and frequency of accidents in those industries, and hence to test and refine his framework. Chapters of his book are devoted to the petrochemical industry, airlines, marine accidents, major construction projects such as dams and mines, and 'exotics', including space exploration and the then-emerging genetic engineering. He concluded that some industries are more prone to catastrophic failure than others. He placed them in a square, a product of his tight/loose coupling and linear/non-linear interaction dimensions (Figure 7.1). Perrow concluded that failure was more likely in technologies characterised by complex interactions and tight coupling, at the top right of the square. As one moves down and left, the inherent risk reduces.

Learning from *Normal accidents*

There are three particular aspects of the study that are relevant in health service research today, namely the substantive findings about safety and failure, the study design and the challenge of producing usable knowledge.

Lesson 1: The study of safety and failure

Twenty-five years on, *Normal accidents* is still in print. As Perrow noted in an afterword in the 1999 edition, the book had been cited in a number of different fields where safety was a central issue, including healthcare. A handful of pioneering studies, including epidemiological studies of the incidence of errors in hospitals in the US (Leape et al, 1991), had produced alarming results. Adverse events – events which harmed patients – were experienced by 6–16% of all hospital patients, and a proportion of these adverse events were fatal. The figures suggested that between 44,000 and

Figure 7.1: Interaction/coupling chart

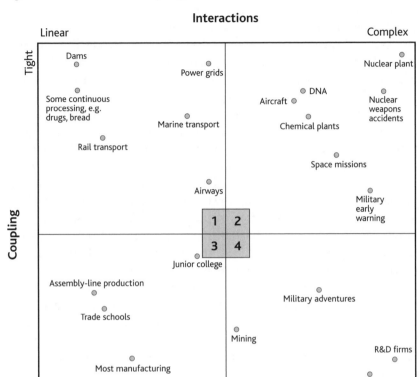

Source: Perrow (1999, fig. 3.1)

98,000 people were dying as a result of preventable adverse events in US hospitals every year.

Normal accidents influenced thinking in the 'safety movement', notably in the seminal Institute of Medicine report *To err is human*, published in 1999. The report set out the normal accidents position in detail, and stated that:

> Accidents are more likely to happen in certain types of systems. When they do occur, they represent failures in the way systems are designed. The primary objective of systems design ought to be to make it difficult for accidents and errors to occur and to minimize damage if they do occur. (p 58)

To err is human was an imaginative response to a serious problem, published by a respected US healthcare organisation. The literature exploded after its publication (Lilford et al, 2006). Viewed through the lens of Perrow's work, however, the vast majority of papers fell into a conceptual trap. Most investigators assumed that accidents in healthcare were isolated events that could be investigated, from which lessons could be drawn and any necessary changes implemented (Shojania et al, 2001; Hoff et al, 2004; Brennan et al, 2005). This assumption has also influenced practice, for example in the importation of root-cause analysis from engineering to trace the clinical action(s) that caused an adverse event.

One consequence of this line of thinking is that little attention has been paid to the nature of healthcare delivery processes and to the ways in which they can fail. Thoughtful writers within the safety field, such as Leape (2009), and in other fields, such as organisation studies (Waring, 2007), are the exceptions that prove the general rule. It is tempting to suggest that the situation reflects the general antipathy to theory, of any kind, in health service research. Yet, as already noted, there seems to have been universal acceptance of reports into high-profile tragedies, such as the Bristol (Kennedy, 2001) and Laming (2003) inquiries. These are case studies in all but name. They provided detailed accounts of events and sought to learn lessons that could help to avoid similar tragedies in the future. Indeed both reports found that, even though key individuals had clearly made mistakes, there were important weaknesses in management and regulation. Escalation could and should have been avoided. Perrow's study helps us, then, by highlighting the paucity of case studies of safety and failure and pointing to one way to redress the balance.

Lesson 2: How to design case studies

As in all case studies, some of the features of the study design were predetermined. Perrow had to undertake a retrospective study: he knew the outcome, an accident, and would need to work backwards to construct an account of the events that led to it. He also realised early on that his intuitions about the cause of the accident differed from those of other investigators, including the official inquiry team. If he wanted to demonstrate that his explanation was better, he would have to discriminate between the candidate explanations.

These fixed features of the study fell a long way short of determining the design of the study, and like everyone else Perrow had to make some design decisions. He made one particularly important decision: to address two questions in parallel. The first was a specific question concerning the reasons why the Three Mile Island accident occurred, and the second a general one about how and why accidents occurred in high-technology organisations in general. The 'twin question strategy' led him to undertake both within case and cross-case comparisons at Three Mile Island.

For the within case comparison, the evidence about the reactor and the control room were different in kind, one derived mainly from engineering records and the other including engineering records, interviews and retrospective expert analysis. Cross-matching the two strengthened confidence in the overall account. Perrow opted to use two different vantage points and then synthesised the two sets of observations. He placed himself in the control room as the accident unfolded, seeking to understand the situation from the perspective of the operators. (Placing himself in the control room at the time, and establishing that the operators could not have understood what was happening in the reactor core, helped Perrow to minimise hindsight bias.) At the same time he 'hovered' above the plant's core and safety systems, which enabled him to understand in broad terms what happened in those systems when the accident began to unfold. He then integrated the two views, so that the reader could see how the operators were responding to developments in the reactor core and safety systems. The Three Mile Island account was further tested by comparison across cases, through the accounts of accidents in other industries. Similar chains of events were observed a wide range of settings, and this increased Perrow's confidence in his theories about normal accidents.

In common with other good case studies *Normal accidents* combined two analytical strategies, which (after Hammond, 1996) we can call correspondence and coherence strategies. A correspondence test is one where the truth or falsity of a claim is judged against the available evidence. For example, the claim that a chemical plant or a hospital ward has an exemplary safety record can be tested empirically. In a coherence test, in contrast, the internal logic of a claim is tested: if the arguments make sense then the claim might be true.

The point of using these two slightly arcane tests is that they shed light on the *process* of arriving at the truth about some or other situation. The most convincing explanation for the events at Three Mile Island, and in other accidents described in the book, was *both* empirically accurate *and* intellectually coherent. The main competing explanation, that the operators simply made mistakes, could be rejected because it failed both tests. Put another way, the tracing of key sequences of events at Three Mile Island and in other major accidents provides a useful means of applying correspondence and coherence tests simultaneously. Indeed, process tracing provided *two* empirical tests, namely that the best account fitted the set of known facts (for example, that buttons were pressed) and also the known *sequence* of events.

Normal accidents is also a good example of the use of a particular approach to theory development. George and Bennett (2006, p 245) argue that:

> An important advantage of typological theorising is that it can
> move beyond earlier debates between structural and agent-centred

theories by including within a single typological framework hypotheses on mechanisms leading from agents to structures and those leading from structures to agents. This allows the theorist to address questions of how different kinds of agents ... behave in and change various kinds of structures.

This is essentially what Perrow did. He developed the coupling–interaction typology, arguing that different technologies had different inherent probabilities of catastrophic failure. He also argued that Three Mile Island and the other accidents he investigated were essentially organisational phenomena, although ones in which the actions of some individuals substantially influenced the course of events. He was interested in large-scale technologies, but took the view that they could be understood only in the context of the organisations that managed and operated them, and of the wider regulatory environment. This point will seem obvious to some readers, but it is worth emphasising that other respected authors focus on safety as a cognitive phenomenon (Reason, 2008) or take the view that organisations are, essentially, machines that are prone to failure (Keller and Modarres, 2005).

Finally in this section, it is important to post a health warning. Rather than follow *Normal accidents* slavishly and assume that accidents in healthcare and nuclear power plants are broadly similar, the lesson is that we should think carefully about the causes of accidents – adverse events – in healthcare. Perrow encourages us to base this understanding on a proper analysis of healthcare *processes*. Accidents occur when usual processes break down in some way. It seems fair to say that we are only just beginning to study the fundamental nature of healthcare delivery seriously. (For example, most representations of care pathways are very schematic, both in practice and in the academic literature.) It may be, for example, that healthcare is neither tightly nor loosely coupled, but a mix of the two: general practice and hospital care are loosely coupled (sometimes effectively uncoupled), while operating theatres and intensive care units are tightly coupled. Or, we may need to find different ways of describing healthcare processes, and how and why those processes can fail.

Lesson 3: Learning from history

Many activities, including clinical audit, incident reviews and – in extreme cases – official inquiries, attest to the importance attached to learning from experience in healthcare, rhetorically at least. These activities are only worthwhile, though, if learning actually occurs and findings and insights lead to changes in clinical practice. Historically, health service researchers have paid relatively little attention to this problem. They have been more concerned with maximising their confidence in research findings – with maximising internal validity. It is no accident that the prospective randomised controlled trial is the method of choice, given its proven value in identifying causal relationships. Other methods, including case studies and all retrospective studies, produce findings with weaker validity and, as a result, are viewed as inferior, to be used only when trials are not feasible.

This would not matter if the uptake of high-quality research evidence from trials and systematic reviews was good, but in practice it has been slow and patchy. There has been a lively debate about ways of bridging the 'translation gap' between health service research and practice (see Dowswell and Harrison, Chapter Seventeen). Indeed, it has dawned on both researchers and their funders that there is an awkward question here: If clinicians cannot translate research findings, why fund the research? Unsurprisingly, the hunt is on for strategies that can bridge the gap, to find ways of transporting findings across the gap and making them digestible to clinicians and managers.

Normal accidents encourages us to wonder whether this is the right way to think about research and development and about learning. If we accept that the challenge is to integrate scientific findings into common-sense practice (Campbell, 1978), those taking on the challenge need to show practitioners how to do it. That is, they need to show how specific findings about safety and failure can be used to change practice out there in messy, real-world settings. The arguments in this chapter suggest that case studies which focus on processes, safety and failure may have a role. They offer practitioners frameworks for making sense of evidence that would otherwise look unconnected; evidence about hand washing here, about equipment maintenance there and so on. Case studies conducted along the same lines as *Normal accidents* balance internal and external validity: they are sufficiently grounded in evidence to be credible, but also produce insights that can be applied generally. On this view, case studies are not a pauper's choice, to be used when experiments cannot be conducted. They fulfil a different, and complementary, role. They contribute to the bridging process between science and common-sense practice, helping practitioners to frame their thinking and to make sense of more detailed findings.

This brings us back to an earlier argument: we need to be confident that we have a good understanding of healthcare processes. This point is highlighted by some of the debates that have developed since *Normal accidents* was first published. For example, some authors have rejected the proposition that organisational processes are always prone to failure, and claim that there are some 'high reliability organisations' (Weick and Sutcliffe, 2007). In another part of the academic woods, Ulrich Beck (1992) and others have developed rather different approaches to thinking about risks, including risks associated with high-technology industries. This reminds us that it makes no sense to rely on a single book, however compelling the arguments it presents. The wider point is that we need to find valid and useful ways of thinking about safety and failure, and to do that we need to set out on the quest for a better understanding of fundamental processes in healthcare.

Concluding comments

Charles Perrow's *Normal accidents* offers three insights to health service researchers. The first is, arguably, the most important. There is a strong tendency to assume that adverse events are caused by individuals doing something wrong, and as a result there has been little serious study of the effects of the organisation and its culture on safety. This is a situation that can and must be remedied if we are to arrive at a proper understanding of healthcare processes and the reasons why they fail. The second insight is that it is possible to produce generalisable findings using case studies, where confidence in the findings is increased by using a number of strategies in concert. The third stems from the fact that health service research faces a major challenge in finding ways of producing usable knowledge and actually getting clinicians and managers to use it. Case studies, of the kind reported by Perrow, may be part of the technical infrastructure for bridging the gap between research and practice, between internal and external validity, and between science and common sense.

Key points

- Charles Perrow's *Normal accidents* sets out detailed accounts of major accidents in organisations managing complex technologies.
- It focuses on the near-meltdown of the Three Mile Island nuclear plant in the US in 1979, but also examines accidents in a number of other industries.
- Perrow developed a general framework for understanding why accidents – and in particular, major accidents – are more common in some industries than others and why there are rare but catastrophic accidents in the nuclear and some other industries.
- Three lessons for health service research are drawn:
  - Case studies have a role in investigations of safety in healthcare processes.
  - *Normal accidents* is an excellent example of a retrospective, inductive, process-tracing case study.
  - There are both possibilities and problems in learning from accidents, and from past events in general.

Further reading

This chapter has focused on three issues raised by Charles Perrow's *Normal accidents.* The first concerns the substantive topic of safety in healthcare systems. A perceptive account of the state of research and practice in this area is provided by:

Brennan, T., Gawande, A., Thomas, A. and Studdert, D. (2005) 'Accidental deaths, saved lives, and improved quality', *New England Journal of Medicine,* vol 353, pp 1405–9.

The second issue concerns case study designs. *Normal Accidents* sits closest to the approach set out in:

George, A. and Bennett, A. (2006) *Case studies and theory development in the social sciences,* Cambridge, MA: MIT Press.

The third issue directs our gaze to the importance of learning from past failures. Any reader who still doubts the force of this point is directed to:

Kennedy, I. (2001) *Learning from Bristol: The report of the public inquiry into children's heart surgery at the Bristol Royal Infirmary 1984–1995,* Cm 5207, London: TSO.
Laming, Lord (2003) *The Victoria Climbié Inquiry,* Cm 5730, London: TSO.

These reports are superb examples of the process of building detailed accounts, showing how tragic events resulted both from the actions – or inactions – of individuals and from the organisational environments they worked in. The technical challenges raised in this chapter can, though, be observed in the reports. Both of them set out recommendations designed to minimise the risk of similar tragedies in the future. Is it clear where the recommendations come from? Could a case study research team have done any better?

References

Beck, U. (1992) *Risk society,* London: Sage.
Brennan, T., Gawande, A., Thomas, A. and Studdert, D. (2005) 'Accidental deaths, saved lives, and improved quality', *New England Journal of Medicine,* vol 353, pp 1405–9.
Campbell, D. (1978) 'Qualitative knowing in action research', in M. Brenner, P. Marsh and M. Brenner (eds) *The social contexts of method,* London: Croom Helm, p 186.
Edgerton, D. (2006) *The shock of the old,* London: Profile Books.
George, A. and Bennett, A. (2006) *Case studies and theory development in the social sciences,* Cambridge, MA: MIT Press.

Hammond, K. (1996) *Human judgment and social policy*, New York: Oxford University Press.

Hoff, T., Jameson, L., Hannan, E. and Flink, E. (2004) 'A review of the literature examining linkages between organizational factors, medical errors and patient safety', *Medical Care Research and Review*, vol 61, pp 3–37.

Institute of Medicine (1999) *To err is human*, Washington, DC: Institute of Medicine.

Keller, W. and Modarres, M. (2005) 'A historical overview of probabilistic risk assessment development and its use in the nuclear power industry: a tribute to the late Professor Norman Carl Rasmussen', *Reliability Engineering and System Safety*, vol 89, pp 271–85.

Kennedy, I. (2001) *Learning from Bristol: The report of the public inquiry into children's heart surgery at the Bristol Royal Infirmary 1984–1995*, Cm 5207, London: TSO.

Laming, Lord (2003) *The Victoria Climbié Inquiry*, Cm 5730, London: TSO.

Leape, L. (2009) 'Errors in medicine', *Clinica Chimica Acta*, vol 404, pp 2–5.

Leape, L. et al (1991) 'The nature of adverse events in hospitalized patients', *New England Journal of Medicine*, vol 324, pp 377–84.

Lilford, R., Stirling, S. and Maillard, N. (2006) 'Citation classics in patient safety research: an invitation to contribute to an online bibliography', *Quality & Safety in Health Care*, vol 15, pp 311–13.

Perrow, C. (1999) *Normal accidents: Living with high risk technologies*, Princeton, NJ: Princeton University Press.

Reason, J. (2008) *The human contribution: Unsafe acts, accidents and heroic recoveries*, Farnham: Ashgate.

Shojania, K.G., Duncan, B.W., McDonald, K.M. et al (eds) (2001) *Making health care safer: A critical analysis of patient safety practices*, Evidence report/technology assessment no 43, Rockville, MD: Agency for Healthcare Research and Quality (AHRQ publication no 01-E058).

Waring, J. (2007) 'Adaptive regulation or governmentality: patient safety and the changing regulation of medicine', *Sociology of Health and Illness*, vol 29, pp 163–79.

Weick, K. and Sutcliffe, K. (2007) *Managing the unexpected: Resilient performance in an age of uncertainty*, San Francisco, CA: Jossey Bass.

eight

Repressed interests: explaining why patients and the public have little influence on healthcare policy: Alford's concepts of dominant, challenging and repressed interests

Stephen Peckham and Micky Willmott

Patient and public engagement has been an enduring theme in UK health policy and practice for many years. Concern about whether the NHS sufficiently considers patient experiences and views began to emerge in the 1960s, with the first patients' organisations being established in the early years of the decade (Lupton et al, 1998; Wood, 2000). Yet in the 1970s Klein refers to the patient as the 'ghost in the machinery' (Klein, 1996). The introduction of Community Health Councils in 1974 was the first formal attempt at patient engagement. But by the 1980s, concerns about the representation of patients' interests remained and began to be expressed as a 'democratic deficit' in the NHS (Cooper et al, 1995; NHSE et al, 1998), and greater interest developed in how to involve patients in service design, evaluation and quality systems (Lupton et al, 1998).

Much of the theoretical discussion about patient engagement has focused on the distinctions between democratic and consumerist modes of engagement. These are characterised by reference to two key analyses, by Arnstein in the 1960s and Hirschmann in the 1970s. Arnstein (1969) visualised the way that public interests are expressed as being like a 'ladder' of engagement, with linear progression from non-involvement (and, in cases, manipulation) through to citizen control. Hirschmann (1970), on the other hand, drew on economics to explain how consumers express their interests through exit, voice and loyalty. It is not our intention here to examine these approaches, as they have been exhaustively explored over the years. Both analyses have strengths and weaknesses, but common to both is that their application often tells little about why patient and public engagement has generally failed to develop in the UK NHS, despite many years of academic, policy and public interest and repeated attempts to reform and enhance engagement. This chapter therefore examines the potential contribution of another analysis which explicitly tackled the question of how repeated attempts to reform a health system did not work but which has been largely neglected in discussions of patient and public engagement.

Robert Alford used a case study approach to determine why attempts at healthcare reform in New York in the 1970s often failed to resolve problems in the health system such as rising costs, staff shortages, poor outcomes and poor quality of care (Alford, 1975, p xi). His argument – set out in the book *Health care politics: Ideological and interest group barriers to reform* – was that embedded structural interests thwarted major reform. He identified three types of structural interests: *dominant, challenging* and *repressed*. He defined these in terms of the extent to which 'interests [are] served or not served by the way in which they "fit" into the basic logic and principles by which the institutions of society operate' (Alford, 1975, p 14). *Dominant* structural interests were those 'served by the structure of social, economic and political institutions as they exist at any given time. Precisely because of this, [they] do not continuously have to organise and act to defend their interests.' *Challenging* interests were 'those being created by the changing structure of society', while *repressed* interests were 'the opposite of the dominant ones.... the nature of institutions guarantees that they will *not* be served unless extraordinary political energies are mobilised' (Alford, 1975, p 14, emphasis in original). Of particular interest here is the fact that Alford characterised the public or community as *repressed interests* with little power as compared to dominant structural interests, exemplified by the medical profession, and challenging structural interests, represented by healthcare administrators. This chapter examines his arguments and discusses whether they are applicable to the situation regarding patient engagement in the UK health system and still relevant today. The chapter is divided into three sections. The first sets out Alford's thesis, the second examines the applicability of his thesis to debates about UK health policy and the third draws lessons about his approach for future case study analysis.

Alford's thesis

The hypothesis underlying Alford's book and which is unpicked gradually throughout the text is set out in the preliminary pages. It is 'that politics serves simultaneously to provide tangible benefits to various elites and symbolic benefits to mass publics, quieting political unrest, deflecting potential demands and blurring the true allocation of rewards' (Alford, 1975, p x). This locates the analysis within debates about pluralist concepts of politics and introduces the case study of reform of the New York health system as a means of addressing questions about the operation of pluralism and market diversity in American society.

Alford expresses surprise at the relative dearth of analysis (up to the point of writing) on health politics, and this might explain why he opts to explore healthcare rather than another sector. He is clear that the analysis does not answer the question how the health system should be organised (Alford, 1975, p 7), but that the case study of perpetual debates about health system problems and reform illustrates his concept of structural interests. The specific puzzle that the book explores is: 'How can the pluralism of interest group competition which results in the fragmentation both of health care and of attempts to plan and reform it be explained?' (p 189).

In chapter 1, Alford argues that existing contemporary diagnoses of the problems facing the New York healthcare system are inadequate. Indeed, he uses quotation marks throughout the text to refer to the 'crisis' in healthcare, demonstrating his reservations about the accuracy of contemporary descriptions. He emphasises that the case study he is concerned with illustrates 'how a complex *system* of organisations handles a *problem*' (Alford, 1975, p 19). He suggests that accounts of the 'crisis' are a political tool that reflects dominant market and bureaucratic interests in the healthcare system. Alford calls these structural interests to differentiate them from interest groups, contending that they are manifestations of interests inherent in society and its institutions, rather than interest groups that consciously collect together to express their interests (p 14). He suggests that structural interests are dominant, challenging and repressed. Although he is careful to state the difference between these, further definition of what he means by interests is inferred rather than defined through the characterisations he uses to populate his typology. He characterises dominant structural interests as 'professional monopolizers', which in this case study are the medical profession. He argues that the principle of professional monopoly is secured within institutional arrangements, such as health system values and norms. Challenging interests are characterised as 'corporate rationalizers', such as healthcare administrators and are 'new' structural interests (p 15) that challenge dominant interests. Alford suggests that dominant and challenging interests represent market and bureaucratic approaches to society (respectively). He suggests that alternatives to these approaches embody critiques of class-based inequalities in society and are repressed. In the case study, these repressed interests are characterised as 'Equal-health advocates' who represent 'the varied interest groups' of the community not covered by either public or private health insurance, the group now known in the US as the uninsured. This suggests that Alford sees this group as synonymous with unmet need, as Checkland et al (2009, p 622) suggest. However, Alford also associates repressed interests with a lack of opportunity for engagement, saying that they have no 'social institutions or political mechanisms' to 'ensure that these interests are served' (Alford, 1975, p 15). He is careful to point out that dominant and repressed structural interests are not always 'in opposition' (p 16), as they may both benefit from some systemic changes.

The case study has clear temporal boundaries and the documents and interview data upon which Alford relies are largely taken from the 1950s to the early 1970s. However, he provides a longer history and context of the health system in New York (Alford, 1975, pp 27–32) in order to reinforce his argument that the notion of a 'crisis' in the healthcare system is perennial. The case study is also bounded by place and context, although, as the book progresses, it is clear that artificial boundaries (for example, administrative jurisdictions) contribute to the difficulties faced in achieving appropriate and accessible health services. Nevertheless, Alford argues that New York is 'not unique' (p 169) and that the issues that affect New York are generalisable to other cities and other sectors.

Two sets of data describing the health system 'crisis' in New York City are presented and analysed in chapters 2 and 3. These provide a detailed account of tensions between the market-based and bureaucratic interpretations of the problems and potential solutions. Alford argues that these are not intended as 'supporting data'; rather, they are 'consistent with the theory' which he propounds (p 190). Chapter 2 presents the plethora of commissions and investigations into the New York health system (and facets of it) which occurred between 1950 and 1971 and summarises 8 of the 23 reports produced in this time. Information on the timing, scope and membership of the commissions and some background to the process that they undertook is provided, although the focus is on the content of the reports. Alford is highly critical of the analyses of the health system provided in these reports. His criticisms include that the investigations rely on subjective, non-specific descriptions of the problems facing New York healthcare, that they lack robust and valid evidence and that they do not draw on previous commissions or experiences. He questions the internal consistency and logic of the reports and suggests that this indicates their bias towards supporting structural interests, specifically the corporate rationalisers. For example, he describes the 'analytic fuzziness' of a 1966 system analysis report as 'a way of concealing acceptance of major system parameters under the guise of abstract theory' (p 51). Alford also indicates how language signifies the inherent bias in these accounts, highlighting the repetition of words such as 'communication', 'cost effectiveness' (p 51) 'fragmentation' (p 56), which he associates with the ideology of corporate rationalisation. Drawing on Edelman's (1971, 1977) notion of symbolic politics, Alford concludes that the commissions and reports are a way of producing 'public quiescence in the face of deeply embedded structural problems in the health system' (p 101).

Alford identifies that the commissions and reports are biased towards secondary care and barely mention the importance of primary healthcare facilities. Chapter 3 therefore provides an account of attempts at a 'bottom-up' initiative to address the lack of primary care facilities in poorer areas of New York. He provides a chronological description of how neighbourhood healthcare facilities were repeatedly over decades raised as a potential solution to a lack of access to primary healthcare in poorer areas in New York, but never quite got off the ground. This allows Alford to more fully introduce an example of repressed interests, embodied by 'equal health advocates', and how existing structural interests are preserved, as he interprets the situation, as a manifestation of the political economy of the US, which favours the market and middle classes (Alford, 1975, p 169).

Having used the New York health system to illustrate his thesis, Alford defends its theoretical generalisability in the remainder of the book – what he calls 'a theoretical synthesis based on assumptions about the functioning of structural interests in a market economy and the way in which state power is appropriate to serve those interests' (Alford, 1975, p 190). In this context, chapter 5 focuses on a more detailed description of dominant and challenging interests (professional monopolists and corporate rationalisers respectively) and how they interact. He emphasises that these interests are 'internally heterogeneous' (p 192) and there may be disputes between groups representing interests (p 15), but that the medical profession is an archetypal example of professional monopolisers. Drawing on Friedson (1970), Alford suggests that the medical profession typifies how 'professionalism provides a way of preserving monopolistic control over services without the risks of competition' (p 199). He suggests that professional monopolists tend to be 'satisfied with the status quo' (p 195) and don't generally propose reform. Corporate rationalisers are presented as the key challengers to the professional monopolisers, and Alford draws on other work (for example, from health economics and law scholars) to argue that they have a different ideology, and material interests which mean that they focus on economic efficiency, 'coordination, integration and planning' (p 205).

Alford acknowledges that professional monopolists' interests might be served by bureaucratic reforms advocated by corporate rationalisers and vice versa, although the two interests are clearly in competition (Alford, 1975, p 217). However, in chapter 6 he describes how the interests of equal-health advocates are generally repressed by both professional monopolists and corporate rationalisers. Although dominant and challenging interests are not weakened by their heterogeneity, Alford suggests that repressed interests, embodied by representatives of the community such as equal-health advocates, are easily 'compromised, soothed or co-opted' (p 218) because of their heterogeneity and because the equal-health advocates who represent them tend not to be stable institutions. The discussion of equal-health advocates and their strategies is relatively short, compared to that of the professional monopolists and corporate rationalisers. This may be partly because of Alford's belief that equal-health advocates were not particularly evident at the time of writing (p 191), and could reflect well-known methodological difficulties in collecting data on the activity of such groups. Alford also cites, though, the need to consider the wider political economy of the US. Therefore the rest of chapter 6 considers the implications of federal politics and interests and how issues such as 'vacillating financial support' for local programmes impact on health systems (p 227), and so Alford acknowledges another ongoing, macro-political debate – that is, the tensions between national and local politics.

The penultimate chapter focuses on the reasons why research and data are neither available nor adequate for exploring why the health system is not satisfactory. Alford suggests that the lack of data highlights difficulties in examining a whole system and also the way in which much research reflects the structural interests in society.

Alford concludes by challenging prevailing notions of pluralism, arguing that pluralism describes the situation of the health system but does not explain the need for it to change (Alford, 1975, pp 256–7). He reiterates that 'the "crisis" of healthcare is *not* a result of the necessary competition of diverse interests, groups and providers in a pluralistic and competitive health economy, nor is it the result of bureaucratic inefficiencies' (p 251). By relating structural interests to fundamental debates about pluralism, Alford contends that problems in the healthcare system cannot be solved using mechanisms available in the health sector because the problems are embedded in the structure of society and are therefore apparent across sectors.

Contemporary relevance

This brief overview provides some interesting insights into Alford's analytical approach but also raises some interesting observations that might look familiar to analysts of UK health policy. Certainly the notion of crisis is one that is familiar to the UK. Alford's suggestion that 'crisis' is, in a way, a perpetual analysis of health systems reflects much political discourse on the NHS since the 1970s. Subsequent reforms, from the late 1970s onwards, have sought to address the 'crisis' in the NHS. Similarly, the tripartite typology that Alford identifies appears familiar, with professionals, managers and patients or the public as key actors. Moreover, tensions between market and bureaucratic models are becoming increasingly apparent in the NHS.

There have been few analyses drawing on Alford's thesis in relation to the UK. In the main, such analyses have focused on applying Alford's concept of structural interests to different professional and managerial groups in the NHS (see North, 1995; Harrison, 1999; North and Peckham, 2001; Checkland et al, 2009). There has been little explicit application of Alford's concept of repressed interests in the UK health system. Indeed, despite the vast UK literature on patient and public engagement, few studies have successfully evaluated the impact of such activity on the health system. Similarly, few studies analyse the institutional arrangements that have been developed within the NHS to foster patient engagement. However, concerns about a 'democratic deficit' in the NHS are long standing (Cooper et al, 1995; NHSE et al, 1998) and so Alford's concept of structural interests might aid understanding of why the interests of patients appear to remain marginal in comparison to other interests in the NHS.

While the representation of patients' interests was partially addressed by the creation of Community Health Councils (CHCs) in the 1970s and attempts to engage people in local commissioning during the 1980s and 1990s, government health policies, particularly in England, have re-emphasised the importance of patient and public involvement in planning and service provision, in addition to the collection of patient satisfaction data (Klein and Lewis, 1976; Moon and Lupton, 1995; Lupton et al, 1998; Milewa et al, 1998). In England, following the NHS Plan (DH, 2000), the Labour government introduced a new system of patient and public involvement to replace CHCs. This involved the creation of a Commission for Patient and Public Involvement in Health in 2003 and Patient and Public Involvement Forums based in NHS Trusts and Primary Care Trusts (PCTs). Patient Advice and Liaison Services – to respond quickly to patients' concerns and demands for information – were also introduced and, more recently, Independent Complaints Advocacy Services. In addition, a general duty on NHS bodies to consult and involve patients and the public was introduced under section 11 of the Health and Social Care Act 2001. All these mechanisms have now been drastically altered with proposals developed in 2007/08 for the establishment of Local Involvement Networks (LINks) and, with the election of the Coalition government, further proposals for strengthening local authority involvement in health. In addition, the creation of Foundation Trusts has raised the prospect of elected boards' being introduced into the governance of local service providers, although actual experience suggests that these forms of wider public representation have remained weak and ineffectual.

Klein and Lewis's (1976) early research on CHCs was, perhaps, the first major study that explored issues of community engagement and engagement mechanisms in the NHS. They found that there were problems related to the representative make-up of CHC boards and also that activity and effectiveness was limited by lack of resources. In a more recent study of CHCs, Moon and Lupton (1995) found that CHCs tended to specialise in resolving resource issues and that while some were challenging in their approach, others appeared to be little more than extensions of the NHS organisations delivering services, playing a supporting role. Harrison et al's (1997) study of mental health and disability groups in the mid-1990s found that NHS and local authority managers often played 'the user card', selectively employing service-user group views to legitimise their own agendas. However, few analyses of patient and public involvement draw on

Alford's thesis, despite its providing a way of analysing the political position of community interests in relation to other interests in the health system.

Two studies have explicitly applied Alford's concept of structural interests in the UK health system. Both of these studies examine groups which represent patients outside the institutional structures of the NHS (for example, LINks) and therefore could be seen as modern, UK equivalents of 'equal health advocate' groups. Wood (2000) draws on Alford in his comparative case study of local patient organisations in one UK city and one US city, using it to highlight the weak position of such patient organisations. He also cites other studies that reflect Alford's findings that patient organisations are *repressed interests*. In a more recent study Baggott et al (2004) explored the role of national health consumer groups in health policy. Their findings suggested that some national groups made some significant contributions to health policy processes. However, they also found that these groups identified the medical profession as an important dominant interest and some groups expressed concern about being co-opted by professional and bureaucratic interests. In their conclusion, Baggott et al (2004) suggest that Alford's typology of interests is not sufficiently nuanced to accommodate differences between community interests, nor the changes in wider political circumstances that had provided for greater patient and public involvement (p 297).

While there seem to be few compelling published examples of how interests are aligned in the UK health context, there is some evidence to suggest that local group activity can lead to changes in service organisation or in decision-making processes in other sectors (for example, Barnes, 1999; Barnes et al, 1999; Harrison et al, 2002). Conversely, there is also evidence that such activity has little or no effect and, as such, 'involvement' policies might be an example of 'symbolic politics' or 'therapy', serving to reassure and to encourage political quiescence (Arnstein, 1969; Edelman, 1971, 1977). Although, as Baggott et al argue, involvement could be interpreted as a form of incorporation, that implies a degree of autonomous power on the part of those co-opted, a sort of micro-level corporatism (Cawson, 1982, 1985; Baggott et al, 2004). Baggott et al also suggest that the new institutions of patient and public involvement (such as LINks) might shape health-consumer group activity in a manner that supports the local health agencies by either shaping public and patient expectations and/or behaviour, and/or actually delivering local services on a subcontracted basis to the specifications of local management. In such circumstances, the new institutions of 'involvement' might be seen as a strategy of incorporation (Marcuse, 1972; Dunleavy and O'Leary, 1987). For example, Harrison et al (2002) found that, even in localities with a strong tradition of 'community development', officials tended to see the 'education' of users to make 'reasonable' service demands as a central objective of involvement, rather than seeing them as representing another set of legitimate interests. The gradual but increasing involvement of patient groups and voluntary organisations in the delivery of health and social care services has changed the context within which such groups operate. Barnes et al (1999) noted how user groups' position as publicly funded service providers militated against their ability to act as pressure groups. While the activity of local patient and public groups might make a significant difference to local policies and services as they become more involved in service planning and delivery this might, at a local level, constitute evidence of the 'hollowing out' of the local state – although, despite the findings of Baggott et al (2004), this is not necessarily true of the central state (Rhodes, 1997). But it is clear that different groups act in different ways and that involvement and influence will, therefore, also be differentiated, suggesting that it is not possible to see all community interests as potentially either *repressed* or *equally repressed*.

More recently, Williamson has argued that, despite changes in institutional arrangements, a greater respect for patient-centred approaches and continued policy interest in patient and public involvement, patient's interests 'are still pervasively repressed' (2008, p 515). Williamson cites patient experiences in relation to referral management, where most attention is focused on the role of managers in streamlining processes and the threat to clinical autonomy. She argues that the interests of patients have had scant attention. Similarly, it is widely recognised that people with long-term conditions (LTCs) experience poor coordination of care, leading to adverse events and increased hospitalisations. International comparisons suggest that the UK lags behind other countries in supporting people with LTCs (Rosen et al, 2007; Schoen et al, 2007). Since the 2001 NHS Plan the government has been committed to improving support for people with LTCs and, in England, set public service agreements in 2005 to reduce emergency bed use and introduce case management for high users of intensive services (DH, 2000, 2004, 2005a, 2005b; Ham, 2009). From a clinical and NHS management perspective, for people with LTCs the emphasis is on developing clinical pathways and care management programmes (Ham, 2009; Wilson et al, 2009). To date there is insufficient evidence of the effectiveness of such approaches in many chronic conditions, or any evidence of significant service-user input influencing the development of pathways (Sulch et al, 2002; Weingarten et al, 2002; Ofman et al, 2004; Singh, 2005; Taylor et al, 2005; McDonald et al, 2006a, 2006b). The evidence from these studies would confirm Baggott et al's (2004) assertion that, as well as differences between policy areas and sectors, there are differences as to which interests are represented within health policy.

Similarly, although patient and public involvement in commissioning has been recognised as desirable since the initial development of NHS purchasing in the 1990s, there is not any significant evidence that such engagement has influenced commissioning decisions (Lupton et al, 1998; Harrison et al, 2002; Chisholm et al, 2007; NPCRDC, nd). The Picker Institute's recent survey found that, while PCTs had a number of mechanisms and defined management responsibilities for patient and public involvement, 'there is a disconnect between these activities and the relatively low expectation that patient, public and community groups will have significant influence on commissioning decisions' (Chisholm et al, 2007). Key barriers identified were difficulties in reaching marginalised, isolated or deprived groups, a lack of understanding among the public of 'commissioning' and a lack of reliable data about patients' experiences. However, when PCTs were asked what approaches they were considering for future engagement, there was a continued emphasis on methods such as formal consultations, patient panels, citizen's juries and surveys rather than on engaging with or involving patients.

Williamson argues that the key focus of debate is still predominantly between corporate rationalisers (the *challenging interest*) and professional monopolisers (the *dominant interest*). Notwithstanding that these two groups are not always clearly defined and that it is at times unclear which occupy the different structural interests (see North, 1995; Checkland et al, 2009), this brief review of contemporary UK literature suggests that it is likely that community interests represented by patient groups, health-consumer groups and the public still characterise *repressed interests* as defined by Alford. As such, Alford's typology of structural interests provides a useful way of analysing the position of patient and public involvement in the UK healthcare system.

Some methodological lessons for health policy analysis

So how does Alford's analysis help us in the analysis of health policy? Clearly, Alford supports a case study approach but demonstrates that case studies should be set within their wider political context. In *Health care politics*, Alford constantly draws on the wider political context of the US healthcare system in his analysis. So perhaps one key message is that politics matter. His approach drew a broader understanding of events, rather than simply focusing on micro aspects of healthcare, such as service use or a specific policy.

Alford's central argument has three broad elements. The first is that bureaucratic and market reforms of healthcare are likely, ultimately, to fail. This is because of their general failure to understand how embedded structural interests operate within healthcare systems. The second is that health policy is affected by an ongoing conflict between dominant and challenging interests. While in his example he showed 'professional monopolisers' as the dominant interest and 'corporate rationalisers' as the challenging interest, Alford was not prescriptive about this and foresaw that different interest groups might occupy these interests (Alford, 1975; North and Peckham, 2001; Checkland et al, 2009). However, his final point was that the community is normally the *repressed interest* and, while both monopolisers and rationalisers may court and collaborate with groups representing these interests, this would be for the benefit of their own interests, too. This appears to be borne out in more recent UK-based studies.

While changes since the 1970s suggest that the patient is no longer the 'ghost in the machinery' of the UK health system, it is clear that, despite significant policy interest in patient and public involvement in the NHS, patients still have little influence over health policy and health services. However, Alford's is neither the only nor perhaps always the most appropriate approach to take to analysing patient and public involvement. For example, approaches such as Grant's (2000) typology of groups as insiders and outsiders in the policy process can aid further exploration of the differences between groups that might represent patients' interests. However, the application of structural interests does illuminate important aspects of the health system and it is unlikely that Alford would have foreseen the diversity within community interests – noted by Baggott et al (2004) – as a problem, as he would have expected the concept of structural interests to be applied in the analysis of specific case studies. Therefore, as a methodological tool employing structural interest theory, it is clearly useful and also provides a useful broader analysis of the position of patient and public interests in health systems.

References

Alford, R. (1975) *Health care politics: Ideological and interest group barriers to reform*, London: University of Chicago Press.

Arnstein, S. (1969) 'A ladder of citizen participation', *Journal of the American Institute of Planners*, vol 35, no 4, pp 216–24.

Baggott, R., Allsop, J. and Jones, K. (2004) *Speaking for patients and carers: The role of health consumer groups in the policy process*, Basingstoke: Palgrave.

Barnes, M. (1999) *Building a deliberative democracy: An evaluation of two citizens' juries*, London: Institute for Public Policy Research.

Barnes, M., Harrison, S., Mort, M. and Shardlow, P. (1999) *Unequal parties: User groups and community care*, Bristol: The Policy Press.

Cawson, A. (1982) *Corporatism and welfare: Social policy and state intervention in Britain*, London: Heinemann.

Cawson, A. (1985) 'Corporatism and local politics', in W. Grant (ed) *The political economy of corporatism*, London: Macmillan.

Checkland, K., Harrison, S. and Coleman, A. (2009) '"Structural interests" in health care: evidence from the contemporary National Health Service', *Journal of Social Policy*, vol 38, no 4, pp 607-25.

Chisholm, A., Redding, D., Cross, P. and Coulter, A. (2007) *Patient and public involvement in PCT commissioning: A survey of Primary Care Trusts*, Oxford: Picker Institute Europe.

Cooper, L., Coote, A., Davies, A. and Jackson, C. (1995) *Voices off: Tackling the democratic deficit in health*, London: Institute for Public Policy Research.

DH (Department of Health) (2000) *The NHS plan: A plan for investment, a plan for reform*, Cm 4818, London: The Stationery Office.

DH (2004) *Choosing health*, London: Department of Health.

DH (2005a) *Supporting people with long term conditions. An NHS and social care model to support local innovation and integration*, London: Department of Health.

DH (2005b) *National service framework for long-term conditions*, London: Department of Health.

Dunleavy, P. and O'Leary, B. (1987) *Theories of the state: The politics of liberal democracy*, London: Macmillan.

Edelman, M. (1971) *Politics as symbolic action*, New York: Free Press.

Edelman, M. (1977) *Political language: Words that succeed and policies that fail*, New York: Free Press and Institute for the Study of Poverty.

Friedson, E. (1970) *Profession of medicine*, New York: Dodd, Mead.

Grant, W. (2000) *Pressure groups and British politics*, Basingstoke: Macmillan.

Ham, C. (2009) 'Chronic care in the English National Health Service: progress and challenges', *Health Affairs*, vol 28, no 1, pp 190–201.

Harrison, S. (1999) *Structural interests in health care: 'Reforming' the UK medical profession*, European Consortium for Political Research joint sessions: Mannheim, 26-31 March 1999, Workshop no 16, 'Success and failure in governance'.

Harrison, S., Barnes, M. and Mort, M. (1997) 'Praise and damnation: mental health groups and the construction of organisational legitimacy', *Public Policy and Administration*, vol 12, no 2, pp 4–16.

Harrison, S., Milewa, T. and Dowswell, G. (2002) *Patient and public involvement in NHS Primary Care: Final report of a Department of Health research study*, Manchester: University of Manchester Department of Applied Social Science.

Hirschmann, A.O. (1970) *Exit, voice, and loyalty*, Cambridge, MA: Harvard University Press.

Klein, R. and Lewis, J. (1976) *The politics of consumer representation: A study of community health councils*, London: Centre for Studies in Social Policy.

Lupton, C., Peckham, S. and Taylor, P. (1998) *Managing public involvement in healthcare purchasing*, Buckingham: Open University Press.

Marcuse, H. (1972) *One-dimensional man*, London: Abacus.

McDonald, P.S., Whittle, C.L., Dunn, L. and de Luc, K. (2006a) 'Shortfalls in integrated care pathways. Part 1: what don't they contain?', *Journal of Integrated Care Pathways*, vol 10, pp 17–22.

McDonald, P.S., Whittle, C.L., Dunn, L. and de Luc, K. (2006b) 'Shortfalls in integrated care pathways. Part 2: how well are we doing?', *Journal of Integrated Care Pathways*, vol 10, pp 23–7.

Milewa, T., Valentine, J. and Calnan, M. (1998) 'Managerialism and active citizenship in Britain's reformed health service: power and community in an era of decentralisation', *Social Science and Medicine*, vol 47, no 4, pp 507–17.

Moon, G. and Lupton, D. (1995) 'Within acceptable limits: health care provider perspectives on community health councils in the reformed British NHS', *Policy and Politics*, vol 23, no 4, pp 335–46.

NHSE, IHSM and NHS Confederation (1998) *In the public interest: Developing a strategy for public participation in the NHS*, London: Department of Health.

North, N. (1995) 'Alford revisited: the professional monopolists, corporate rationalisers, community and markets', *Policy and Politics*, vol 23, no 2, pp 115–25.

North, N. and Peckham, S. (2001) 'Analysing structural interests in primary care groups', *Social Policy and Administration*, vol 35, no 4, pp 426–40.

NPCRDC (National Primary Care Research and Development Centre) (nd) *PCT surveys*, Manchester: NPCRDC.

Ofman, J.J., Badamgarav, E., Henning, J.M., Knight, K., Gano, A., Levan, R.K. et al (2004) 'Does disease management improve clinical and economic outcomes in patients with chronic diseases? A systematic review', *American Journal of Medicine*, vol 117, pp 182–92.

Rhodes, R.A.W. (1997) *Understanding governance: Policy networks, governance, reflexivity and accountability*, Buckingham: Open University Press.

Rosen, R., Asaria, P. and Dixon, A. (2007) *Improving chronic disease management*, London: King's Fund.

Schoen, C., Osborn, R., Doty, M.M., Bishop, M., Peugh, J. and Murukutla, N. (2007) 'Toward higher-performance health systems: adults' health care experiences in seven countries', *Health Affairs*, vol 26, no 6, pp 717–34.

Singh, D. (2005) *Which staff improve care for people with long-term conditions? A rapid review of the literature*, University of Birmingham: HSMC and the NHS Modernisation Agency.

Sulch, D., Evans, A., Melbourn, A. and Kalra, L. (2002) 'Does an integrated care pathway improve processes of care in stroke rehabilitation? A randomised controlled trial', *Age and Ageing*, vol 31, pp 175–9.

Taylor, S., Bestall, J., Cotter, S., Falshaw, M., Hood, S., Parsons, S. et al (2005) *Clinical service organisation for heart failure (Review)*, Oxford: The Cochrane Collaboration.

Weingarten, S.R., Henning, J.M., Badamgarav, E., Knight, K., Hasselbad, V., Gano, A. et al (2002) 'Interventions used for patients with chronic illness – which ones work? Meta-analysis of published reports', *British Medical Journal*, vol 325, pp 925–33.

Williamson, C. (2008) 'Alford's theoretical political framework and its application to interests in health care now', *British Journal of General Practice*, vol 58, no 552, pp 512-16.

Wilson, P.M., Bunn, F. and Morgan, J. (2009) 'A mapping of the evidence on integrated long term condition services', *British Journal of Community Nursing*, vol 14, no 5, pp 202–6.

Wood, B. (2000) *Patient power? Patients associations in Britain and America*, Buckingham: Open University Press.

Part Three

'Safe in our hands': conflicts and challenges (1980s and 1990s)

The second group of case study chapters deals with the period of the 1980s and 1990s. To a large extent, this period shaped most clearly the configuration of interests, ideas and institutions that we see in the NHS today. Thatcher's assertion that the NHS was 'safe in our [that is, the Conservative government's] hands' (http://news.bbc.co.uk/1/hi/1888158.stm) reflected a political pragmatism in the 1980s that recognised the saliency of the NHS among the electorate. Nonetheless, Thatcher never quite escaped the claim that the Conservative government had 'damaged' the NHS, a charge that David Cameron sought to nullify ahead of the 2010 general election. The chapters in this section explore the conflicts and challenges of major reforms, starting with managerialism and including the introduction of the internal market. Each examines the health policy process through the lens of case studies of books or official reports.

Fraser Macfarlane and colleagues (Chapter Nine) examine the Griffiths Inquiry of 1983 in order to explore the introduction of general management in the NHS. They chart the ways in which managers have become an established member of the NHS 'tribe'. Although management was seen as a solution to many NHS ills (notably by the Griffiths Inquiry), in recent years, it has become increasingly seen as part of the problem. Managers have been portrayed in unflattering ways that are redolent of the critiques of their pre-Griffiths bureaucratic colleagues. Moreover, the Griffiths reforms introduced a form of managerialism that set a pattern for later reforms, notably marketisation and competition in the 1990s and subsequently.

During the 1980s, AIDS emerged as a major public health policy 'problem' which governments (in the UK and elsewhere) were generally ill equipped to handle. The formulation of policy in response to the exogenous shock represented by AIDS is examined by David Evans (Chapter Ten). He uses Berridge's (1996) book to view this policy process and to reflect upon subsequent policy developments.

David Wainwright and Michael Calnan (Chapter Eleven) examine the Audit Commission's report (1996) on GP fundholding. Fundholding was, arguably, one of the more divisive policy initiatives associated with the 1991 internal market reforms because, some claimed, it fostered a two-tier approach within the NHS. However, the involvement of GPs in commissioning decisions has become more widely accepted, and indeed forms the core of the 2010 health reforms of the Coalition government.

While it is claimed that GPs are central to the 2010 reforms, the legacy of the 1948 settlement whereby GPs became independent contractors, semi-detached from the NHS, remains a potent factor in shaping policy.

The final two chapters in this section explore two case studies in highly influential books both within and beyond the health policy field. David Hughes (Chapter Twelve) traces the study by David Hunter (1980) of two health boards. However, it is Hunter's methods and their subsequent impact across health policy that are notably significant. Louise Locock and Sue Dopson (Chapter Thirteen) draw on Pettigrew and colleagues' (1992) study of organisational change in the NHS. Like Hughes, they trace its influence in shaping a generation of research.

References

Audit Commission (1996) *What the doctor ordered: A study of GP fundholders in England and Wales*, London: HMSO.

Berridge, V. (1996) *AIDS in the UK: The making of policy, 1981–1994*, Oxford: Oxford University Press.

Hunter, D.J. (1980) *Coping with uncertainty: policy and politics in the National Health Service*, Letchworth: Research Studies Press.

Pettigrew, A.M., Ferlie, E. and McKee, L. (1992) *Shaping strategic change: Making change in large organizations: the case of the National Health Service*, London: Sage.

nine

The 1983 Griffiths Inquiry

Fraser Macfarlane, Mark Exworthy and Micky Willmott

Introduction

Managers now appear to be a permanent fixture in the NHS landscape but they are relatively recent recruits into the NHS 'family'. It is now just over 25 years since they first appeared, having either been transformed from NHS administrators or recruited from outside the service. Nowadays, managers account for 2.7% of the 1.3 million-strong NHS workforce (NHS Confederation, 2008).

The seminal moment for the NHS was the Griffiths Inquiry report (DHSS, 1983), which introduced general management at all levels within the service. This arguably provided a turning-point at which NHS management was transformed. Indeed, without 'Griffiths', it is fair to surmise that NHS management would not look or act like it does today. This chapter seeks to reflect on 'Griffiths' as a case study and the introduction of general management after a period of over 25 years of reflection. It aims to trace the background to the changes as well as to set out the impact of general management in the shorter and longer terms. We argue that Griffiths was a result of a radical change in public sector organisation – moving from a consensus approach to an approach with formal management, indicative of the new public management which was sweeping across the public sector in the 1980s. We have selected this example to illustrate aspects of contemporary policy making, namely, that radical change is possible and that it can happen quickly and without too much disruption in service delivery. Griffiths also provides a baseline against which subsequent public management reforms (especially those in the NHS) can be gauged. For example, Griffiths proposed greater involvement of the public and clinicians in running NHS organisations. It could also be argued that the Griffiths changes were visionary, as such themes (for example, marketisation) evolved over a period of 25 years.

In writing this chapter, we cannot complain that there has been a shortage of material from which to draw. Since 1983, a huge amount of research has been undertaken looking at Griffiths and its impact. In a recent review of the literature (see Exworthy et al, 2009), almost 450 documents were found that were relevant to Griffiths and NHS general management. At least

100 documents describe empirical research (although some report the same research). Common research methods used were questionnaires/surveys (at least 25 documents) and interviews with managers and other stakeholders (at least 20 documents), although sample sizes were often small. The volume of research on the introduction of general management led Cox (1991) to wryly suggest that 'The DGM [District General Manager] or UGM [Unit General Manager] who has not been included in some sociologist's or management specialist's sample must be feeling very left out!' (p 96).

The Nuffield Trust and King's Fund have both published at least eight reports and funded original research in this field. There are also documents from within the NHS (for example, Glennerster et al, 1988; Silver, 1996). Literature on the impact of the Griffiths Report (DHSS, 1983) was most prolific in the late 1980s and early 1990s. The general growth in literature reflects the growing preoccupation with management throughout the existence of the NHS, because 'organisational structure and managerialism have been seen as part of the solution to the problems of the NHS' since the 1970s (Cox, 1991, p 94).

There are many examples of empirical studies evaluating the impact of Griffiths and the introduction of general management. Indeed, there have been several systematic reviews of these studies (for example, Harrison et al, 1992). However, the studies (n=27) were completed before the next major structural change in the NHS, namely the introduction of the internal market in 1991, and may have missed the wider impact of Griffiths for this significant managerial change. Added to this rich field of evidence is a range of autobiographical or biographical writing by managers themselves (for example, Busset et al, 1987; Edwards, 1993), although little of this focuses on the Griffiths reforms. Nevertheless, the Griffiths Report and these studies of its impact continue to be referenced in historical accounts of the NHS and its development (for example, Klein, 2006; Greener, 2008). There is therefore a significant gap in assessing Griffiths against the wider panoply of policy reforms in the NHS and NHS managers' perspectives on it as a key transition in the evolution of NHS management.

Along with archival analysis and history, we present Griffiths as a case study because it focuses on the ongoing implications of a specific policy, thereby providing a way to delineate the phenomenon about which to collect evidence (Van Wynsberghe and Khan, 2007, p 2; Yin, 2003, p 5). The use of Griffiths as a case study allows the evolution of NHS managers' roles to be tracked, because individual careers are 'a sequence of work role transitions' (Gunz, 1989, p 225) and these transitions should be viewed within a 'longer career narrative' and broader context (Cohen and Mallon, 2001, p 52).

Antecedents of the Griffiths Inquiry

Money and the funding of the NHS have been a perennial problem. Day and Klein (1983) put forward a strong argument that in the years prior to the Griffiths Inquiry, ministers had been pursuing a 'receding mirage' that the NHS could stretch ever-tightening resources by improving the quality of management within the service. In 1971, the Secretary of State for Health (Keith Joseph) put forward plans to reorganise the NHS and promote effective management. He argued that: 'the importance of good *management* in making the best use of resources can hardly be overstated' (DHSS, 1971; emphasis added). Subsequent Secretaries of State have also turned their attention to management and improving its quality. (Indeed, Andrew Lansley echoed his predecessors by calling for 'strong management' in the NHS [West, 2010]).

Harrison and Wood (1999) point out that, in 1983, the UK government attempted to commission an inquiry into NHS 'manpower' [*sic*]. The person first offered its chair declined, and ultimately Sir Roy Griffiths was approached. He initially declined on the grounds that if there were problems with the size and cost of the workforce, these were probably only symptoms of problems with the wider management of the NHS. He would be only part of this review if it were changed to focus on NHS management. If the NHS were to continue, wider problems of funding and organisation would need to be addressed, he argued.

The Griffiths Inquiry (DHSS, 1983) has been presented as evidence of a shift in fiscal policy and political ideology that was associated with the Conservative government elected in 1979 (Greener, 2001, p 636; Klein, 2006, p 101). However, the change it symbolises illustrates how the existing order in the healthcare arena had already come to be questioned (Klein, 2006, p 101). In particular, there was a drive to devolve decision making and to distance accountability from government and to move it towards local public organisations (Klein, 2006, p 101). Greer and Jarman (2007) suggest that general management developed 'alongside the longstanding increase in the political salience and central management of the NHS' (p 11).

The Inquiry symbolised the shift in interest from the structure to the dynamics or the way in which the NHS should be managed (Packwood, 1997, p 93; Klein, 2006, p 105). As Packwood (1997) notes, this is linked to persistent debates about 'which and whose, values should shape the organisation, those rooted in individual practice or in broader service provision' (p 93).

Policy analysis in the early 1980s included debates about the desirability of general management. For example, Hunter (1984) suggests that arguments for general managers and away from consensus management were 'well rehearsed' before Griffiths (p 93). Although, as Harrison et al (1990, p 76) note, the introduction of general management was not the 'product of any systematic empirical study of the NHS' and the antecedents were 'multiple and complex'. They note that 'occupational politics' were particularly important. Indeed, it has been argued that the Inquiry may have been at least partially prompted by concerns about management of personnel emerging from pay disputes that occurred in 1982 (Stowe, 1988, in Klein, 2006, pp 116, 137).

The Griffiths Inquiry

The Inquiry into NHS administration was commissioned in February 1983 by Secretary of State for Health Norman Fowler and was chaired by Sir Roy Griffiths (then managing director of Sainsbury's supermarket). The aims of the Inquiry were to:

- review management incentives
- examine ways in which NHS resources were used and controlled and
- advise the Secretary of State of any further action required (Sherman et al, 1983, p 196).

As Griffiths later said himself:

> We were asked not to make any recommendations which would require legislation. The background to the setting up of the Inquiry was the tremendous parliamentary questioning on the waste and inefficiency in the Service. We were not at the outset asked to write a report, and the impression given was that we should simply advise at appropriate meetings, the whole exercise taking say a day a month for about eight months. (Griffiths, 1992, p 61)

Therefore, the focus was on reviewing management action to secure value for money and efficiency (Hunter, 1984, p 91). The style of Inquiry was distinctive, because it was conducted quickly (in six months), informally (it did not take formal submissions) and the Inquiry team was small, comprising just four people (Klein, 2006, p 117). The members of the team were:

- Roy Griffiths (Chairman): Deputy-Chairman and Managing Director of Sainsbury's
- Michael Bett: Board Member for Personnel, British Telecom
- Jim Blyth: Finance Director, United Biscuits
- Sir Brian Bailey: Chairman, Health Education Council, Chairman, TV South West, Ex-Chairman of South Western Regional Health Authority.

There is evidence of the debates about what the Inquiry would recommend and comments about the process (for example, Halpern, 1983, p 832). Evidence from major stakeholders also shows that it was a significant event at the time, which people felt would have a practical impact on people's jobs and a potential impact on NHS culture (Hyde and Wilson, 1983; HSSJ, 1983). Debates about the efficiency and costs of healthcare administration were a significant political issue, highlighted at the Conservative Party conference by the Secretary of State for Health (Sherman, 1983, p 1248), whose comments were picked up by national newspapers (*Guardian*, 1983a, p 2).

The report was published in November 1983 and combined 'diagnosis [of the issues] with prescription' (Harrison et al, 1990, p 81). The Inquiry's findings largely agreed with prevailing criticism of the NHS, which was that consensus management was 'inefficient, wasteful of resources and lacking in professional management and direction' (Merali, 2003, p 549) and 'institutionalised stagnation' (DHSS, 1983, quoted in Harrison et al, 1990, p 78). Although the analysis of the issues was not new, the 'blunt language' (Klein, 2006, p 118) it used meant that its description of the problem became (in)famous, epitomised by the statement that: 'if Florence Nightingale were carrying her lamp through the corridors of the NHS today she would almost certainly be searching for the people in charge' (in Klein, 2006, p 118).

The key recommendation of the report was that consensus management (operating in the NHS since 1974) should be replaced by general management in order to improve systems of control and review (Pollitt et al, 1991, p 62). The report advocated that daily decision making should happen at a local level, supported by a 'strong general management board' at the centre to ensure the devolution of power with clear lines of accountability (Rivett, 1998, p 354). General managers would be responsible and accountable for 'making things happen' at each unit, district and regional level of the NHS, and the report proposed an overall reduction in the number of staff involved in decision making and implementation (Rivett, 1998, p 354).

Reflecting on the report nine years later, Griffiths highlighted a significant point:

> One important prelude to the recommendations: we believe that a small, strong general management body is necessary at the centre (and that is almost all that is necessary at the centre for the management of the NHS) to ensure that responsibility is pushed as far down the line as possible, i.e. to the point where action can be taken effectively. At present devolution of responsibility is far too slow because the necessary direction and dynamic to achieve this is currently lacking. (Griffiths, 1992, p 62)

The report also proposed that the NHS, through these managers, should be more cognisant of the users of its services, as a 'good business' is aware of its customers (Sir Roy Griffiths, quoted in *Guardian*, 1983c, p 26) although mechanisms for achieving this were not suggested (Pollitt et al, 1991, p 63). However, little literature has subsequently been found that has analysed this aspect of the report.

The Inquiry did not recommend the wholesale transfer of administrators into management roles. Rather, clinicians were encouraged to take on managerial roles. This seems to have often been overlooked in the early years of (general) management, as the relations between managers and clinicians were often fraught with conflict (Exworthy and Halford, 1999). The entry of people from industries outside the NHS, including former military personnel, was also advocated (for example, Alleway, 1985).

As well as implications for regional and local NHS organisations, the report had consequences for the Department of Health and Social Security (DHSS), which was required to implement the report's recommendations. The development of a Supervisory Board was aimed at reducing the 'perceived fragmentation in the policy-making and management process' (Pollitt et al, 1991, p 62). There was a recommendation that within the DHSS and the existing statutory framework, a Health Services Supervisory Board and a full-time NHS Management Board should be established.

At a more local level, District Chairmen should plan for all day-to-day decisions to be taken in the main hospitals. This represented a clear intention to devolve management nearer to the patient. It was also recommended that clinicians should be involved more closely in this management process, while balancing the need for clinical freedom. In particular, Griffiths was keen that clinicians should participate fully in decisions about priorities for the use of resources. More emphasis was also placed on 'proper' estate management, with measures to introduce a more commercial approach to planning and management.

Another notable and interesting recommendation was that the Management Board and Chairmen should ensure that patients were central to the approach of management in planning and delivering services for the population as a whole. In particular, they were to determine how well the service was being delivered at a local level by obtaining the experience and perceptions of patients and the community, using techniques such as market research. It was also suggested that more should be done to promote realistic public and professional perceptions of what the NHS could and should provide as the best possible service within the resources available.

Immediate reaction to 'the Griffiths prescription' and its implementation

Newspapers reported that the inquiry called for NHS management to have 'more thrust at all levels' (Webster, 1983, p 5) and an editorial agreed with the central criticism made in the report that the NHS lacked leadership and the 'implicit assumption of the report that an organisation which does not know where the buck stops is likely to keep passing it' (*Guardian*, 1983b).

Media coverage from the period notes the 'mixed reaction' to the Inquiry (Webster, 1983, p 5) and the tone with which general management was received varied by constituency group. Indeed, there is evidence that the Secretary of State for Health anticipated this response, particularly from 'vested interests' in the NHS (Cross, 1983, p 2). However, the government welcomed the report (Rivett, 1998, p 354), albeit belatedly (Harrison et al, 1990, p 64).

Allen (1986) and Banyard (1988) note the differing attitudes towards general management between occupational groups and trade unions. Rivett states that there were 'gleeful shouts of triumph' from administrators (1998, p 355). Learmonth (2005) recalls the 'heady period after the release of the NHS Management Inquiry' and that 'many of the individuals who came to be called managers were themselves deeply committed to what they believed were the new ideals of general management even though most had previously been known as administrators' (p 619).

This reception was despite the experience of some practical difficulties relating to changes in pay and conditions as a result of the shift to general management (Alleway, 1987). The reaction of other NHS stakeholders to the Griffiths Report was more equivocal. Nurses were defensive about losing their position in decision making and doctors seemed to be ambivalent (Rivett, 1998). Although Allen (1986) noted low morale following the changes, a survey by Banyard (1988) found that just over half (53%) of managers regarded general management as a 'favourable innovation'.

As might be expected, interest in the Griffiths reforms was not confined to the people affected and media commentators. There were numerous commentaries and analyses of the content of the report and the concept of general management (see, for example, Hunter, 1984). Some of these are opinion pieces based vicariously on assumptions and ideology, and not necessarily on empirical evidence. Although there were problems with the implementation of the Inquiry's recommendations for management at the national executive level, they were fully implemented at lower levels (Klein, 2006, p 118). This is despite evidence of concern about the short time-scale for implementation, in particular, the identification and recruitment of the new 'general managers' (Harrison et al, 1992, p 57).

The first health authority general manager, a former administrator, was appointed in July 1984 – the first of 1,800 managers to be engaged (Timmins, 1984). By February 1986, 60% of District General Managers and Regional General Managers were ex-NHS administrators, 19% were doctors, 10% were nurses and only 8% came from outside the NHS (Petchey, 1986, quoted in Cox, 1991). Similar figures are cited for 1987, when the majority (61%) of managers were former administrators or NHS finance personnel, 25% were clinical professionals (mostly doctors) and 12% were from outside the NHS (Klein, 2006, p 120). An early analysis suggested that most of the 'outsiders' were former military professionals who had taken early retirement and whose forces pension supplemented the 'poor NHS salary', which was thought to have deterred professionals from the private sector, who were initially targeted (Alleway, 1985).

Early analysis and studies describe reactions to the reforms and reflect uncertainties about the practicalities of implementation (for example, Dearden, 1985; Alleway, 1987; Templeton College, 1987a, 1987b; Stewart, 1988). For example, a study of the practical aspects of implementing general management was commissioned by the NHS Training Authority in the mid-1980s and presented in a series of publications by Templeton College (1987a, 1987b).

Evidence suggests that the overall impact of the changes was mixed (Ham, 1999, p 31). The speed and extent of general management implementation varied and it was found that implementation varied across different areas and among different occupational groups (Banyard, 1988; Pollitt et al, 1991). However, it has been suggested that this depended on the different resources available (Banyard, 1988), while others have not found any link between material and workforce resources and implementation of general management (Harrison et al, 1992). Indeed, it has also been suggested that the quality of relationships in areas before Griffiths was a stronger determinant of the success of general management than was resource availability (Harrison et al, 1992). Pollitt et al (1991) found that, regardless of the variance in improvements, there was almost always substantial change at senior level. Rivett (1998) argued that Griffiths' reforms were set to a timetable that was 'managerially unrealistic' (p 356) and Harrison et al (1992) noted that the managers with most experience were critical of the speed of change demanded (p 57).

Marnoch (1989) found that, despite a greater 'cost consciousness' as a result of the Griffiths reforms, budgeting, resource management and consumer responsiveness were less successfully implemented. Indeed, throughout the literature, there is little reflection on whether patients and the public noticed the changes and little evidence of the impact on their experience of healthcare, even though Griffiths had emphasised the need for greater responsiveness to patients and the public.

Longer-term impact of general management after Griffiths

The impact of the Griffiths Report is well described in contemporary literature (for example, Day and Klein, 1983; Sherman, 1984) and in retrospective analyses (for example, Packwood, 1997; Rivett, 1998; Webster, 1998). Indeed, Griffiths (1992) published his own analysis of the impact of the reforms. In it, he argued that the report 'forced the professions themselves to rethink their position' (p 65), which, he felt, they had done. However, he was concerned that the introduction of general management should not result in 'yet another profession in the National Health Service to work in parallel with other professions' (p 65). There are many empirical studies evaluating the impact of Griffiths and the introduction of general management, although they differ greatly in terms of size, scope and methodological rigour (Harrison et al, 1992). As well as literature examining the short-term impact and medium-term implications of general management, eight longitudinal studies analysing NHS management have been found (Packwood, 1997; Learmonth, 1998; Rivett, 1998; Wall, 2001; Harrison and Lim, 2003; Nolan and Carlisle, 2006; Saunders, 2006; Robson, 2007).

In addition, nine examples of biographical or autobiographical writing by managers have been identified (for example, Busset et al, 1987; Edwards, 1993), along with several descriptive accounts of managers' careers (for example, Wall, 2001; Holmes, 2007). However, it is not possible to say how representative this literature is of the experiences of managers, as the items tend to be written by senior managers with privileged access to publications; the views of middle managers and/or managers whose careers have been less successful or high profile are less well known. As Learmonth (2001, p 422) notes, it is important to consider that accounts from managers tend only to report successes.

It is also not clear from these studies whether and how the Griffiths changes affected the culture of the NHS. This may be because many of the studies that aimed to assess the impact of the introduction of general management were relatively short-term projects and focused on the process of implementation and the beliefs and reactions of key stakeholders at the time. In a review of the 'first wave' of post-Griffiths ethnographies, Hughes (1996) notes that studies did not find any attempts to shape culture and said little about the 'symbolic facets of management' (p 294) because they were too early to pick up the cultural dimension, and pressure from funders encouraged a synoptic view. This reinforces the importance of this project in taking a longer-term perspective.

Pollitt et al (1991) presented a three-fold criticism of the Griffiths report:

• Griffiths applied a model of managerialism founded on distrust, whereas the consensus model of working required trust.

- Griffiths failed to offer a convincing analysis of the relationship between running the NHS and the political system within which it is set.
- Griffiths did not adhere to management theory, seeing managers as 'technicians', and disregarded the 'art of management' (p 79).

It could be argued that, to some extent, the Griffiths report had only cosmetic consequences on the role of NHS managers as 'the re-labelling from administrator to manager that was licensed by the NHS Management Inquiry was not one that necessarily altered the substance of administrators'/managers' activities' (Learmonth, 2005, pp 625–6).

Studies which analyse NHS management over a longer period (for example, Harrison and Lim, 2003) temper suggestions that there was 'managerial revolution' in the NHS in the 1980s (Hughes, 1996, p 294); indeed Webster notes that there was a post-Griffiths 'management war' (1998, p 168). Goodwin (1998) contends that studies of NHS management from before 1991 and onwards tend to show similar conclusions, with a common theme of the impact of the increasing pressures of the external environment and government and a shift from internal to external management, described as a 'move from maintenance management to the management of change with greater leadership of public services' (p 22). He argues further that there is now a compromise 'with general management retained but operating within a framework of planning, collaboration and partnership' (Goodwin, 1998, p 24).

Klein (2006) also offers a long view, concluding that NHS managers are no longer trying to break the institutional stalemate that Griffiths identified but have instead become a stakeholder in their own right, a member of the NHS 'tribal club' which might be as much a barrier to reform as a facilitator. On reflection, the relationship between managers and clinicians may now be seen as a strategy of 'collusion'. This has been described in detail elsewhere and appears to be a pragmatic approach to a potentially difficult situation (see Kitchener and Exworthy, 2008 for further debate on these strategies).

This literature reinforces Greener's (2001) assertion that most policy reforms 'are not as radical as the rhetoric of the time suggested' (p 642), and that 'for all its radical intent' (p 639). Yet, Griffiths was a 'step to further change' (Webster, 1998). Studies of the impact of the Griffiths Report are a reminder that change is slow and incremental and that policy initiatives are not always wholly implemented, nor are they the only way to shape the culture of organisations.

In addition, we argue that Griffiths set in train a set of processes which, together with other reforms, have had far-reaching consequences for the NHS and managers working within it. The Griffiths reforms were part of the wave of new public management that transformed the structure and process of the NHS after the 1980s. They paved the way for further managerial reforms. These include the purchaser–provider split of the NHS quasi-market, self-governing Trusts and, latterly, Foundation Trusts, and closer links with the private/commercial sector. Conceptually, new public management has evolved, some argue, in two distinct ways, affecting, first, managers and second, NHS organisations.

First, Currie et al (2008) argue that in recent years entrepreneurial managers have emerged within the public sector. Linked to the modernisation agenda of the Blair premiership (1997–2007), entrepreneurialism has been closely associated with a shift of emphasis from management to leadership (Newman, 2005). While aspects of entrepreneurialism are not new in the public sector, there has been greater emphasis on risk taking, innovation and pro-activity (Currie et al, 2008, p 989). Certainly, the policy of granting autonomy to Foundation Trusts has been closely associated with the three characteristics that Currie and colleagues identified (Exworthy and Frosini, 2008).

Second, could the Griffiths Inquiry, with the introduction of general management practices also have had a major impact on the organisational form and organisational memory? Pollitt (2009) has put forward the hypothesis that post-bureaucratic forms of organisations perform less well than traditional bureaucracies in the areas of organisational memory and learning experience. The introduction of NHS general managers not only added another stakeholder to the NHS but was part of a set of processes that have been called post-bureaucracy (Hoggett, 1996; Pollitt, 2009). The consequences of post-bureaucracies include accelerated staff turnover and organisational change.

Regarding staff turnover, two aspects are worth noting here. First, there is a growing body of evidence that suggests that general managers with no organisational memory, including those who joined the NHS from 'outside' organisations, have seldom been successful (Exworthy et al, 2009). The successful general managers, it could be argued, were those who had the organisational memory and could build on their learning experience. These were the ones who had been part of the NHS bureaucracy. The second aspect is the average period in office for Chief Executives, which, in acute Trusts, is approximately two years four months (Sergeant, quoted in Foreword to Hoggett-Bowers, 2009, p 2); this equates to about 700 days.

As the NHS and other public services have embraced the new public management agenda and moved towards post-bureaucracy, there is a danger that, with rapid staff turnover, this memory will be lost – not least because of the introduction of contracted-out services, variable contracts and part-time and temporary working practices. Career structures have changed, with managers 'jumping from organisation to organisation, from public sector to private sector and back, in order to get on' (Pollitt, 2009, p 200). The implication is that modernisation of the organisational form has led to a collective forgetfulness and an inability to learn.

As regards organisational change, there has been growing frequency of major organisational change. Goodwin (2006) argues that 'The time intervals between episodes of major structural reforms have progressively diminished to the point that the NHS risks becoming caught up in a vortex of permanent upheaval' (p 186). This permanent revolution is, arguably, precisely the intention of the recent NHS reforms, that is, to create a self-sustaining and continuous process prompted by decentralised agents (individuals and organisations) operating within a (quasi-)market logic (Stevens, 2004; Allen, 2006).

While there is some dispute about the emergence and extent of post-bureaucracy in the NHS, it is apparent that many recent trends rely upon a cadre of managers responsible for shaping the strategic and operational activities of organisations and health systems. This would not have been possible without the Griffiths reforms.

Summary: Griffiths' legacy

The Griffiths Inquiry is a useful case study that serves as a lens through which to regard the development of NHS management (and indeed, broader public management). The case study draws on existing archival and empirical evidence as well as contemporary data (from interviews with NHS managers) to highlight the impact of policy shifts on NHS managers. Case study design ensures that phenomena are viewed in context (Yin, 2003) and the focus on the Griffiths Inquiry provides a context for understanding the evolution of NHS management. The Griffiths Inquiry illustrates how concepts such as career transitions (Fouad and Bynner, 2008), entrepreneurialism or post-bureaucracy can be applied. It is also a methodological device to provide focus and elicit managers' perceptions of change and how they 'make sense of their careers as they unfold through time and space, attending to ... the holistic nature of career as well as to specific career transitions' (Cohen and Mallon, 2001, pp 48–9). The case study offers insights into wider institutional changes relating to the structure of the NHS. Of course, not all of Griffiths was implemented. While the issue of public involvement remains problematic (Florin and Dixon, 2004), there have recently been significant steps in introducing clinician (executive) leadership (Kitchener, 2000). The shift from management to leadership has been instrumental in fostering greater clinical involvement in management decision making across the NHS (Gray and Harrison, 2004).

In short, as a case study, the Griffiths Inquiry illustrates the ways in which radical change was possible at a particular moment, that change did happen relatively quickly and that it was implemented without too much disruption in service delivery. The consequences of such reform continue to be felt today.

References

Allen, D. (1986) 'Trials and tribulations of fledgling DGMs', *Health Service Journal*, vol 96, no 4994, p 494.

Allen, P. (2006) 'New localism in the English National Health Service: what is it for?', *Health Policy*, vol 79, nos 2–3, pp 244–52.

Alleway, L. (1985) 'Military manoeuvres in the NHS', *Health Service Journal*, vol 95, no 4967, pp 1192–3.

Alleway, L. (1987) 'Manager's pay: fight for a slice of the cake', *Health Service Journal*, vol 97, no 5065, pp 986–7.

Banyard, R. (1988) 'How do UGMs perform?', *Health Service Journal*, vol 98, no 5110, pp 824–5.

Busset, A., Crail, R., Griffiths, P., Hewitson, P., Horner, J., Parker, V., Randall, A. and Wall, A. (1987) *On being a general manager*, Manchester: University of Manchester Department of Community Medicine.

Cohen, L. and Mallon, M. (2001) 'My brilliant career? Using stories as a methodological tool in careers research', *International Studies of Management and Organisation*, vol 31, no 3, pp 48–68.

Cox, D. (1991) 'Health service management – a sociological view: Griffiths and the non-negotiated order of the hospital', in J. Gabe, M. Calnan and M. Bury (eds) *The sociology of the Health Service*, London: Routledge, pp 89–114.

Cross, D. (1983) 'Fowler set to unveil new management style for hospitals', *The Times*, 25 October, p 2.

Currie, G., Humphreys, M., Ucbasaran, D. and McManus, S. (2008) 'Entrepreneurial leadership in the English public sector: paradox or possibility?', *Public Administration*, vol 86, no 4, pp 987-1008.

Day, P. and Klein, R. (1983) 'Two views on the Griffiths Report. The mobilization of consent versus the management of conflict: decoding the Griffiths Report', *British Medical Journal*, vol 287, no 6407, pp 1813–16.

Dearden, R. (1985) 'The development of general management', *Hospital and Health Services Review*, vol 81, no 4, pp 163–4.

DHSS (Department of Health and Social Security) (1971) *National Health Service reorganisation: Consultative document*, London: DHSS.

DHSS (1983) *NHS Management Inquiry Report* (The Griffiths Report), London: DHSS.

Edwards, B. (1993) *The National Health Service: A manager's tale*, London: Nuffield Trust.

Exworthy, M. and Frosini, F. (2008) 'Room to manoeuvre? Explaining local autonomy in the English National Health Service', *Health Policy*, vol 81, nos 2–3, pp 204–12.

Exworthy, M. and Halford, S. (eds) (1999) *Professionals and the new managerialism in the public sector*, Buckingham: Open University Press.

Exworthy, M., Macfarlane, F. and Willmott, M. (2009) *NHS transitions: Taking the long view*, London: Nuffield Trust.

Florin, D. and Dixon, J. (2004) 'Public involvement in health care', *British Medical Journal*, vol 328, pp 159–61.

Fouad, N. and Bynner, J. (2008) 'Work transitions', *American Psychology*, vol 63, no 4, pp 241–51.

Glennerster, H., Owens, P. and Kimberley, A. (1988) *The nursing management function after Griffiths: A study in the North West Thames region*, London: LSE and NW Thames Regional Health Authority.

Goodwin, N. (1998) 'Leadership in the UK NHS: where are we now?', *Journal of Management in Medicine*, vol 12, no 1, pp 21–32.

Goodwin, N. (2006) 'Healthcare system strategy and planning', in K. Walshe and J. Smith (eds) *Healthcare management*. Maidenhead, Open University Press, pp 183–200.

Gray, A. and Harrison, S. (eds) (2004) *Governing medicine: Theory and practice*, Buckingham: Open University Press.

Greener, I. (2001) 'The ghost of health services past revisited', *International Journal of Health Services*, vol 31, no 3, pp 635–46.

Greener, I. (2008) 'Decision making in a time of significant reform', *Administration and Society*, vol 40, no 2, pp 194–20.

Greer, S. and Jarman, H. (2007) *The Department of Health and the civil service. From Whitehall to department of delivery to where?*, London: Nuffield Trust.

Griffiths, R. (1992) 'Seven years of progress: general management in the NHS', *Health Economics*, vol 1, no 1, pp 61–70.

Guardian (1983a) 'NHS administrative costs lower than in other countries', 24 October, p 2.

Guardian (1983b) Editorial: 'The Sainsbury Prescription', 26 October, p 12.

Guardian (1983c) 'Fowler brings in manager for restructured health service', 26 October, p 26.

Gunz, H. (1989) 'The dual meaning of managerial careers: organizational and individual levels of analysis', *Journal of Management Studies*, vol 26, no 3, pp 225–50.

Halpern, S. (1983) 'The quality quiz', *Health and Social Service Journal*, 14 July, pp 832–3.

Ham, C. (1999) *Health policy in Britain. The politics and organisation of the National Health Service*, 4th edn, Basingstoke: Palgrave.

Harrison, S. and Lim, J. (2003) 'The frontier of control: doctors and managers in the NHS 1966 to 1997', *Clinical Governance*, vol 8, no 1, pp 13–18.

Harrison, S. and Wood, B. (1999) 'Designing health service organization in the UK, 1968 to 1998: from blueprint to bright idea and "manipulated emergence"', *Public Administration*, vol 77, no 4, pp 751–68.

Harrison, S., Hunter, D.J. and Pollitt, C. (1990) *The dynamics of British health policy*, London: Unwin Hyman.

Harrison, S., Hunter, D., Marnoch, G. and Pollitt, C. (1992) *Just managing: Power and culture in the National Health Service*, London: Macmillan.

HSSJ (*Health and Social Service Journal*) (1983) 'Hands off the units', 3 November, p 1310.

Hoggett, P. (1996) 'New modes of control in the public service', *Public Administration*, vol 74, no 1, pp 9–32.

Hoggett-Bowers (2009) *NHS chief executives: Bold and old*, London: Hoggett-Bowers.

Holmes, M. (2007) *History in the making: An oral history of the healthcare manager role*, London: Institute for Healthcare Management.

Hughes, D. (1996) 'NHS managers as rhetoricians: a case of culture management?', *Sociology of Health and Illness*, vol 18, no 3, pp 291–314.

Hunter, D.J. (1984) 'NHS management: is Griffiths the last quick fix?', *Public Administration*, vol 62, pp 91–4.

Hyde, A. and Wilson, M. (1983) 'A model for management', *Health and Social Services Journal*, 3 November, p 1309.

Kitchener, M. (2000) 'The bureaucratisation of professional roles: the case of clinical directors in UK hospitals', *Organization*, vol 7, no 1, pp 129–54.

Kitchener, M. and Exworthy, M. (2008) 'Models of medical work control: a theory elaboration from English general practice', in L. McKee, E. Ferlie and P. Hyde (eds) *Organising and re-organising: Power and change in health-care organisations*, Basingstoke: Palgrave, pp 209–23.

Klein, R. (2006) *The new politics of the National Health Service*, 5th edn, London: Longman.

Learmonth, M. (1998) 'Kindly technicians: hospital administrators immediately before the NHS', *Journal of Management in Medicine*, vol 12, no 6, pp 323–30.

Learmonth, M. (2001) 'NHS Trust chief executives as heroes?', *Health Care Analysis*, vol 9, no 4, pp 417–36.

Learmonth, M. (2005) 'Doing things with words: the case of "management" and "administration"', *Public Administration*, vol 83, no 3, pp 617–37.

Marnoch, G. (1989) 'After the culture shock', *Health Service Journal*, vol 99, no 5180, pp 1500–1.

Merali, F. (2003) 'NHS managers' views of their culture and their public image: the implication for NHS reforms', *International Journal of Public Sector Management*, vol 16, no 7, pp 549–63.

Newman, J. (2005) 'Network governance, transformational leadership and the micro politics of public service change', *Sociology*, vol 39, no 4, pp 717–34.

NHS Confederation (2008) 'Key statistics on the NHS', available at: www.nhsconfed. org/issues/about-1857.cfm.

Nolan, A. and Carlisle, D. (2006) 'A brief history. Heading for half century', *Health Service Journal*, vol 116, no 5999 (Supplement), pp 3–6.

Packwood, T. (1997) 'Analysing changes in the nature of health service management in England', *Health Policy*, vol 40, no 2, pp 91–102.

Pollitt, C. (2009) 'Bureaucracies remember, post-bureaucratic organizations forget?', *Public Administration*, vol 87, no 2, pp 198–218.

Pollitt, C., Harrison, S., Hunter, D.J. and Marnoch, G. (1991) 'General management in the NHS: the initial impact 1983–88', *Public Administration*, vol 69, no 1, pp 61–83.

Rivett, G. (1998) *From cradle to grave: 50 years of the NHS*, London: King's Fund.

Robson, N. (2007) 'Adapting not adopting: 1958–74. Accounting and managerial "reform" in the early NHS', *Accounting, Business and Financial History*, vol 17, no 3, pp 445–67.

Saunders, G. (2006) *Themes that emerge from fifty years of the English Management Training Scheme*, Coventry: NHS Institute.

Sherman, J. (1983) 'Fowler turns tables to give administrators rough ride', *Health and Social Service Journal*, 20 October, p 1248.

Sherman, J. (1984) 'The fear of Fowler clones', *Health Service Journal*, vol 94, no 4923, p 1348.

Sherman, J., Black, T. and Halpern, S. (1983) 'Manpower checkout', *Health and Social Service Journal*, 17 February, pp 196-7.

Silver, R. (1996) *Managing to care: The work, achievements and frustrations of managers in the NHS*, Birmingham: National Association of Health Authorities and Trusts.

Stevens, S. (2004) 'Reform strategies for the English NHS', *Health Affairs*, vol 23, no 3, pp 37–44.

Stewart, R. (1988) *Postscript to the Templeton series on district general managers*, Oxford: NHS Training Authority.

Templeton College (1987a) *Study no 1: DGMs and chairmen: A productive relationship?*, Oxford: Oxford Centre for Management Studies and NHS Training Authority.

Templeton College (1987b) *Study no. 5: Managing with doctors: Working together?* Oxford: Oxford Centre for Management Studies and NHS Training Authority.

Timmins, N. (1984) 'NHS staff split on proposals to appoint managers', *The Times*, 12 January, p 2.

van Wynsberghe, R. and Khan, S. (2007) 'Redefining case study', *International Journal of Qualitative Methods*, vol 6, no 2, pp 1–10.

Wall, A. (2001) *Being a health service manager: Expectations and experience. A study of four generations of managers in the NHS*, Maureen Dixon essays series on health service organisations, London: Nuffield Trust.

Webster, C. (1998) *The National Health Service: A political history*, Oxford: Oxford University Press.

Webster, P. (1983) 'NHS management needs more thrust at all levels, report says', *The Times*, 26 October, p 5.

West, D. (2010) 'Lansley tells Confed: NHS needs strong management', *Health Service Journal*, 24 June, www.hsj.co.uk/home/nhs-confed-2010/lansley-tells-confed-nhs-needs-strong-management/5016380.article.

Yin, R.K. (2003) *Case study research: Design and methods*, Thousand Oaks, CA: Sage.

ten

AIDS in the UK: The making of policy, 1981–1994 (Berridge, 1996): a case study in British health policy

David Evans

Context

What is a case study in British health policy? Like other authors in this volume, I pondered this question when invited by the organisers to suggest a case study to discuss at the symposium that led to this book. It was clear to me that there was no simple definition or set of criteria that I could apply. So I reflected on those examples of policy analysis of specific 'cases' that had contributed to the development of my own understanding of the complexities of the policy process. Among several texts I considered, Andrew Pettigrew and colleagues' (1992) *Shaping strategic change* stood out as a significant influence on my thinking early in my research career, in particular by helping me to see how conceptual models can help make sense of what at first sight appear to be complex and unique policy examples (see Locock and Dopson, Chapter Thirteen). In the end, however, I chose a very different type of book, Virginia Berridge's (1996) *AIDS in the UK: The making of policy, 1981–1994*, despite its being more usually found on the history shelves rather than in the policy section of libraries.

Why choose this work of contemporary history as my health policy case study? Partly, it was because of the personal impact it had on me at the time. I had been working in HIV/AIDS prevention in the late 1980s and early 1990s, and this book helped to make sense of the complex reality of the unique historical moment that I had lived through. More generally, although I had not reread it since its publication in 1996, I had a strong memory of the quality of the writing and the real insight it gave me into the inner (and usually hidden) workings of the UK health policy process. While it was only a decade and a half old, I regarded it as a 'classic' work, and it seemed worthwhile revisiting such a classic and judging whether or not it had stood the test of time. That it was written as contemporary history, not as health policy, within a different academic tradition and conventions, seemed to me to make it more worthwhile in contributing to the development of a broad understanding of what might constitute case studies in British health policy.

On rereading the book I was also interested to note that on five occasions Berridge herself uses the term 'case study' (Berridge, 1996, pp 2, 195, 213, 284, 285). In none of these instances is she describing her book or the methodological approach to research that underpins it. Rather, on each occasion she uses the term to flag up a particularly interesting aspect of the policy process. Berridge's first use of this term is typical of the others:

> The response to AIDS brought into play the medic-bureaucratic tradition of health policy making in Britain, operating in conjunction with political support. AIDS was, from that perspective, a case-study in the continuities of power, despite an apparent 'Thatcher revolution' in government. (p 2)

Implicitly then, a case study in this usage is an episode of policy making that exemplifies themes with wider relevance that the observant researcher can learn from, rather than a particular methodological approach to historical or policy research.

As the book makes clear, AIDS emerged in the 1980s as a new policy problem in the UK. The first cases of the not-yet-named acquired immune deficiency syndrome were recognised in gay men in New York in mid-1981, with the first case in the UK following late in the same year. For the next few years there was intense debate over its cause, in particular whether it was directly due to an infectious organism. Initially, policy makers in the UK and elsewhere showed little interest in responding to the emerging epidemic. By 1983, however, increasing evidence of heterosexual transmission and the infection of people with haemophilia through blood products was raising alarm bells in policy circles, the media and, more widely, among the public. Confirmation in 1984 that a virus (later called HIV) was the causative agent for AIDS and could be sexually transmitted or blood borne, and the development in 1985 of a blood test for HIV, meant that HIV became a policy problem that the UK government could no longer ignore. At the very least, the government had to decide whether to introduce routine testing and, if so, in what settings and within what parameters. The evidence of blood-borne transmission, fanned by alarmist media coverage, raised huge public concern about the safety of blood supplies. A series of key policy decisions followed. These included the introduction of routine testing in the UK Blood Transfusion Service and additional voluntary testing through genito-urinary medicine clinics and GP practices, but HIV/AIDS was not made a notifiable disease, nor would there be legislation to criminalise its sexual transmission. Each of these decisions raised the profile of AIDS as a policy problem and necessitated further policy decisions, for example, on the extent to which the government would support 'safer sex' education within existing health education programmes or (controversial) harm-minimisation strategies such as needle exchange schemes for injecting drug users.

Writing in 2010, it is difficult to recapture the media scare-mongering, the public anxiety and (for a short time) the sense of crisis within UK policy. As Berridge recounts, it was one of the few historical moments when policy makers were interested in historical research, specifically in what lessons could be learned from earlier 20th-century efforts to control other sexually transmitted infections (Berridge, 1996, p 4). Out of this historical moment was born an international network of historians, sociologists, policy analysts and activists working to capture and learn from the history of AIDS. In the UK, the Nuffield Provincial Hospitals Trust funded the AIDS Social History Programme at the London School of Hygiene and Tropical Medicine, with the medical sociologist Phil Strong as its initial director. Virginia Berridge was then appointed as co-director. Berridge and Strong published an edited collection, *AIDS and contemporary history*, in 1993, among a number of other publications, before the programme was subdivided into history and sociology, with books in the two areas planned by Berridge and Strong respectively. Strong died unexpectedly in 1995 and only the history book was published, as *AIDS in the UK*.

Critique

In reassessing *AIDS in the UK*, I have applied two sets of criteria. First, I have critiqued the text using the same appraisal criteria that I would apply to any health policy case study. There is of course no formally agreed set of criteria for assessing the quality of policy analysis, but I adopted the Critical Appraisal Skills Programme (CASP) checklist for assessing the quality of qualitative research papers (Public Health Research Unit, 2006), which I have found a very useful appraisal tool for qualitative policy research. I recognise that this approach may be viewed as somewhat problematic, in that I am assessing scholarship in one discipline against the standards of another, but all such boundaries and definitions are to some extent artificial and permeable, and if I am to make the case for *AIDS in the UK* being a relevant case study of British health policy, then it is against the standards of policy research that it must be tested.

Second, I have looked for evidence of impact. Assessing impact in these days of the UK Research Excellence Framework is, of course, both topical and contested. In principle, I would have liked to have examined impact in the policy world as well as the academic world, but without the resources to conduct primary research and talk to policy makers (as Berridge herself did for *AIDS in the UK*), it is very difficult to assess the impact on policy. There is, of course, an extensive literature on the complex and often indirect relationship between research and policy (Weiss, 1979; Duke, 2001; Young et al, 2002; Wells, 2007), and historical research such as this is, arguably, even less likely than contemporary policy research to have a directly observable impact in the policy world.

In terms of academic impact, I have looked at two main indicators. First, I have sought to identify *AIDS in the UK*'s initial impact in terms of book reviews. For longer-term impact, I then looked at subsequent citations, not simply in terms of crude numbers (which can be a simplistic and deceptive indicator) but, in particular, in terms of the extent to which the book's central arguments and analytical framework have been accepted and built upon by subsequent scholars or debated and critiqued.

In order to identify citations I searched for 'AIDS in the UK: the making of policy' in Google Scholar from 1996 (date of the book's publication) until 2010 (the date this review was completed). In addition, I used my university library to check for citations in relevant books that would not have made it into online databases. Thus, this was by no means a full, systematic literature review but, given the constraints of unfunded research, it was as comprehensive as I could make it.

In searching for relevant book citations, I needed to consider what fields I would include as relevant. AIDS policy in the UK is of potential relevance to a number of disciplines and geographies. Thus, one might look for an impact on AIDS policy literature in the UK, Europe, the developed world or globally. Alternatively, one might seek impact in texts on UK AIDS policy, sexual health policy, health policy, social policy or public policy. Clearly, one might need to examine both contemporary policy and historical texts. Finally, within health policy, one might reasonably seek an impact on distinct but related areas of health, for example illegal drug use. Again, although not wholly comprehensive, I soon found what qualitative researchers might regard as saturation. I established, for example, that very few post-2000 UK social policy texts cover AIDS in more than a brief sentence or two, if at all, and with few if any references to primary sources on AIDS. In critiquing *AIDS in the UK*, I want to look at four key questions asked by the CASP appraisal criteria:

- Was there a clear statement of the aims of the research?
- Was the research design appropriate to address the aims of the research?
- Is there a clear statement of findings?
- How valuable is the research?

Establishing the clarity of aims is relatively easy. Although the book has no section explicitly labelled 'aims', the first three pages of the Introduction provide a comprehensive statement of aims. Running through the Introduction, there are several separate passages which collectively give a strong indication of what the book is about. Thus, early on we have the following statement:

> There has been a unique opportunity to study the British response from the early days of the policy reaction, to collect interim recollections before they become too encrusted with the patinas of justification, mythology, even nostalgia. There is a possibility of capturing that 'real vibrant sense of history as happening just around the corner'. (p 2)

On the next page the aims of this book are distinguished from other works of the same period that were concerned with the cultural history of AIDS:

> This account focuses on issues which have influenced government policy-making, on policy rather than on the wider cultural ramifications of AIDS. (p 3)

Finally, this aim of understanding the process of policy making is linked with a wider aim, to contribute to understanding the nature of historical enquiry:

> It focuses on the general issues of the construction and definition of AIDS over time as a policy problem, and the relationship between science and the definition of policy, especially through the changing meaning of AIDS. In doing so, the book also aims to examine the way in which the study of AIDS has thrown light on the nature of historical enquiry and its role in the study of contemporary policy concerns. (p 3)

Thus, by the end of the Introduction, the aims of the book are clear: it is primarily to tell the story of the history of the AIDS policy process in the UK from 1981 to 1994 from the multiple perspectives of key policy stakeholders, and secondarily to contribute to an understanding of the role history can play in the study of policy. Thus, the first of my CASP criteria has been met.

The next CASP question concerns the appropriateness of the research design for the research questions. And here we have a significant challenge. As with most historical works, there is no research design or methods section. There is, it is true, a 'Frameworks of interpretation' section in the Introduction, but this mainly locates the author's position within contemporary analytical debates on AIDS and does not provide even a summary of the research methods. Information on the methods of data collection is sparse and dispersed through the Introduction, other chapters and the extensive notes. It is clear that the main methods of data collection were oral history interviews and documentary analysis. Further, we know that in those days, before the UK Freedom of Information Act, Berridge's access to official documents was severely limited by the 30-year rule. But there is much about research design and methods that we are simply not told. We learn little, for example, about recruitment and sampling of informants. How did Berridge decide whom to talk to? How many of the people she approached agreed or declined to be interviewed? Was there any systematic bias in non-respondents? Similarly, we know very little about the interview process. Were respondents asked open, semi-structured or structured questions? Were the questions based on pre-existing theories? Finally, we know little about the process of analysis. Were interviews analysed thematically? Was the validity of the analysis tested in any way? Indeed, were the transcripts coded at all? From the perspective of the CASP criteria, therefore, there is insufficient methodological detail and we are unable to come to an assessment of whether the research design is appropriate for the research questions. This, then, is a significant omission if we want to consider the book as a health policy case. This having been said, however, it must be noted that it is not traditional in historical scholarship such as this to include methods sections in books, so it is unreasonable to expect it here from a historian such as Berridge. And set against the lack of methodological detail must be the richness of the primary data presented in the book.

In terms of the next CASP criterion, the clear presentation of findings is one of the real strengths of *AIDS in the UK*. Berridge identifies four phases of the policy response:

1981–85 Policy making from below
1986–87 Wartime emergency
1987–89 Normalisation and chronic disease
1990–94 The re-politicisation of AIDS.

In 'policy making from below', Berridge describes how groups outside the normal policy-making circles (and gay groups in particular) were drawn into positions of policy influence. This was a time of voluntarism and self-help among the gay community that was first affected by AIDS, but also among the emergent scientific, clinical and epidemiological AIDS specialisms. Despite the political and media pressure for a punitive response, a liberal consensus was legitimised by medical and scientific expertise.

Berridge then recounts how a period of 'wartime emergency' followed the realisation that AIDS could affect the wider community. 'This was collective fear not of the mass alone, but at the elite opinion-forming levels of society' (p 83). Politicians then publicly and dramatically intervened. There was an intensive mobilisation of the mass media via the famous 'Don't die of ignorance' campaign. AIDS was officially established as a high-level national emergency. But the crisis response was a continuation of the liberal consensus rather than one of quarantine or stigmatisation.

The third phase, of 'normalisation', is identified by Berridge as following the slowing rate of growth of the epidemic and the transformation of AIDS into another chronic disease for which palliative treatments were now available. In this phase new professional experts replaced the self-help volunteers of the earlier phases and the AIDS voluntary sector became increasingly remote from the corridors of power.

The final phase, of the 're-politicisation of AIDS', is described by Berridge as a time of shifting policy alliances, with inner and outer circles of influence. AIDS was at the same time being mainstreamed and marginalised. The outer circle invoked the re-gaying of AIDS as an objective. At the same time an anti-AIDS alliance emerged that questioned the AIDS orthodoxy.

This is, of course, a very brief summary of a lengthy and detailed analysis based on the empirical evidence of extensive interviews with key policy stakeholders throughout these four phases. I found it convincing at the time, and equally so on rereading it a decade and a half later. In terms of the final CASP question, about the value of the work, Berridge's work seems to me to be invaluable for understanding the UK AIDS policy process, with many of the lessons generalisable to the wider UK policy process. Few case studies give you such a detailed insight into the fundamental decision-making processes shaping a major new area of policy making, nor evidence of their analysis with such extensive empirical data.

Contemporary reflection

In reflecting on the critical question of the overall value of *AIDS in the UK*, I want consider both its initial reception and its longer-term impact on scholarship. I would have liked to have looked at the impact on policy as well, but this was never likely to be easy to uncover and document with regard to a historical work, particularly one focused on AIDS after AIDS slipped down the UK policy agenda from the mid-1990s.

In terms of initial impact, I tracked down 11 contemporaneous book reviews. Three were in more journalistic publications (*Guardian, New Statesman and Society* and *Times Higher Education Supplement*), while 8 were in peer-reviewed academic journals. Unsurprisingly, several were in historical journals (*Social History of Medicine, Medical History, Contemporary British History*), while the others were mainly in health and medical journals (*British Medical Journal, Journal of the Royal Society of Medicine, Trends in Microbiology, Drugs: Education, Prevention and Policy*). There was one review in a sociology journal (*Contemporary Sociology*) but, perhaps significantly, none that I could find in the main UK-orientated social policy journals.

The initial critical response as expressed in these book reviews was overwhelmingly positive. Six of the authors were entirely complimentary (Coutinho, 1996; Loudon, 1996; Stewart, 1996; Turney, 1996; Bowling, 1997; Weindling, 1997). Ann Bowling (1997), a prominent health service researcher, was typical in her review: '*AIDS in the UK* is a highly skilful and immensely readable historical analysis of AIDS policy, and an example of historical research at its best and most readable.' The equally eminent medical historian Paul Weindling (1997) was similarly admiring: 'Carefully and intelligently researched, this analytical and succinct overview of the evolving perceptions of AIDS constitutes a fundamental historical account and is of contemporary relevance as AIDS policies further evolve.'

Other authors were largely positive but also included some degree of criticism or qualification. While praising the book as 'supremely well written' and making a 'significant contribution,' the sociologist Karen Booth (1997) commented that 'the sociologist who is looking for breakthrough theories either on policy making or on the political construction of AIDS will be disappointed'. Similarly, Dodds (2000) while commending Berridge's 'detailed account', argues that she fails to problematise key issues. Jeffrey Weeks (1996) described the book as 'judicious', 'an important and valuable book' with rich and revealing empirical detail; but Weeks then suggests that 'judiciousness also has its limitations', and that 'what is lost is a sense of extreme cultural and sexual – as well as, often, personal – crisis that shaped the actions of many of the main actors', Daniel Fox (1997) judges the book as 'the most exhaustive and persuasive study to date of policy making for the AIDS/HIV epidemic in any country', but also comments that 'many readers will disagree with particular emphases and interpretations'. Finally, while describing *AIDS in the UK* as a 'must' read, De Cock (1997) is concerned that the book does not give enough attention to the global epidemic or to the 10% of AIDS cases occurring in black Africans in the UK.

In terms of the book's longer-term academic impact, the evidence from the number of citations is mixed. Google Scholar shows a respectable 106 citations as of October 2010, which is far less than the impressive 433 citations for the other case study I considered examining (Pettigrew et al, 1992), but many more than for other historical texts on UK sexual health policy, such as Davidson's (2000) social history of venereal disease in 20th-century Scotland.

There is clear evidence of the work's impact in the history of medicine literature. The book is cited as early as 1999 in Dorothy Porter's *Health, civilisation and the state: A history of public health from ancient to modern times* (1999). Davidson (2000) references Berridge's book several times in his book and follows her analysis of the development of the 'liberal consensus' in AIDS policy. I personally have cited *AIDS in the UK* in a chapter on the history of sexually transmitted infection policy in England (Evans, 2001), in which I, like Davidson, largely follow her analysis regarding AIDS policy. Berridge's work is more extensively cited in Sheard and Donaldson's (2006) account of the history of the Chief Medical Officer, where there is an extensive discussion drawing on *AIDS in the UK*, with numerous references to it. Yates (2002) draws on the book in his history of British drug policy, 1950–2001. Berridge herself has, quite appropriately, referenced her own work in a number of subsequent historical pieces (for example, Berridge, 2000; Berridge, 2003; Berridge et al, 2006).

There are, however, other history of medicine texts that cover AIDS in the UK and so might have been expected to cite Berridge but do not do so. Peter Baldwin's (2008) chapter on the history of AIDS in the industrialised world includes Britain as one of a number of countries under review, but does not reference Berridge's book, despite *AIDS in the UK* arguably being a more appropriate source for his points regarding Britain than the two British references he does use. General histories of medicine in Britain cover AIDS only briefly or not at all. Anne Hardy's (2001) history of health and medicine in Britain since 1860 only briefly mentions AIDS, with no references to Berridge or indeed to any other sources on AIDS. Webster's (2001) textbook for the Open University similarly covers AIDS very briefly, with no citations, although Berridge's book is listed in the bibliography. General social histories of the UK which cover the 1980s also commonly do not cover AIDS policy (for example, Pugh, 1999; Benson, 2005).

There are similarly mixed results with regard to impact in the policy literature. Increasingly, general social or health policy texts either omit discussion of AIDS or provide only a limited synopsis, with no citation of any primary research (for example, Hunter, 2003; Dean, 2006; Baldock et al, 2007; Orme et al, 2007; Alcock, 2008; Harrison and McDonald, 2008; Bochel et al, 2009). Relatively few policy texts focus on UK sexual health policy, but even those that do, such as Burtney (2004), only briefly mention AIDS, with no references to Berridge or other specific research on AIDS policy.

In those comparatively few texts where AIDS policy is given more attention, the extent to which Berridge is cited remains variable. Rudolf Klein (2006) covers UK AIDS policy in the fifth edition of his own classic, *The new politics of the NHS*. But Klein chooses to reference his own earlier article (Day and Klein, 1989) on UK AIDS policy rather than to cite Berridge's book. Others, including myself (Evans, 1999, 2006) and Baggott (2000), treat *AIDS in the UK* as a standard text to cite on UK AIDS policy at the time, particularly in order to give a framework for periodisation of the policy response. Brown (2000) draws on Berridge extensively to inform his study of AIDS, risk and social governance. Duke (2001) makes two references to Berridge's book in a paper on UK prison drug policy, drawing on her analysis of the development of the liberal consensus on HIV/AIDS and harm minimalisation.

More intriguing still are those authors who appear to make use of Berridge's periodisation but do not attribute it to her. Rosenbrock et al (2000) outlined four phases of AIDS policy, from exceptionalism to normalisation, with some overlap in concept with Berridge but no reference to her periodisation (although her book is cited later in the paper, with regard only to normalisation). Similarly, Freeman (2000) has an extensive discussion of AIDS policy in Western Europe, with a specific focus on UK policy, and provides a periodisation of AIDS policy that is consistent with *AIDS in the UK*. Despite his work's being published four years after Berridge's, however, he does not reference the book but cites only an earlier 1992 article by Berridge and Strong. Steffen (2004) writes on AIDS and health policy responses in Europe and describes four phases which strongly echo Berridge's four phases, but does not cite Berridge in this part of the article (though she does briefly cite *AIDS in the UK* at a later point in her paper).

It is impossible, of course, to determine the extent to which the periodisations by Rosenbrock et al, Freeman and Steffen were or were not influenced by Berridge's earlier articulation of UK AIDS policy periodisation. Concepts like these can emerge independently in different places at the same time, or can be transmitted informally through conference discussions and meetings and so lose their attribution to any particular author. What can be said with more certainty is that where other authors have cited Berridge and discussed her analysis of UK AIDS policy, they have tended to agree with her. With the exception of the very limited criticism summarised earlier in some initial book reviewers, no subsequent writer that I have found has challenged the fundamental lines of analysis of *AIDS in the UK*.

A final area to consider is the impact the book has had on methodology. Berridge herself, of course, has written extensively on the value of historical methods for the study of contemporary health policy, and her chapter on historical research for a health services research text (Berridge, 2001), unsurprisingly, uses *AIDS in the UK* as a helpful example. Bowling (2009) similarly highlights Berridge's book as an example of documentary research in her own widely read health services research methods book.

Returning to my original questions about what constitutes a case study in British health policy and the enduring value of Berridge's book, my conclusion is that *AIDS in the UK* has stood the test of time and represents an important and illuminating example of a case study in British health policy. If the book has a significant failing from a health policy perspective, it is a lack of detailed and explicit discussion of methodology. Other than this, however, it is an exemplary book which demonstrates the generalisable learning that can flow from a well-conducted health policy case study (even if it is not presented as one). Not only does it make sense of AIDS policy making in the UK in the period under study (1981–94), but it anticipates the subsequent focus of policy to normalise AIDS as yet another chronic disease, at least in the UK, where access to anti-retroviral treatment is universal. Although few policy makers or policy analysts are interested in UK AIDS policy now, were they to be so, *AIDS in the UK* would remain a key text for understanding current policy on AIDS.

The book has not perhaps had the impact it deserves, largely because of the rapid decline of AIDS as a policy problem in the UK since the mid-1990s. Subsequently the policy focus on AIDS has shifted largely to the developing world. Contemporary policy problems arising from AIDS in developing countries are somewhat different from those faced by the UK in the 1980s, in particular those related to ensuring that people living with HIV receive anti-retroviral treatment in financially challenged health systems that are not currently able to provide universal healthcare. However, aspects of Berridge's analysis are still very relevant. The alliances that Berridge explores between activists, clinicians and civil servants are as important in international AIDS policy as they were in the UK. And *AIDS in the UK* demonstrates the importance of examining short-term policy 'crises' such as the advent of AIDS in the UK in the context of longer-term continuities, in particular the long-standing policy consensus on a 'liberal', non-coercive approach to sexually transmitted infections. Moreover, given the importance of private philanthropic foundations such as the Bill and Melinda Gates Foundation within current global AIDS policy communities, Berridge's book is a reminder that such philanthropy has yet to be critically examined in the historical context of its role in 20th-century public health.

It is a shame if, as appears to be the case, *AIDS in the UK* has been pigeon-holed as a book on the history of AIDS policy and has not been used as a case study to contribute to developing a wider understanding of the health policy process in the UK. There is much that the policy world can learn from the case of AIDS in the UK about how new policy problems emerge, how policy communities form, and seek to influence policy, and how governments respond to these emerging policy drivers. *AIDS in the UK* remains as relevant as a case study of British health policy today as it was when published in 1996. Moreover, its illustration of the value of a case study of current health policy by a contemporary historian is not unique. The History and Policy collaboration (co-founded by Berridge) has published over 100 papers on its website by historians seeking to inform current UK public policy. As with *AIDS in the UK*, it is very difficult to assess the impact of this wide body of historical work on policy decisions. But, as Weiss and many others have argued, research seldom influences policy in a simple, linear way; just as likely is the 'enlightenment model' of influence, where 'it is the concepts and theoretical perspectives that social science research has engendered that permeate the policy-making process' (Weiss, 1979). Without alluding explicitly to 'theory' (to which many historians have something of an aversion) *AIDS in the UK* does in fact contribute to building policy theory around key concepts such as policy communities, science–policy relationships and models of the policy process. Berridge and her colleagues in History and Policy have demonstrated the potential of historical research to contribute to the understanding of contemporary policy, and *AIDS in the UK* remains a classic example of how to conduct a case study in British health policy.

References

Alcock, P. (2008) *Social policy in Britain*, 3rd edn, Basingstoke: Palgrave Macmillan.

Baggott, R. (2000) *Public health: Policy and politics*, Basingstoke: Macmillan.

Baldock, J., Manning, N, and Vickerstaff, S. (2007) *Social policy*, 3rd edn, Oxford: Oxford University Press.

Baldwin, P. (2008) 'Can there be a democratic public health? Fighting AIDS in the industrialised world', in S.G. Soloman, L. Murard and P. Zylberman (eds) *Shifting boundaries of public health: Europe in the twentieth century*, Rochester: University of Rochester Press.

Benson, J. (2005) *Affluence and authority: A social history of twentieth century Britain*, London: Hodder Arnold.

Berridge, V. (1996) *AIDS in the UK: The making of policy, 1981–1994*, Oxford: Oxford University Press.

Berridge, V. (2000) 'AIDS and patient support groups', in R. Cooter and J.V. Pickstone (eds) *Companion to medicine in the twentieth century*, London: Routledge, pp 687–701.

Berridge, V. (2001) 'Historical research', in N. Fulop, P. Allen, A. Clarke and N. Black (eds) *Studying the organisation and delivery of health services: Research methods*, London: Routledge, pp 140–53.

Berridge, V. (2003) 'Post-war smoking policy in the UK and the redefinition of public health', *Twentieth-Century British History*, vol 14, no 1, pp 61-82.

Berridge, V. and Strong, P. (eds) (1993) *AIDS and contemporary history*, Cambridge: Cambridge University Press.

Berridge, V., Christie, D. and Tansey, E. (2006) *Public health in the 1980s and 1990s: Decline and Rise?*, London: Wellcome Trust Centre for the History of Medicine.

Bochel, H., Bochel, C., Page, R. and Sykes, R. (2009) *Social policy: Themes, issues and debates*, Harlow: Pearson.

Booth, K. (1997) Book review: 'AIDS in the UK: the making of policy', *Contemporary Sociology*, vol 26, no 6, pp 714–15.

Bowling, A. (1997) Book review: 'AIDS in the UK: the making of policy', *Drugs: Education, Prevention and Policy*, vol 4, no 1, pp 95–7.

Bowling, A. (2009) *Research methods in health: Investigating health and health services*, Maidenhead: McGraw Hill/Open University Press.

Brown, T. (2000) 'AIDS, risk and social governance', *Social Science & Medicine*, vol 50, no 9, pp 1273–84.

Burtney, E. (2004) *Young people and sexual health: Individual, social and policy contexts*, New York: Palgrave Macmillan.

Coutinho, R. (1996) Book review: 'AIDS in the UK: the making of policy', *British Medical Journal*, vol 312, no 7040, p 1236.

Davidson, R. (2000) *Dangerous liaisons: A social history of venereal disease in twentieth-century Scotland*, Amsterdam: Editions Rodopi.

Day, P. and Klein, R. (1989) 'Interpreting the unexpected: the case of AIDS policy making in Britain', *Journal of Public Policy*, vol 9, no 3, pp 337–53.

De Cock, K. (1997) Book review: 'AIDS in the UK: the making of policy', *Trends in Microbiology*, vol 5, no 3, pp 124–5.

Dean, H. (2006) *Social policy*, Cambridge: Polity Press.

Dodds, C. (2000) Book review: 'AIDS in the UK: the making of policy', *Social History of Medicine*, vol 13, no 1, pp 190–1.

Duke, K. (2001) 'Evidence-based policy making? The interplay between research and the development of prison drugs policy', *Criminal Justice*, vol 1, no 3, pp 277–300.

Evans, D. (1999) 'The impact of a quasi-market on sexually transmitted disease services in the UK', *Social Science & Medicine*, vol 49, pp 1287–98.

Evans, D. (2001) 'Sexually transmitted disease policy in the English National Health Service 1948–2000: continuity and social change', in R. Davidson and L. Hall (eds) *Sex, sin and suffering: Venereal disease and European society since 1870*, London: Routledge, pp 237–52.

Evans, D. (2006) '"We do not use the word crisis lightly ...": sexual health policy in the UK', *Policy Studies*, vol 27, pp 235–52.

Fox, D. (1997) Book review: 'AIDS in the UK: the making of policy', *Medical History*, vol 41, no 4, pp 514–15.

Freeman, R. (2000) *The politics of health in Europe*, Manchester: University of Manchester Press.

Ham, C. (2004) *Health policy in Britain: The politics and organisation of the National Health Service*, Basingstoke: Palgrave Macmillan.

Hardy, A. (2001) *Health and medicine in Britain since 1860*, Basingstoke: Palgrave.

Harrison, S. and McDonald, R. (2008) *The politics of healthcare in Britain*, London: Sage.

Hunter, D.J. (2003) *Public health policy*, Cambridge: Polity Press.

Klein, R. (2006) *The new politics of the NHS*, 5th edn, Abingdon: Radcliffe.

Loudon, I. (1996) Book review: 'AIDS in the UK: the making of policy', *Journal of the Royal Society of Medicine*, vol 89, no 9, pp 531–2.

Orme, J., Powell, J., Taylor, P. and Grey, M. (2007) *Public health for the 21st century: New perspectives on policy, participation and practice*, Maidenhead: Open University Press.

Pettigrew, A., Ferlie, E. and McKee, L. (1992) *Shaping strategic change: Making change in large organizations: the case of the National Health Service*, London: Sage.

Porter, D. (1999) *Health, civilization and the state: A history of public health from ancient to modern times*, London: Routledge.

Public Health Research Unit (2006) *10 questions to help you make sense of qualitative research*, Oxford: PHRU.

Pugh, M. (1999) *State and society: A social and political history of Britain 1870–1997*, London: Arnold.

Rosenbrock, R., Dubois-Arber, F., Moers, M., Pinell, P., Shaeffer, D. and Setbon, M. (2000) 'The normalisation of AIDS in Western European countries', *Social Science & Medicine*, vol 50, no 11, pp 1607–29.

Sheard, S. and Donaldson, L. (2006) *The nation's doctor: The role of the Chief Medical Officer, 1855–1998*, London: Radcliffe Publishing.

Steffen, M. (2004) 'AIDS and health-policy responses in European welfare states', *Journal of European Social Policy*, vol 14, no 2, pp 165–81.

Stewart, H. (1996) 'AIDS in the UK: the making of policy', *Guardian*, 5 July, Features, p 16.

Turney, J. (1996) Book review: 'AIDS in the UK: the making of policy', *Times Higher Education Supplement*, no 1254, p 27.

Webster, C. (2001) *Caring for health: History and diversity*, Buckingham: Open University Press.

Weeks, J. (1996) Book review: 'AIDS in the UK: the making of policy', *New Statesman and Society*, vol 9, no 396, p 41.

Weindling, P. (1997) Book review: 'AIDS in the UK: the making of policy', *Contemporary British History*, vol 11, no 2, pp 171–2.

Weiss, C. (1979) 'The many meanings of research utilization', *Public Administration Review*, vol 39, no 5, pp 426–31.

Wells, P. (2007) 'New Labour and evidence based policy making, 1997–2007', *People, Place & Policy Online*, vol 1, no 1, pp 22–9.

Yates, R. (2002) 'A brief history of British drug policy, 1950–2001', *Drugs: Education, Prevention and Policy*, vol 9, no 2, pp 113–24.

Young, K., Ashby, D., Boaz, A. and Grayson, L. (2002) 'Social science and the evidence-based policy movement', *Social Policy & Society* vol 1, no 3, pp 215–24.

eleven

What the doctor ordered: the Audit Commission's case study of general practice fundholders

David Wainwright and Michael Calnan

On 19 January 2011 the UK's Coalition government presented to Parliament the Health and Social Care Bill (DH, 2011a), which contained plans for health service reform so radical in scope that an editorial in *The Lancet* claimed that they would spell 'the end of the NHS' (*Lancet*, 2011). Central to the proposed reforms was the plan to delegate responsibility for commissioning 'the great majority of NHS services' to local GP consortia, announced in a White Paper six months prior to the Bill. Both critics and supporters were keen to compare it with the GP fundholding model that flourished between 1991 and 1997 (LeGrand, 2010; Toynbee, 2010; Wainwright, 2010). However, the government pointed out that the new model was not simply a recreation of general practitioner (GP) fundholding and signalled its intention to 'learn from the past' (DH, 2010, p 28). This chapter elucidates what can be learned from the past by taking the fundholding initiative of the 1990s as a case study. The Audit Commission's (1996) report on fundholding is a central element, but we have also broadened the case study to include evidence from other studies and consideration of the impact this evidence has had on policy. We begin by going back to the 1980s to explore the context that gave rise to fundholding.

The policy context

Description of the fundholding mechanism

The principle behind GP fundholding is a simple one: give GPs a budget to buy health services for their patients, it is argued, and they will use their bargaining power to achieve improvements in quality of care, waiting times and value for money (Butler, 1992).

Initially this principle was enacted modestly. Only practices with a patient list greater than 9,000 were allowed to join the scheme and the cost to the practice was capped at £5,000 per patient. The range of services that fundholders were able to purchase was also limited to outpatient diagnostic tests, practice prescriptions, non-medical practice staff and a limited range of hospital procedures in ophthalmology; ear, nose and throat; thoracic surgery; operations on the cardiovascular system; general surgery; gynaecology; and orthopaedics – which amounted to around 20% of the healthcare budget. In order to join the scheme practices had to prove that they possessed sufficient managerial and technical competence. Crucially, any savings made by the practice had to be reinvested in patient care rather than used to boost doctors' pay, although expenditure on practice buildings legally became part of the GPs' equity that could be realised on retirement, providing a modest financial incentive for GPs to join the scheme.

By April 1993 some of these constraints had been eased. The minimum list size was reduced to 7,000 (later to 5,000) and a range of community services were added to the purchasing budget. Over time, more substantial changes were introduced, including total purchasing and primary-care led commissioning; smaller practices joined forces to form multi-funds, some of which covered up to 300,000 patients; and Health Authorities devised new ways of involving GPs in their own commissioning role, through locality planning (Mays et al, 2001). These developments took the model some way from its initial, practice-based focus and posed a problem for evaluation, so our analysis is limited to fundholding as it stood at the time of the Audit Commission's report in 1996. Although changes had been made by this time, the approach remained essentially the same as that introduced in 1991.

The political and philosophical origins of the fundholding model

Fundholding may have been tacked on to the 1990 reforms as an afterthought and its implementation may have been tentative and piecemeal, but it origins lie in the most fundamental ideological divide of the 20th century (Wainwright, 1998). A central driver of the reforms was the belief that a market-style mechanism would be a better way of allocating goods and services than the social planning model that had been applied to the NHS since its inception in 1948 (Butler, 1992). No longer would the interests of patients be subordinated to the diktat of remote bureaucrats or indifferent hospital doctors, it was claimed. Instead, patients would have a powerful advocate who understood their needs and had the bargaining power to ensure that those needs were optimally met.

The NHS was born into a very different political climate in which top-down social planning was seen as a way of overcoming the inefficiency and inequity of a system that had previously combined private care, insurance schemes and charitable provision. The experience of centralised state planning in the war years suggested that it was possible for government to manage healthcare resources directly in order to achieve policy objectives. Support for social planning was a part of the post-war consensus around the role of government and the welfare state. Indeed it was a Conservative government that introduced a 10-year planning cycle into the NHS in its 1974 reforms.

Despite the apparent consensus, planning has long been criticised on the grounds that it is impossible to assess the likely costs and benefits of all options for change, or to accurately predict what the outcome of a plan will be, and that the planners' ability to implement the optimal solution will inevitably be undone either by a combination of structural and cultural constraints or because of sabotage by vested interests. More trenchantly, Hayek (1944) argued that social planning must inevitably lead to bureaucratic tyranny, with the preferences of the consumer being subordinated to the judgement of the planner and the use of coercive measures to ensure that the plan is adhered to.

From the late 1970s Hayek's views became increasingly influential in Conservative politics and it was claimed that, by replacing the market mechanism with bureaucratic planning, the welfare state had subordinated its clients to the exercise of professional power and generated gross inefficiency (Harris and Seldon, 1979; Green, 1988). By the 1980s the post-war consensus was crumbling and state planning was increasingly seen as outdated and unworkable.

Implicit in the critique of planning is an assertion of the superiority of incremental decision making and the free market. Lindblom (1959) argued that corporate decision making was more accurately characterised as 'disjointed incrementalism' than as rational planning. Instead of taking the most rational route to a desired outcome, organisational decision making typically entails dispute and negotiation between different interest groups, which tends to undermine blueprint planning. Instead, managers are obliged to make small incremental changes at the margins, allowing interested parties to negotiate a mutually agreeable response to each small change. This is seen not only as a more accurate depiction of what actually happens, but also as a more desirable model of decision making, allowing for greater innovation and avoiding the necessity for concentration of power or the use of coercive measures to enforce the plan. Critics have also argued for local decision making over bureaucratic centralism. E.F. Schumacher (1974) proposed that large corporations should transform themselves into a loose confederation of quasi-autonomous units in order to generate the entrepreneurial innovation he associated with small-scale companies.

The critique of planning came at a time when the post-war programme of nationalisation and state planning was increasingly associated with economic stagnation and poor-quality goods and services. In this climate the New Right argued that the decisions of the entrepreneur were more responsive to consumer demands than were those of the bureaucratic planner, for whom 'only human kindness, not the much stronger and more dependable spur of self-interest, assures that they will spend the money in the way most beneficial to the recipients' (Friedman and Friedman, 1980, p 147). It was this intellectual climate based on the critique of state planning and the putative benefits of incremental decentralised decision making that fomented the quasi-market reforms introduced in 1990.

Given the political climate and the New Right's rhetorical commitment to the free market, it is perhaps surprising that the reforms introduced in 1990 were not more radical. Private healthcare had coexisted with the NHS since its inception, but the reforms did little to encourage a shift from public to private provision. Though billed as 'market reforms', the NHS and Community Care Act 1990 established only an internal or quasi-market in which one arm of the state (the health authorities and fundholders) was enabled to purchase services from another arm of the state (NHS Trusts) (DH, 1989).

Rather than directly empowering the patient, the reforms were based on the principle of advocacy, in which a professional purchaser would act on behalf of the patient. General practitioners' close proximity to patients meant that they were putatively much better placed than health authority commissioners to purchase on the patient's behalf. Thus, by constructing the GP as patient champion, the addition of fundholding to the reforms substantially boosted their claimed market orientation.

Controversy over the scheme

From the moment the reforms were announced they sparked controversy and dispute (Butler, 1992). A wide range of professionals and organisations opposed the reforms, principally the British Medical Association (BMA), which launched a £3 million propaganda campaign (Butler, 1992).

In April 1989 a meeting of the Conference of Local Medical Committees unanimously condemned the reforms, but although its leaders were opposed to them, the profession itself was increasingly divided between staunch opponents and a growing number of practices that saw the changes either as an inevitability or as an opportunity. While the campaign waged by the BMA and other bodies was winning the battle for public opinion, it failed to draw any concessions from the government or to stem the increasing number of practices expressing an interest in fundholding. By the summer of 1991 the BMA's campaign had run out of steam and was likened by one commentator to a bull that had charged the toreador, missed, and now did not know what to do (Smith, 1991, p 74).

While the BMA's campaign failed to hinder the implementation of fundholding, its rhetoric forged a web of meaning through which expectations about the consequences of fundholding were shaped and articulated, providing a road map for those interested in evaluating the fundholding initiative. Thus, the language of 'cream-skimming', 'transaction costs', 'financial stability of hospitals', 'doctor–patient relationship', 'quality improvements', 'cost-effectiveness', and 'two-tier health care' provided the point of departure on the road to discovering whether fundholding was working.

Early claims of benefits and disadvantages

Fundholding was introduced without any official provision for evaluation. Indeed, the Secretary of State for Health, Kenneth Clarke, claimed that it would be a sign of weakness to resort to the advice of academics in this way (Robinson, 1993). The breach was initially filled by a series of relatively modest studies, principal among which was a programme of seven research projects commissioned by the King's Fund to evaluate the reforms. One of the projects, led by Howard Glennerster, explored the consequences of fundholding for efficiency and equity by studying practices in three regions (Glennerster et al, 1992, 1993, 1994, 1996).

On the efficiency side, Glennerster et al found evidence that although GPs were not well placed to use their purchasing power to lever broad strategic changes, 'they were best at attacking the micro-level inefficiencies and the insensitivities of the monopolistic hospital mentality' (1993, p 100). For example, fundholders had levered faster return of laboratory tests, coaxed consultants out of their hospitals to run clinics in local surgeries and appointed practice-based staff, such as physiotherapists and counsellors, to meet the needs of their patients. The capacity to channel savings on their drugs budgets into other services provided a potent incentive for fundholders to economise on their prescribing. However, these efficiencies and improvements came at a cost. Compared with the block contracting of health authorities, the micro-level negotiations of fundholders proved rather expensive, an estimated 4–5% of budget, compared with 3% for the District Health Authorities. This raises a fundamental question concerning the efficiency of the fundholding model: Do the efficiency gains outweigh the higher administrative costs? Glennerster et al felt that they probably did, but were unable to give the definitive answer.

Turning to issues of equity, Glennerster et al found little evidence of cream-skimming, that is, the tendency for practices to refuse to take on patients who were likely to prove costly, such as the elderly. This had been a problem with health maintenance organisations in the US (Weiner and Ferris, 1990), but the different incentives and imperatives of fundholding were sufficient to safeguard against this, and, as Glennerster et al (1993) observed, if the problem did arise, then the funding formula could be tweaked to ensure that practices received additional funding for patients who were likely to incur above-average costs. Similarly, many had predicted that making GPs aware of the costs of treatment would damage the doctor–

patient relationship by encouraging GPs to withhold treatment in order to save money, but a study by Coulter and Bradlow (1993) found that the rate of referrals to outpatients was the same for a matched sample of fundholding and non-fundholding practices.

Harder to discount was the claim that fundholding would lead to a two-tier service, with fundholding practices receiving a higher budget than non-fundholders and their patients benefiting from better services and preferential treatment (Coulter and Bradlow, 1993). Several early qualitative studies of fundholding gave credence to this view (Duckworth et al, 1992; Newton et al, 1993; Corney, 1994), but this was not borne out by Glennerster et al, who found some evidence that the reverse was true. The claim that fundholders had been able to lever better-quality services and preferential treatment for their patients had greater traction, but, as Glennerster observed, this inequality was a problem of transition that argued for a rapid extension of the benefits of fundholding to all practices, rather than for scrapping the reform (Glennerster et al, 1994).

The work of Glennerster and other early evaluators of fundholding began the slow process of moving the policy debate on from the speculation and rhetoric that had accompanied the introduction of the scheme. However, little of this early research was quantitative or employed quasi-experimental designs, leading one commentator to note that by 1995 much of the evidence on fundholding was 'qualitative or impressionistic, sometimes purely anecdotal in nature' (Coulter, 1995, p 234). Coulter went on to list the difficulties faced by those wanting to mount evaluative studies: lack of clarity regarding the objectives against which fundholding might be evaluated; difficulties in attributing the cause of observed changes to the fundholding model, when so many other initiatives had been implemented contemporaneously; difficulty in selecting control or comparator groups; selection effects (early fundholders were far from representative); and knowing when to evaluate changes, given the evolutionary nature of the reforms.

It was this lacuna that the Audit Commission's review set out to fill by providing an extensive, objective and rigorous review of the costs and benefits of the programme.

The Audit Commission study

Scope and aims

As well as assessing the costs and benefits of fundholding and the extent to which it delivered value for money, the Audit Commission's review also sought to assess the potential of fundholding and make recommendations as to how this potential might be fully realised. This approach differs subtly from a formal policy evaluation, in that the fundholding model is largely taken as given and the emphasis is on the performance of fundholders and what can be achieved within the model, with recommendations for future development. In the Preface, comparisons with non-fundholding practices and assessing the impact of fundholding on NHS Trusts are eschewed, although several comparisons with non-fundholders appear in the report and one of the five chapters concerns NHS Trusts.

Method

The Audit Commission's report was based on an extensive data-collection exercise. Two national surveys of all fundholding practices in England and Wales were conducted. Other sources of data included: financial profiles based on returns from NHS regions; information supplied by local auditors of Family Health Service Authorities (FHSAs) and fundholders; and a survey of multi-funds and consortia. Qualitative interviews were also conducted during site visits to 56 practices in 15 FHSAs (covering a spread of early and late entrants to the scheme), representatives from the 15 FHSAs and 12 Trusts across England and Wales (in areas of high, medium and low fundholding coverage).

Ideally, fundholders would have been directly compared with non-fundholders, but because practices had self-selected into the scheme (rather than being randomly selected and matched with a set of non-fundholding controls) they differed from other practices in a number of key ways, rendering comparisons largely invalid. Similarly, comparisons could not be made with health authorities, because the two models of purchasing were subject to different rules. Finally, the Audit Commission faced the difficulty of establishing causality between the fundholding model and the benefits achieved by practices. Many of the initiatives launched alongside fundholding, for example the waiting list initiative, involved the combined efforts of practices, Trusts and health authorities, making it difficult to unpick who should take the credit for success.

Despite these limitations, the Audit Commission's review of fundholding was more extensive and wide ranging than any previous attempt to evaluate the scheme (Waite and Cornwell, 1996). After years of speculation, political posturing and small-scale or methodologically weak studies, the Audit Commission's study promised to provide an authoritative account of the costs and benefits of fundholding.

Main findings

The Audit Commission's review found that fundholders had used their purchasing power to generate an estimated £206 million in efficiency savings. However, by the end of 1994/95 fundholding practices had received £232 million to cover the costs of management, clerical equipment and computing (to which must be added management and transaction costs accrued by health authorities and Trusts). On the face of it, fundholding had not been a financial success, although, even if fundholding was a more expensive method of commissioning, the question remained as to whether these additional costs were justified by improvements in the quality of services. The review found many examples of quality improvements achieved by some fundholders, including:

- Closer focus on individual needs: better management of waiting lists and more timely/informative communication from consultants – in particular, quicker discharge letters, enabling the GP to put in place community services.
- Better-quality services: there was evidence that hospitals were consulting fundholders on the quality of services and that fundholders were specifying quality standards that must be met, under the threat of switching provider.
- More effective healthcare: some fundholders were conducting self-audits of referrals and prescribing, leading to the development of guidelines and shared care agreements with consultants. Some fundholders were using contracts with providers to specify evidence-based guidelines; however, 'most fundholders [were] not making full use of the increasing body of knowledge about clinical effectiveness to change the way they commission' (p 26). More typically, fundholders tended to purchase practice-based services that were popular with patients but whose effectiveness (at the time) was largely unproven – for example, physiotherapy and counselling – because, as generalists, they could not keep up with the evidence base in all specialities.
- Increased efficiency: the £206 million in efficiency savings achieved by fundholders came from their ability to manage their contract portfolio to purchase more activity at less cost; for example, by reducing inappropriate outpatient follow-up appointments, increasing day surgery rates, shifting to cheaper providers and by better prescribing. Some fundholders had achieved a reduction in repeat outpatient appointments in some specialities by specifying the ratio of new to repeat attendances in their contract, but it was a mixed picture. Also, it is questionable whether this improvement was entirely attributable to fundholding; health authorities had achieved similar results and providers were also keen to do this. Interestingly, none of the fundholders questioned by the Audit Commission had switched providers purely to buy at lower prices; rather they were driven more by waiting times and by relationships with consultants. On average, fundholders spent less on prescribing than did non-fundholders, but this difference was only significant for first-wave fundholders.

- Wider choice for patients: many fundholders gave freedom of referral as their key reason for joining the scheme – fundholders were able to refer where they liked, whereas non-fundholders had to refer where the health authority told them to. However, the Audit Commission found no evidence that patients had moved to fundholding practices in order to access this benefit. Moreover, none of the fundholders visited had made major changes to where it referred, and they mostly maintained pre-fundholding referral patterns. Although small changes at the margins had been made, for example using a private provider temporarily in order to clear a cataract waiting list, the majority (55%) had made changes to just one or two services, most commonly pathology and physiotherapy.
- Developing services nearer to patients: there was some evidence of fundholding leading to increased provision of therapeutic services in the practice, for example counselling, physiotherapy, dietetics, chiropody, and of consultant outpatient clinics being conducted in the practice or a community hospital. However, health authorities were also keen to achieve some shift of services from District General Hospitals to community hospitals or primary care, again making it difficult to attribute this improvement directly to fundholding.

In short, the Audit Commission found evidence that many fundholders had achieved efficiency gains and improvements in the quality of care, even if these changes tended to be small scale and incremental, rather than broad strategic developments. Importantly, there were wide variations in the extent to which these benefits had been achieved. For example, early entrants to fundholding appeared to have achieved much more than those that joined the scheme in subsequent waves, perhaps reflecting a tendency for larger, better-organised and more enthusiastic practices to join early. This finding is important, because it shifts the evaluative focus away from whether the fundholding model per se is capable of achieving benefits and towards the more vexed question of what needs to be done to enable practices to make the most of the opportunities offered by fundholding. It was this question of implementation that the Audit Commission addressed in the closing chapters of its report.

A key factor was the extent to which fundholders invested in managerial capacity and expertise. The fundholding budget included an allowance for management, but not all practices had used this to pay for an experienced manager and many did not actively manage their budgets. There was wide variation in the extent to which GPs themselves became involved in management; some became over-involved in the minutiae of fund management, while elsewhere practice managers were inappropriately left to make strategic decisions. Good practice entailed a structured approach to needs assessment and prioritisation, which was then translated into purchasing plans that stated how the fund would be used to achieve specific benefits for patients, but less than half of fundholders did this. One in six practices had no fundholding plan, and where plans did exist they were often of poor quality or out of date. Budget management was also patchy, with one in five practices overspent in 1994/95.

A market–style solution to this problem might have involved developing stronger financial incentives for GPs to become more effective purchasers and buy in expert managers. However, the Audit Commission eschewed this approach and recommended extending the regulatory role of health authorities. Management of fundholding passed from the defunct FHSAs to the newly formed Health Authorities (HAs), in April 1996. The new HAs were given responsibility for producing joint commissioning strategies that tied fundholder purchasing in with HA commissioning; setting fundholders' budgets and paying invoices; performance review and monitoring; and helping to develop fundholders' management and purchasing skills. These regulatory powers marked a shift in the rhetoric around fundholding, away from notions of incrementalism and the delegation of power, and towards an older rhetoric of central planning and accountability.

This tension between fundholding practices keen to retain their freedom to purchase as they saw fit and HAs equally eager to regulate their activity is a manifestation of a fundamental ideological divide between the market mechanism and state planning (Wainwright, 1998). The centrifugal force of the market mechanism was throwing decision-making power outwards, to achieve the benefits of incrementalism, but at the same time the centripetal force of bureaucracy was drawing power back to the centre in order to regulate the system. The UK was still governed by a Conservative government that, rhetorically, remained committed to the free market, but in practice gravity was slowly reasserting itself.

Few would argue with the claim that purchasing requires skills that develop over time, or that HAs could have a role to play in supporting the development of those skills, but the Audit Commission's recommendations for strengthening accountability and introducing an accreditation system went some way beyond support:

> ... standards could be strengthened by introducing new targets, or raising the existing ones [...] Failure to comply should lead the way to a graduated system of penalties and public warnings and ultimately, to removal from the scheme. (p 97)

The state telling the buyer what to do and taking away their right to buy if they did not toe the line was some way from the market mechanism that inspired the fundholding scheme and, as the Audit Commission acknowledged, might undermine the innovation and autonomy that the scheme had set out to achieve:

> The problem with strengthening the accountability arrangements in this way is that it risks replacing ground-level innovation and freedom with health authority control, contradicting the principles of devolution. (p 97)

Ultimately, this tension lies beyond the scope of evaluation and raises fundamental principles of a political nature, and it led the Audit Commission to conclude, on an ambivalent note:

> Two fundamental questions of principle remain unresolved: when, if at all, should it be possible to contest fundholders' purchasing decisions? And who should have that authority? (p 98)

The Audit Commission's review went some way towards assessing the costs and benefits of fundholding and identified the problems of managerial expertise and cultural change that had hindered its implementation. What it could not do was resolve the ideological tension between market-style incrementalism and state planning. It was ideological conviction that had led to the introduction of fundholding. Would ideology also dictate its future, or would the Audit Commission's findings shift the debate towards evidence-based policy making?

The impact on policy

The immediate response

The response to the Audit Commission's review began even before the report was published. Commenting on a leaked draft, the *Independent* newspaper described the findings as a 'devastating indictment of the government's flagship health care scheme' (Brown, 1996). *The Lancet*, under the headline, 'Not what the UK health ministers ordered', concluded that 'The cost of the scheme has far outweighed the efficiency savings and few GPs have succeeded in purchasing more effective treatment for their patients' (Dean, 1996, p 1545). The *British Medical Journal* offered an equally pessimistic interpretation; an editorial titled 'The problems of fundholding' concluded that 'the commission's report makes gloomy reading for those who would like to believe that fundholding is the answer to the NHS's problems' (Stewart-Brown et al, 1996, p 1312). The editorials in *The Lancet* and the *BMJ* also referred to some of the gains made by fundholders, but the overall impression given was that of an expensive experiment that had failed to achieve much.

Whether these commentaries were fair is a moot point. Certainly, they did not distinguish between the merits of the fundholding model, that is, what it was capable of achieving, and the problems of implementation, that is, enabling and incentivising GPs to realise those potential achievements. The focus of the Audit Commission's review was on ways in which the benefits achieved by some fundholders could be extended to all, but the reception by the professional journals was that of another nail in the coffin of an already moribund initiative.

New Labour and the abolition of fundholding

Under Tony Blair's leadership, New Labour had largely shorn itself of any ideological opposition to quasi-market mechanisms (Flynn, 2007). Nor was the Labour government, elected to office in May 1997, averse to continuing policy initiatives inherited from the previous Conservative administration (Kay, 2002). However, opposition to fundholding had become totemic for Labour in the run-up to the 1997 general election; it had become a symbol of all that was wrong with Conservative health policy, a shared belief that united the party and provided a relatively simple means by which the new government could distance itself from the previous administration.

The extent to which fundholding had become a point of polarisation between Labour and the Conservatives is apparent in the House Commons debate on the Audit Commission's findings (*Hansard*, 1996). Alan Milburn (a future Secretary of State for Health under Labour) asked Gerald Malone, the Conservative Minister of State for Health, 'How does he justify wasting £260 million a year on red tape for fundholding when it produces no gains for patients?' In response the Minister claimed that the Audit Commission's report showed that fundholding had benefited over half of the population and that 'GP fundholders will understand that it is the Labour party's intention to abolish them if it ever comes to power, as will the 53 per cent of the population who benefit from GP fundholding.' The exchange is a prime example of the extent to which an ostensibly objective policy evaluation can generate diametrically opposed interpretations when filtered through the prism of party-political rhetoric. For the Conservative government, the Audit Commission's report was a ringing endorsement of its policy, but for the Labour opposition it confirmed its belief that fundholding must go.

Labour's manifesto for the 1997 general election pledged to replace fundholding with a more collaborative model in which practices would work together to influence the commissioning process. Crucially, practices would no longer hold a budget with which to buy services but would merely have an 'indicative budget', and commissioning would be done at the level of the locality rather than the practice – a move which one wag likened to Stalin's forced collectivisation of the kulaks. On coming into office in May 1997, Labour immediately suspended entry to the fundholding scheme, following this with a White Paper (DH, 1997) that announced the scrapping of fundholding and the internal market (although the separation of provision and commissioning was retained) and the establishment of 500 Primary Care Groups (PCGs), each of which would cover a population of around 100,000, from April 1999 onwards. Over time, the PCGs were aggregated into much larger Primary Care Trusts (PCTs), many of which were as big as the HAs they eventually replaced. By the turn of the century, the model of the GP buying services for his practice and using that purchasing power to drive down costs and improve quality had disappeared.

GP commissioning consortia: fundholding revisited?

Despite the Labour Party's hostility to fundholding when in opposition and its decision to scrap the scheme shortly after taking office, the detail of its policy statements betrays a more equivocal stance. For example, the White Paper proposing the abolition of fundholding stated that 'the Government wants to keep what has worked about fundholding, but discard what has not' (DH, 1997, p 33). However, the PCGs and later PCTs were slow to engage in this process and it was not until 2004 that the government announced its plans to implement practice-based Commissioning (PBC) in its *NHS Improvement Plan* (DH, 2004). Commentators at the time saw this announcement as a return to the fundholding model (Hawkes, 2004).

In fact, PBC remained significantly different to fundholding. GPs would have only an *indicative* budget rather than actual control over the purse strings and contracts would continue to be let by PCTs. If anything, PBC had even weaker incentives for GPs; efficiency savings were still to be reinvested in patient care, but only 70% of savings would accrue to the practice, with the remainder appropriated by the PCT. Not surprisingly, the scheme was slow to take off and suffered from ineffective and bureaucratic governance by the PCTs; lack of managerial capacity and capability; lack of reliable data; and, more fundamentally, a lack of clarity over how the scheme should actually work (Curry et al, 2008; Coleman et al, 2009; Wood and Curry, 2009). Despite the government's attempt to reinvigorate PBC through a new vision document in 2009 (DH, 2009), it continued to flounder in the run-up to the election of May 2010, and even the government's primary care tsar, David Colin-Thomé, disparagingly branded it 'a corpse not for resuscitation' (quoted in Hawkes, 2009).

In the run-up to the 2010 election, the Conservative Party debated a return to direct budget holding by GPs, and it included a commitment to this in its election manifesto (The Conservatives, 2010, p 46), and again immediately after the election in the Coalition's plan for government (HM Government, 2010). These initial proposals lacked detail and it was not until a White Paper on health was published in July 2010 that the full extent of the proposals became clear (DH, 2010).

The diagram in Figure 11.1 shows the structure of the reformed health service proposed in the 2010 White Paper. Strategic Health Authorities and Primary Care Trusts would be abolished, with responsibility for commissioning 'the great majority of NHS services' passing to local GP commissioning consortia, (small groups of practices with a pooled commissioning budget). The consortia would be accountable to a new NHS Commissioning Board that would also have responsibility for commissioning residual services such as dentistry and pharmacy.

The proposals described in the 2010 White Paper went much further than the earlier fundholding model. The range of services for which GP consortia would have responsibility was to be much greater; accounting for 80% of the health budget, rather than the 20% for which fundholders had responsibility. In the 1990s practices could choose whether to opt into fundholding or not, giving rise to a heated controversy about the creation of a two-tier NHS. This time all practices would be obliged to join commissioning consortia, thereby avoiding the two-tier issue.

The model proposed in the 2010 White Paper may have been more radical than fundholding, but was it radical enough to unleash the efficiencies and

Figure 11.1: The structure for GP commissioning proposed in the 2010 White Paper

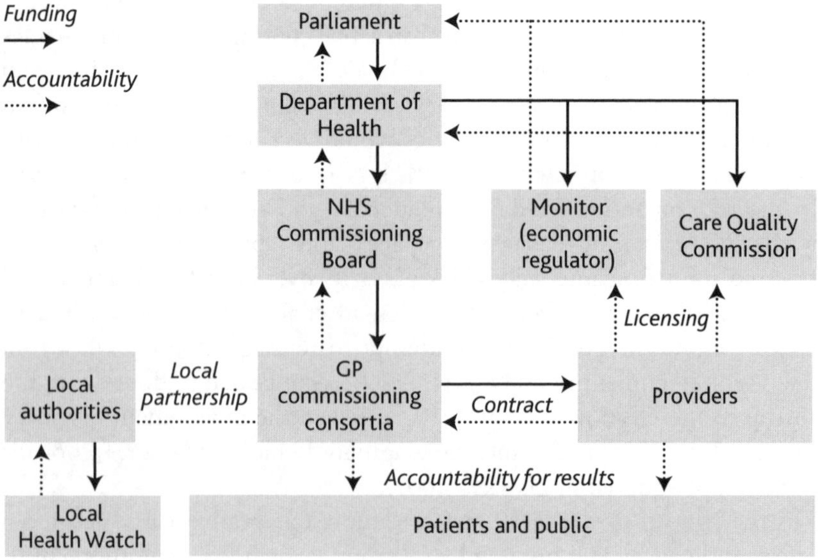

Source: DH (2010)

quality improvements that fundholding had promised, but only partially delivered? In order to reduce management costs and manage financial risk GP consortia would need to comprise several practices; however, if they were too large they would lose their local focus and the influence of individual practices over their consortium would be diluted. More importantly, the proposals said little about how GPs would be incentivised to engage in the process of making efficiency savings or improving the quality of services. The new NHS Commissioning Board would oversee their activities; Monitor (the independent regulator of NHS Foundation Trusts) would play a role in promoting competition and regulating prices; and there would be patient and public involvement in commissioning; however, these are all rather bureaucratic methods of regulation, rather than market-style incentives.

A truly market-orientated approach would enable GP commissioners to profit from the efficiency savings they managed to achieve, perhaps pocketing 10% of savings, with the remaining 90% to be reinvested in improving patient care. This would provide a potent incentive for GPs to save money and might prove tempting to a Conservative government committed to reducing Britain's record budget deficit while maintaining the quality of public services. However, rather than sharpening the market mechanism, the Coalition government was soon obliged to dilute its proposals.

Throughout the autumn of 2010 opposition to the proposed reforms gathered pace and included exchanges between the Conservative Minister for Health and the British Medical Association that were redolent of the bad old days of fundholding. By April 2011, Prime Minister David Cameron announced the government's intention to 'pause, listen, reflect and improve' the planned reforms. Under the chairmanship of Steve Field the 'NHS Future Forum' conducted an eight-week consultation exercise, publishing its findings in June (NHS Future Forum, 2011a). While recognising the need for reform and the desirability of GPs taking responsibility for the financial and quality consequences of their clinical decisions, the Future Forum report called for substantial changes to the content and pace of change. The revised structure recommended by the Future Forum is illustrated in Figure 11.2.

Key recommendations include:

- Replacing the proposed GP commissioning consortia with clinical commissioning consortia that include nurses, hospital doctors and allied health professionals as well as GPs and managers.
- Giving council-based health and wellbeing boards a role in the commissioning of local services, including the right to refer commissioning plans back to clinical commissioning consortia.
- Extending the role of the NHS Commissioning Board so that it sets the parameters for choice and competition, for example, promoting integration of health services and social care and stating how competition

Figure 11.2: The framework for choice and competition: underpinning choice within the system

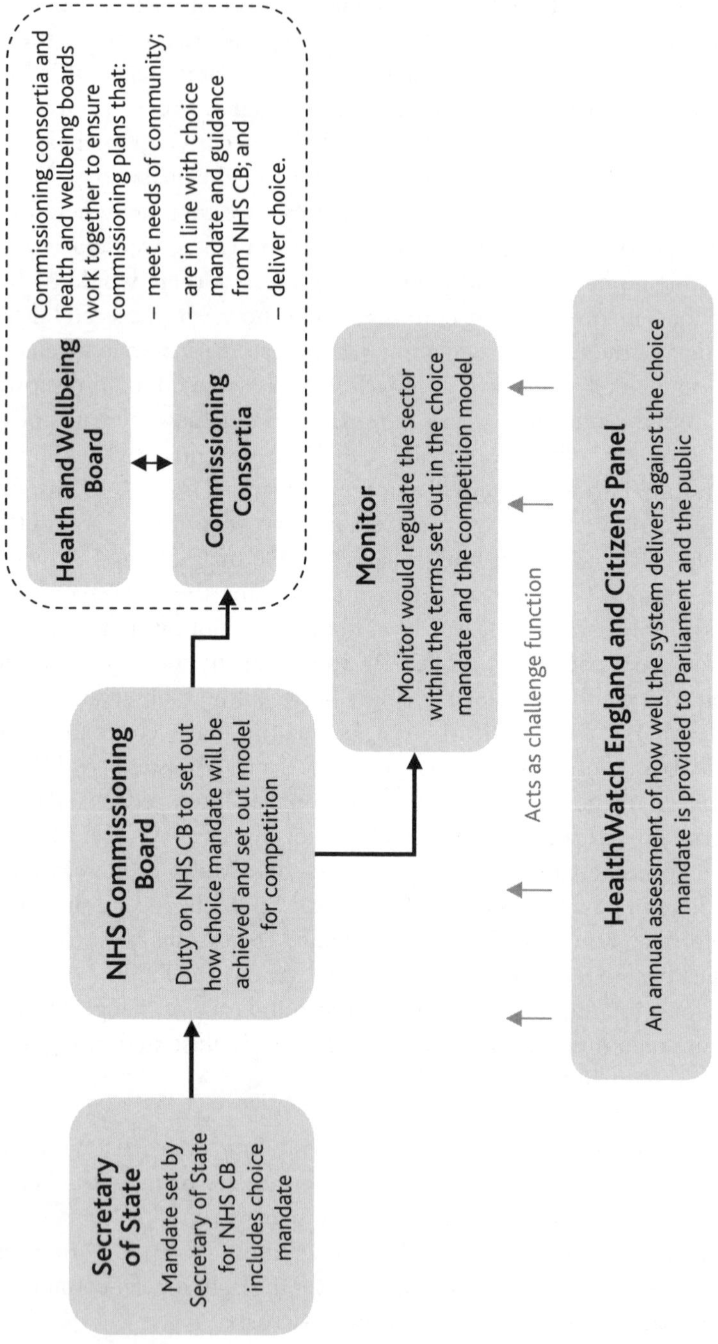

Secretary of State

Mandate set by Secretary of State for NHS CB includes choice mandate

NHS Commissioning Board

Duty on NHS CB to set out how choice mandate will be achieved and set out model for competition

Health and Wellbeing Board

Commissioning Consortia

Commissioning consortia and health and wellbeing boards work together to ensure commissioning plans that:
- meet needs of community;
- are in line with choice mandate and guidance from NHS CB; and
- deliver choice.

Monitor

Monitor would regulate the sector within the terms set out in the choice mandate and the competition model

Acts as challenge function

HealthWatch England and Citizens Panel

An annual assessment of how well the system delivers against the choice mandate is provided to Parliament and the public

Source: NHS Future Forum (2011b)

should be used. Commissioning consortia would then work within this framework.

- Safeguarding the use of competition. The primary duty of Monitor should no longer be to promote competition as an end in itself, but to promote patients' interests and the integration of services.

In its response to the Future Forum report the government accepted all of the key recommendations (DH, 2011b). Some commentators have speculated that these concessions may be purely tactical and that a future administration might gradually reintroduce the more radical measures proposed in the 2010 White Paper, but for the time being, the policy pendulum appears to have once again swung away from the incremental decision-making inherent in the fundholding model, back towards strategic planning and centralised governance. The question remains as to whether this more bureaucratic approach will yield the efficiency gains and quality improvements that a market-style mechanism might have generated.

Conclusion

GP fundholding originated in the neo-liberal critique of state planning and the belief that a quasi-market mechanism would lead to the more efficient and effective use of healthcare resources. The model was implemented and then abandoned without formal recourse to evaluation or the evidence base. Claims and counter-claims for fundholding were often impressionistic or ideological and it was, arguably, political rhetoric that determined its rise and fall.

In the midst of the experiment the Audit Commission's report emerged as the most extensive and systematic attempt to appraise the model. What emerges from its findings is a snapshot of a policy that was capable of achieving significant gains in efficiency and improvements in services, but which was hampered by poor implementation and reluctance on the part of GPs to fully realise the opportunities before them. The Audit Commission responded to its own findings by proposing a series of recommendations that would have increased the regulation of fundholders by HAs. However, within a year of the report's being published the New Labour government had swept away fundholding. The last decade has seen a series of attempts to rekindle fundholding without actually delegating budgetary control to practice level.

This case study illustrates some of the limitations of the 'naïve rationalist' model of evidence-based policy making (Russell et al, 2008). The Audit Commission conducted the most extensive and rigorous appraisal of the original fundholding model that we have. Yet its findings had little direct impact upon policy making, at least in the short term, when its findings were used as ammunition to fuel the political rhetoric of the government and its critics. In the longer term, arguably, the Audit Commission's review has diffused into the subsequent policy debate. As a result of its inquiries, we know that fundholding can generate efficiency savings; that its administrative costs outstripped these gains; that further and perhaps substantially greater gains could be made if GPs could be motivated to fully engage with the process. More than anything, the Audit Commission's report described vignettes illustrating the fundholder's ability to lever tangible benefits that had not been achievable before, for example, consultants agreeing to run outpatient clinics in the practice, or laboratory services agreeing to return the results of diagnostic tests more quickly. Ten years on, these vignettes continue to exercise the imagination of policy makers and politicians as they strive for that elusive model that will generate the efficiency of the market and the rational strategy of the social plan.

References

Audit Commission (1996) *What the doctor ordered: A study of GP fundholders in England and Wales*, London: HMSO.

Brown, C. (1996) 'Fundholding: GPs cannot cope', *Independent*, 13 May, available online: www.independent.co.uk/news/fundholding-gps-cannot-cope-1347055. html.

Butler, J. (1992) *Patients, policies and politics: Before and after Working for Patients*, Buckingham: Open University Press.

Coleman, A., Checkland, K.H., Harrison, S.R. and Dowswell, G.G. (2009) *Practice-based commissioning: Theory, implementation and outcomes. Final report*, Manchester: NPCRDC.

Conservatives, The (2010) *Invitation to join the government of Britain: The Conservative Manifesto 2010*, London: Conservative Party.

Corney, R. (1994) 'General practice fundholding in South East Thames RHA: the experience of first wave fundholders', *British Journal of General Practice*, vol 44, pp 34–7.

Coulter, A. (1995) 'Evaluating general practice fundholding in the United Kingdom', *European Journal of Public Health*, vol 5, no 4, pp 233–9.

Coulter, A. and Bradlow, J. (1993) 'Effect of NHS reforms on general practitioners' referral patterns', *British Medical Journal*, vol 306, pp 433–7.

Curry, N., Goodwin, N., Naylor, C. and Robertson, R. (2008) *Practice based commissioning: Reinvigorate, replace or abandon?*, London: The King's Fund.

Dean, M. (1996) 'Not what the UK health ministers ordered', *The Lancet*, vol 347, pp 1545.

DH (Department of Health) (1989) *Working for Patients*, Cm 555, London: HMSO.

DH (1997) *The new NHS: Modern, dependable*, London: The Stationery Office.

DH (2004) *The NHS improvement plan: Putting people at the heart of public services*, Cm 6268, London: The Stationery Office, available online: www.dh.gov.uk/en/Publicationsandstatistics/Publications/PublicationsPolicy/AndGuidance/DH_4084476.

DH (2009) *Clinical commissioning: Our vision for practice-based commissioning*, available online, www.dh.gov.uk/en/Publicationsandstatistics/Publications/PublicationsPolicyAndGuidance/DH_095692.

DH (2010) *Equity and excellence: Liberating the NHS*, London: TSO, available online: www.dh.gov.uk/en/Publicationsandstatistics/Publications/PublicationsPolicyAndGuidance/DH_117353.

DH (2011a) *Health and Social Care Bill*, London: House of Commons, available online: www.publications.parliament.uk/pa/cm201011/cmbills/132/11132.i-v.html.

DH (2011b) *Government response to the NHS Future Forum report*. London: TSO, available online: www.dh.gov.uk/prod_consum_dh/groups/dh_digitalassets/documents/digitalasset/dh_128227.pdf.

Duckworth, J., Day, P. and Klein, R. (1992) *The first wave: A study of fundholding in general practice in the West Midlands*, Bath: Centre for the Analysis of Social Policy, University of Bath.

Flynn, N. (2007) *Public sector management*, 5th edn, London: Sage.

Friedman, M. and Friedman, R. (1980) *Free to choose*, Harmondsworth: Penguin.

Glennerster, H., Chen, A. and Bovell, V. (1996) *Alternatives to fundholding. WSP/123, Welfare State Programme*, London: LSE/STICERD.

Glennerster, H., Matsaganis, M. and Owens, P. (1992) *A foothold for fundholding*, Research Report 12, London: King's Fund Institute.

Glennerster, H., Matsaganis, M., Owens, P. and Hancock, S. (1993) 'GP fundholding: wild card or winning hand?', in R. Robinson and J. Le Grand (eds) *Evaluating the NHS reforms*, London: King's Fund Institute, pp 74–107.

Glennerster, H., Matsaganis, M. and Owens, P. with Hancock, S. (1994) *Implementing GP fundholding: Wild card or winning hand?*, Buckingham: Open University Press.

Green, D.G. (1988) *Everyone a private patient*, London: Institute of Economic Affairs.

Hansard (1996) House of Commons debate on fundholding, 18 June 1996, vol 279, cols 669–70.

Harris, R. and Seldon, A. (1979) *Over-ruled on welfare*, London: Institute of Economic Affairs.

Hawkes, N. (2004) 'GPs head back to the future', *The Times*, 6 October, available online: www.timesonline.co.uk/tol/news/uk/health/article490965.ece.

Hawkes, N. (2009) 'Are the Conservatives serious?', *British Medical Journal,* vol 339, pp 1174.

Hayek, F.A. (1944) *The road to serfdom*, London: Routledge & Kegan Paul.

HM Government (2010) *The Coalition: Our programme for government*, available online: www.direct.gov.uk/prod_consum_dg/groups/dg_digitalassets/@dg/@en/documents/digitalasset/dg_187876.pdf.

Kay, A. (2002) 'The abolition of the GP fundholding scheme: a lesson in evidence-based policy making', *British Journal of General Practice*, vol 52, pp 141–4.

Lancet, The (2011) 'The end of our National Health Service', vol 377, p 353.

LeGrand, J. (2010) 'GPs and the future of the NHS', *Guardian*, Letters, 10 July.

Lindblom, C.E. (1959) 'The science of muddling through', *Public Administration Review*, vol 19, pp 79–88.

Mays, N., Wyke, S., Malbon, G. and Goodwin, N. (eds) (2001) *The purchasing of health care by primary care organizations: An evaluation and guide to future policy*, Buckingham: Open University Press.

Newton, J., Fraser, M., Robinson, J. and Wainwright, D. (1993) 'Fundholding in the Northern Region: the first year', *British Medical Journal*, vol 306, pp 375–8.

NHS Future Forum (2011a) *Summary report on proposed changes to the NHS*, available online: www.dh.gov.uk/prod_consum_dh/groups/dh_digitalassets/documents/digitalasdig/dh_127540.pdf.

NHS Future Forum (2011b) *Choice and competition delivering real choice*, available online: www.dh.gov.uk/prod_consum_dh/groups/dh_digitalassets/documents/digitalasset/dh_127541.pdf.

Robinson, R. (1993) 'Introduction', in R. Robinson and J. Le Grand, *Evaluating the NHS reforms*, London: King's Fund Institute, pp 1–12.

Russell, J., Greenhalgh, T., Byrne, E. and McDonnell, J. (2008) 'Recognising rhetoric in health care policy analysis', *Journal of Health Service Research and Policy*, vol 13, no 1, pp 40–6.

Schumacher, E.F. (1974) *Small is beautiful: A study of economics as if people mattered*, London: Abacus Sphere.

Smith, J.R. (1991) 'The BMA in agony', *British Medical Journal*, vol 303, p 74.

Stewart-Brown, S., Gillam, S. and Jewell, T. (1996) 'The problems of fundholding', *British Medical Journal*, vol 312, pp 1311–12.

Toynbee, P. (2010) 'The NHS may not survive this volcano of ideology', *Guardian*, 6 July.

Wainwright, D. (1998) 'Disenchantment, ambivalence and the precautionary principle: the becalming of British health policy', *International Journal of Health Services*, vol 28, no 3, pp 407–26.

Wainwright, D. (2010) 'GPs and the future of the NHS', *Guardian*, Letters, 10 July.

Waite, R.K. and Cornwell, J. (1996) 'Audit Commission's report was based on large samples and up to date data', *British Medical Journal*, vol 313, p 1548.

Weiner, J. and Ferris, P. (1990) *GP budget holding in the UK: Lessons from America*, Research Report No 7, London: King's Fund Institute.

Wood, J. and Curry, N. (2009) *PBC two years on: Moving forward and making a difference?*, London: King's Fund.

twelve

Coping with uncertainty: Policy and politics in the National Health Service (Hunter, 1980)

David Hughes

The chapter discusses David Hunter's classic case study of resource allocation after the 1974 NHS reorganisation, *Coping with uncertainty: Policy and politics in the National Health Service* (Hunter, 1980). Hunter's research follows the well-established sociological tradition of basing case analysis on the longitudinal study of social processes in one or more formal organisations, in this instance following the activities of key participants in two Scottish health boards over two financial years. A shorter account of the same study appeared in the inaugural issue of the journal *Sociology of Health & Illness* (Hunter, 1979).

The study: administrative politics in the era of consensus management

Hunter's book takes us back to a time before the Griffiths general management reforms and the NHS internal market, when funding of services depended on short-term plans and annual revenue allocations. In the Scottish context, money was passed down from the Scottish Home and Health Department (SHHD) to the 15 health boards and thence to the districts and service units. The allocation to the boards was based on the Scottish Health Authorities Revenue Equalisation (SHARE), a Scottish equivalent of the English Resource Allocation Working Party formula, which aimed to promote greater geographical equity. Hunter's study is concerned with how the boards used these monies, and in particular with the degree of local discretion boards had in sharing out development funds (DFs). Most services were financed on the basis of 'historic uplift' of existing budgets, with changes in patterns of provision generally limited to a small percentage of activity supported by new monies – the so-called DFs. Development funding was thus crucially important as the main mechanism for bringing about changes in the pattern of services. This was a pressing policy issue in the mid-1970s, given the perceived lack of equity in service provision across sectors and the evident problems in redirecting funds from acute care to the so-called Cinderella services. While the gap between national policy intentions and local spending patterns was well known, the dearth of empirical research meant that the mechanisms of resource allocation within boards remained hidden. It was unclear whether the imbalances in funding arose 'from power relations within health boards (for instance the medical dominance of decision making by prestigious specialties), whether they emanate[d] from a desire not to disturb vested interests, or whether they exist[ed] because of the uncertainties of the environment' (Hunter, 1980, p 43).

Hunter examined these issues in two boards and their constituent districts in the two financial years running from April 1975 to April 1977. DFs had particular significance as the only new money in a system where it was extraordinarily difficult to reallocate funds from mainstream budgets. Under the financing system of the day the greater part of the revenue allocation was already committed on a historic basis (there were no 'zero-based reviews'), so that service changes depended on the availability of growth monies at the margin. Consequently Hunter opted to focus his investigations on use of DFs, concentrating specifically on that part of the budget used to fund staff (the recurring revenue allocations). He reasoned that decisions taken in this area dictated the direction in which the service moved, whether, for example, by funding more community-based health visitors and nursing auxiliaries for domiciliary care or by increasing numbers of hospital nurses.

While some politicians of the period, such as Enoch Powell (1967), considered the NHS to be over-centralised, Hunter found that the boards possessed significant decision-making autonomy in shaping new service developments. A plethora of 'directives' from the centre did not translate into the kind of centralised direction seen in more recent times, because of both the lack of a clear chain of command and the countervailing influence of powerful professionals in the hospitals (Klein, 1974; DHSS, 1983). This was the era of 'consensus management', when, in the view of many commentators, the need to gain agreement from representatives of competing interest groups hampered decision making and resulted in stasis or, at most, incremental change. Hunter's data suggested that while the environment did make change difficult, the area and district boards nevertheless functioned to allow significant service developments to occur, for example, in the area of community services.

The study explores the internal working of the boards in terms of 'administrative politics', a concept which directed attention to interactions between organisations as well as the decisions of individual actors. While decisions were heavily constrained by competing interests, and shaped by standard operating procedures (SOPs) and routines, administrators were often able to skirt around difficulties by anticipating the arguments of the different interest groups and charting a passage acceptable to all sides. Under conditions of uncertainty, actors developed a range of coping strategies based on decision rules, routines and SOPs that rendered decision making manageable.

Hunter describes how the administrators of the mid-1970s found themselves choosing between 'more of the same' or 'new directions'. They had to decide whether to plug gaps in over-stretched services or engineer a major change in the pattern of services, as in most years they did not have sufficient resources to do both. This often came down to the difference between short-term tactics – fire-fighting – and longer-term strategy. It was sometimes possible to compromise in order to fund elements of both, but Hunter suggests that in practice a good proportion of DFs went to relieve pressures arising from existing services. The flare-up of a crisis in mainstream services might well require switching DFs from planned developments.

In this environment, administrators were often caught in a dilemma about whether to spread DFs thinly so that all the competing parties got something ('fair shares') or to support a few major developments with full funding (priority setting). Both health boards in Hunter's study tended to pursue the 'fair shares' strategy. This was partly a way of managing risk, since the approach avoided the unwelcome possibility of investing the bulk of DFs in a handful of developments which were then seen to be unsuccessful. But it also reflected the difficulty of gaining agreement for large-scale investments. Where large amounts of DFs went into a single service it was usually in response to a crisis, such as overspending on the nursing budget, rather than a planned reallocation of resources.

Decision making was hemmed in by both external and internal constraints. Poor coordination with local authority social services was a perennial problem that led to a failure to integrate services in the areas of elderly care, mental illness and learning disabilities, and put pressure on acute services because of 'bed blocking' by long-stay patients. Local actors were also constrained by the requirements of national policy initiatives, in areas such as family planning and junior doctors' pay, that were imposed top-down by the SHHD. In good years national policies were supported by earmarked allocations from the centre, but in the period of financial retrenchment studied by Hunter, health boards were expected to meet the costs from within the DF allocation, reinforcing a perception among the board officers that the SHHD became more interventionist in lean times. Generally, Hunter portrays the Scottish health service as less centralised and interventionist than the English NHS. Nevertheless, he shows how the SHHD exerted a powerful indirect influence, both through guidance and rules on conditions of service and through informal contacts within administrative and professional networks. Here Hunter (1980, p 161) detected a 'mixture of centralising and decentralising tendencies' that in outline appears surprisingly similar to the combination of contrary forces – the 'centralised decentralisation' –

detected by contemporary students of British public services (for example, Vincent-Jones, 2006; Exworthy et al, 2010).

The internal constraints affecting the health boards included a further array of factors that limited freedom of action – historic patterns of service funding that could not be readily changed, spending commitments arising from past service developments, the rigid timetable of the annual funding cycle, the shortcomings of official data, and the need to enter a formal consultation process when certain kinds of service changes were contemplated. Hunter also draws attention to the well-documented problems of moving forward with unanimous decisions within the consensus management system, and the recurrent issue of finding an arbitrator when district officers could not agree on a particular order of priorities. Referring disputes upwards to the area officers might resolve an issue, but only at the cost of raising questions about the competence of the district staff and giving away their devolved authority to make district-level decisions. Hunter concludes that reluctance to pass on too many issues to the area executive group (AEG) pushed district staff towards compromise solutions and the 'fair shares' approach to DFs. This tendency was reinforced by the fragmented nature of decision making in NHS organisations with multiple divisions and complex management structures. In boards with responsibility for overseeing many services and specialities, the decision makers found themselves having to choose between developments that were almost all highly rated but non-commensurable, so that (in current parlance) they continually found themselves 'choosing between apples and oranges'.

Hunter describes how, in the absence of objective criteria or formal decision tools, the decision makers employed a range of practical coping strategies to manage the demands of this uncertain environment. These were, essentially, attempts to use practical conceptions of equity and reciprocity to justify the 'fair shares' approach. They were often reduced to a series of rule-of-thumb questions. Who has done all right so far? Who has had too much in relation to the rest? Who has over- or underspent? Who will be hurt least? The 'fair shares' approach tended to slow major service changes and perpetuate existing patterns of service delivery. It left little space for the more strategic assessment of needs of the kind envisaged in rational systems theory accounts of NHS planning processes.

Overall, the picture that emerges from Hunter's work is one of incrementalism qualified by the occasional local deal that brings about a bigger, step change in a service. This is a version of incrementalism that gives due weight to the micro-politics of organisations and the agency of actors. Even in the era of consensus, the boards were deeply political organisations where resource allocation depended on negotiations between coalitions of sectional interest groups and where good outcomes depended on the ingenuity of organisational actors to balance pressures and constraints and keep the system operating.

Theory and methods

Hunter's study represents a rare moment at the end of the 1970s when medical sociology met health services research. It was written at a time when, although several important qualitative studies of clinical decision making were appearing, comparable studies of administrative decision making remained thin on the ground. Ron Brown's (1979) study of the implementation of the 1974 NHS reforms in Humberside did contain some qualitative case material, but drew on the literature of public administration and change theory rather than health sociology. Brown's associates, Haywood and Alaszewski (1980), used some of this same case material in a second book that focused more on power and decision making and also influenced Hunter's thinking (he cited the work as forthcoming under the title *The NHS – Who rules?*). Chris Ham was writing up his case study of the Leeds Regional Hospital Board (Ham, 1981), based largely on documentary sources, but Hunter remained unaware of this work until after *Coping with uncertainty* was in print. With rare exceptions, such as Taylor's (1977) case study of a controversial health board decision, sociological ethnography had not yet been applied to this domain. Hunter's study introduced new sociological concepts and methods of sociological fieldwork to organisations and issues that before had been examined mainly at a distance. The study uses a mix of observation, interviews and documentary analysis to get inside the 'black box' of healthcare organisations and examine constraints, coping strategies and the scope for individual agency via direct engagement with administrators and professionals.

In terms of conceptual approach, Hunter considers the fit of his data against theories from the mainstream policy literature such as rational systems analysis, incrementalism, 'muddling through' and more politically oriented writing that feeds into his preferred framework of 'administrative politics'. Along the way he discusses the insights of Heclo on administrators' puzzlement and uncertainty, Allison on 'bureaucratic politics', Wildavsky on 'aids to calculation', and March and Simon on 'the organisational and social environment' of decisions. Significantly, the influence of contemporary British micro-sociological studies comes through in the more interpretive and phenomenological cast that Hunter gives to these theories. Thus, he argues that 'rationality takes on a multi-faceted perspective where each individual, or group, in an organisation may believe that he, or they, are acting rationally in maximising his, or their own interests', so that rationality has a subjective and relational character (Hunter, 1980, p 60). The study was unusual in placing primary emphasis on participants' own explanations of why things happened or did not happen. It also introduced concepts such as 'decision rules' and routines that had become current in other Scottish studies of the period. Hunter completed the research as a doctoral student at the University of Edinburgh, but there was an obvious influence from sociologists such as Rex Taylor, Alan Davis, Phillip Strong, Gilbert Smith and David May at the MRC Institute of Medical Sociology in Aberdeen, who were busily applying similar concepts to decision making at other levels of the health and social care system (Payne et al, 1981; van Teijlingen and Barbour, 1996). Thus, the study broke new ground by utilising a sophisticated, micro-sociological analysis to understand a domain where macro or middle-range theories originating from public administration or political science had predominated (for example, Maddox, 1971; Brown, 1973; Draper and Smart, 1974; Heidenheimer et al, 1976; Barnard and Lee, 1977).

The British micro-sociological studies of this period were heavily influenced by American interactionist writers who had used fieldwork methods to study healthcare settings (Becker et al, 1961; Roth, 1963; Strauss et al, 1964; Roth and Douglas, 1983 – the latter partially carried out in Aberdeen). Researchers in this tradition emphasised the importance of gathering first-hand information derived from direct observation and participation. Although Hunter's theoretical borrowings from interactionist theory were limited, he opted for a similar fieldwork strategy and thus adopted an approach that had long been associated with case study research. The link between fieldwork methods and the exemplary case goes back to the early Chicago School studies of the 1920s (Bulmer, 1986; Abbott, 1999) and remained strong in the neo-Chicagoan interactionist studies that were influencing British medical sociology by the 1970s (Fine, 1995). The typical Chicagoan researcher engages closely with research subjects to study a given locale or setting over an extended period of time and uses the case as a building block for inductive theory generation (Platt, 1992; Ragin and Becker, 1992). Although Hunter does not dwell on this legacy, both these features are present in his study.

Hunter states that an overriding obstacle confronting almost any study of real-world resource allocation is 'the near impossibility of being able to capture all the multifarious elements that comprise any decision process in a complex organisation' (p 67). His solution to this problem was to collect data via a fieldwork-based study which combined a large component of observation with interviews and documentary analysis. While acknowledging that attendance at formal meetings might not capture the informal backdrop to decisions – the chat over coffee or the meeting in the corridor – Hunter proceeds on the basis that 'what was captured really happened but not all that happened was necessarily captured'. In fact, by the standards of the mixed-methods studies of today, Hunter's observations were quite extensive. He obtained permission to attend all meetings relating to the allocation of DFs in the two boards. These spanned the four levels of the AEGs, the district executive groups (DEGs), the professional advisory committees and the policy and resources committees. The AEG was the core committee in which area-level officers – the Secretary, Treasurer, Chief Administrative Medical Officer and Chief Area Nursing Officer – conducted administrative business, sometimes assisted by colleagues in other functional or professional roles. The DEG included a similar line-up of post holders at the (lower) district level. Hunter's plan was to concentrate on health board Alpha in the first year of the study and then complete observations in the following financial year in both Alpha and Beta boards.

As has become common in this type of study, the observations were supplemented by interviews, in Hunter's case completed with the committee participants, as well as overseeing civil servants from the SHHD. These were open-ended and based on an *aide-mémoire* guide rather than a formal interview schedule, so as to allow variation in light of respondents' different roles and the different stages of the annual cycle. The fieldwork approach, involving spending time in organisations, also allowed a variety of informal contacts – chats over lunch or coffee and so on – which Hunter describes as a 'particularly rich source of data' (p 71). Finally, the case studies included analysis of board reports, committee papers, minutes and memoranda relating to DFs. Hunter used a second-stage questionnaire administered to the remaining 13 Scottish health boards to assess the generalisability of the case study findings. The latter strategy has been employed in several later studies, including research in the 1990s by this author.

Interestingly, Hunter's study ran into a problem only too familiar to present-day researchers when a worsening NHS financial climate made it necessary to modify the original study design. The deteriorating state of public finances in the mid-1970s led to a virtual freeze on development monies in Year 2 of the study, forcing a mid-stream change of approach. The original plan to concentrate on the allocation of DFs in Alpha in Year 1, and both health boards in Year 2, was cast into doubt when it became clear that there would be little to observe regarding DFs in the second year. The focus on health board meetings in both areas changed to cost savings and the preservation of the most essential developments. This meant that internal deliberations took a different form, so that the research now centred on meetings that were less routinised and systematic. The focus of the case study shifted from how health boards operated in a period of steady growth to how they coped with financial crisis. As happens frequently in real-world studies, the planned comparisons and the logic of widening the focus of the original single case study to assess its generalisability broke down to a large extent as the working of the NHS system changed. However, as we shall see, the study generated a range of theoretical propositions that, in the present author's view, have applicability well beyond the specifics of two Scottish health boards operating in the mid-1970s.

Case studies and the broad HSR programme

Hunter's study came to be seen as an exemplar of the type of qualitative evaluation that fitted within the broad vision of health services research (HSR) championed in a Rock Carling Monograph by Raymond Illsley (1980a), the then director of the Aberdeen MRC Institute of Medical Sociology. Illsley oversaw a research programme that ranged from large-scale cross-sectional surveys and cohort studies to micro-studies of the doctor–patient consultation and health visitors at work (van Teijlingen and Barbour, 1996). This was at a time when the Social Science Research Council had not yet been reconstituted as the ESRC and the hegemony of evidence-based medicine still lay in the future. It was a period when medical sociology was still flying high and qualitative studies had an acknowledged place in the research armamentarium. But Illsley was perceptive enough to anticipate the challenging times ahead, and used the monograph to articulate a defence of social science in HSR. He highlighted the limitations of the randomised controlled trial (RCT) and argued that trials needed to be supplemented by other forms of evaluation. In practice, Illsley suggested, the feasibility of experimental research in real-world health service settings was limited by inability to control inputs and exclude extraneous influences, as well as considerations of ethics, opinion, policy or administration. In an NHS environment characterised by constant changes, researchers needed to be willing to combine methods flexibly and to include case study designs in their methodological armoury. Hunter's study was prominent among Illsley's chosen examples of this 'illuminative' type of evaluation. Illsley points approvingly to Hunter's focus on *process*, his close engagement with research subjects over an extended period (two years) and his use of varied data sources.

> In practice his case studies do evaluate the process by which policy is implemented both against the objectives of policy and against implicit assumptions about the rationalist nature of the implementation process. The data are not cut and dried in the tradition of the natural sciences, instead they trace and reflect what is and must be a fragmented, complex process ... The data have to be put together and the process reconstructed with various forms of logical analysis but also with judgements about the relative weight and influence of actors and items. The study, therefore, goes well beyond the normal purpose of a trial which is to confirm or deny a hypothesised relationship between input and output derived from

> pre-existing theory ... The task of relating an input (development funds) to an output (a resource allocation) produces simultaneously an explanatory model of how the system works [...] I consider that, as scientific attention turns from laboratory conditions and drug or operative intervention to the study of health services and policy change, where formal trials are impractical or unrevealing, sociological research of this kind will become increasingly for evaluating purposes necessary. (Illsley, 1980a, p 135)

Illsley was ahead of his time in recognising the importance of implementation studies – that 'policy in action is composed by its interpretation by professional and administrative staff' (1980a, p 156), so that resource allocation decisions need to be understood against the background of the different interests of separate organisational groupings and the negotiations between them. Again, in Hunter's study he saw something of the shape of things to come. We shall, Illsley (1980b, p xviii) wrote, 'have to rely more heavily in future on similar studies to achieve that understanding of "process" which is so important to the dynamics and outcome of policy implementation'.

The Aberdeen approach remains enormously influential in British medical sociology and, because of its engagement with other disciplines, also had an impact on the broader field of HSR. Hunter's study is often seen as part of that corpus of work. Undoubtedly there is a close connection, and even in his Edinburgh days Hunter had approvingly cited Illsley's (1975) call for a broad empirical research programme. He was to move across to Aberdeen two years later, though as head of a unit for the study of elderly care services in the Department of Community Medicine rather than the MRC Unit.

Though probably unknown to many of today's younger generation of researchers, Hunter's study can be seen as the prototype for an important stream of qualitative case studies of NHS management, based on intensive fieldwork in chosen organisational settings, that continues to the present time. Writing in the silver anniversary issue of the journal *Sociology of Health & Illness*, Lesley Griffiths (2003) traces Hunter's influence on a series of more sociologically influenced studies in this domain. One of the most significant cross-overs of ideas came when Hunter's erstwhile Aberdeen colleague Phillip Strong combined with Jane Robinson at the University of Warwick to undertake a study of the implementation of the Griffiths general management reforms that shared many of the features of the earlier study (Strong and Robinson, 1990). The authors coined the term 'policy ethnography' to describe a form of applied qualitative research that engages closely with NHS management work to explore events from the perspectives of participants.

Policy ethnography, as defined by Strong and Robinson, is not written for an academic audience alone. It recognises that its subjects – managers and professionals – are experts in the field in which they work, and therefore it employs a sense-making framework shared with subjects – not discovered by the ethnographer. This shapes the nature of data collection so that the research interview is framed as a dialogue rather than a scripted set of questions linked to an agenda determined by the researcher. Importantly, Strong and Robinson responded to the funding agencies' concern with representativeness and generalisability by opting for a 'big picture' account of events in a large number of NHS organisations and settings, rather than 'thick description' of social process in a small number of settings. The focus shifted from repeated observations of a setting over time to widely spread interviews and one-off observations of management meetings across a large system. This pragmatic choice resulted in a turn away from traditional cases studies in favour of fieldwork that dipped into a range of settings and provided snapshots of action rather than sustained engagement.

Many of the studies of the last two decades seek to strike a balance between in-depth case studies and the synoptic approach. Some, like Flynn et al's (1996) study of contracting for community health services, are closer to the Strong and Robinson version of policy ethnography. Other studies, such as those completed by a second Warwick research group (Pettigrew et al 1992; Ferlie, 1994; Bennett and Ferlie, 1994, 1996) put more emphasis on case studies and the study of social process in selected settings, though usually without the degree of engagement over time of Hunter's original study (see Locock and Dopson, Chapter Thirteen). My own work with Griffiths and McHale (for details see Hughes, 2007) also favoured something closer to the Hunter fieldwork model, concentrating observational fieldwork on just two commissioners, but with second-stage interviews with the remaining commissioning health authorities in Wales.

During this same period Hunter himself pursued a highly successful and influential career, moving first to the King's Fund Institute and then to the Nuffield Institute for Health at Leeds University and the University of Durham. Working within a team that also included Stephen Harrison, Christopher Pollitt and Gordon Marnoch, he completed major studies of the implementation of the Griffiths reforms and the NHS resource management initiative (Pollitt et al, 1988; Harrison et al, 1990; Pollitt et al, 1990, 1991; Harrison et al, 1992) (see Macfarlane et al, Chapter Nine). This body of work draws more on political science and public policy than the sociological studies mentioned earlier, and has helped to introduce the fieldwork approach to a wider readership in those disciplines. Again, however, the studies tend to aim for wide coverage and supplement interviews with limited case studies, generally, as Marinetto suggests in Chapter Two, of a small-scale, localised and highly episodic nature.

Contemporary relevance

Hunter's study remains highly relevant as perhaps the earliest British example of a genre of qualitative case studies of policy implementation in action that usefully complements more conventional health policy and HSR studies. As one of the few studies of NHS management work that utilises in-depth case studies, involving ongoing engagement with subjects over a substantial time period, Hunter's study provides an attractive alternative model to the small-scale case studies often completed today. Commentating on the dangers of truncated ethnography, the famous anthropologist Bronislaw Malinowski (1922, p 7) wrote that 'there is all the difference between a sporadic plunging into the company of natives and being really in contact with them'. It might be said that, in striving for the synoptic view of a large range of settings, many recent policy ethnographies achieve only superficial contact with managers and professionals, and a poorer understanding of social process than was provided by the early Scottish study.

The quest for the big picture is, in my view, a pragmatic response to the pressure from funding agencies and academic reviewers for representativeness and generalisability (see Chapter One), and here too Hunter's study touches on possible solutions that should interest contemporary researchers. In essence, his study pursues a twin-track approach. In line with the micro-sociological tradition on which it draws, it argues that valuable theory can be derived from a single case, and – implicitly – that this theory can be tested through replication and falsification (in future case studies). But at the same time, Hunter's two-stage design of case studies, followed by a survey of all Scottish health boards, helps to set his qualitative findings in context, and addresses the generalisability issue in more conventional HSR terms. Surprisingly few contemporary researchers employ this simple yet effective strategy of combining in-depth case studies with wider survey data. Too many opt instead to combine a survey with an over-large number of small, truncated case studies. Where small research teams present eight, ten or even more case studies within the constraints of a three-year study, the adequacy of observations and understanding of social processes inevitably suffers.

Interestingly, the larger research teams supported under some recent UK funding initiatives may be making the inclusion of substantial case studies more feasible, since bigger teams can cover more settings and thus partially address the representativeness issue (see Chapter One). Hunter himself is part of a group investigating health inequalities policies across the devolved administrations of the UK, which incorporates a strong case study component (Blackman et al, 2009, 2010; Smith et al, 2009). His former collaborator, Harrison, led a recent project examining practice-based commissioning (PBC) in England which incorporated substantial fieldwork in case study settings (Checkland et al, 2009a, 2009b; McDonald et al, 2009; Coleman et al, 2010). Although the project followed the trend I have criticised by including the high number of 10 PBC sites (over the two phases of the study), the availability of a large team made it possible to collect a larger corpus of data than is typical of synoptic studies of this type. Thus they completed 131 interviews with participants and conducted 130 formal observations, as well as analysis of associated documentation (Coleman et al, 2009). My own team's recent comparative study of NHS service contracting in England and Wales also retains a strong case study focus with just two English and two Welsh cases studies completed over two annual contracting cycles (Hughes et al, 2011).

Although the specifics of the resource allocation system that Hunter studied have passed into history, that pre-internal market period has been given additional contemporary relevance by the ending of the purchaser/provider split in Scotland and Wales. At a time when few serving NHS managers can remember the old health authorities and closer integration between planners and service units, a re-examination of how things worked in those far-off days of consensus management, as well as the later Griffiths phase, may help policy makers to avoid repeating past mistakes. My recent research in Wales suggests that many contemporary NHS managers talk of 'integration' and the move to unified health boards without any real comprehension of the internal tensions that existed both in the consensus management period and in the brief phase of general management that preceded the 1990s market reforms. Hunter's study offers a fascinating account of the dynamics of separate interest groups and segmented organisations in the context of an integrated NHS. It directs attention to the micro-political processes via which participants squabbled over resources and reached practical solutions on how to allocate them. Although many aspects of NHS structure and culture have moved on from that time, I suspect that this may not be a million miles from how things operate in Wales and Scotland in the near future.

References

Abbott, A. (1999) *Department and discipline: Chicago sociology at one hundred*, Chicago: University of Chicago Press.

Barnard, K. and Lee, K. (eds) (1977) *Conflicts in the National Health Service*, London: Croom Helm.

Becker, H.S., Geer, B., Hughes, E.C. and Strauss, A.L. (1961) *Boys in white: Student culture in medical school*, Chicago: University of Chicago Press.

Bennett, C. and Ferlie, E. (1994) *Managing crisis and change in health care: The organizational response to HIV/AIDS*, Buckingham: Open University Press.

Bennett, C. and Ferlie, E. (1996) 'Contracting in theory and in practice: some evidence from the NHS', *Public Administration*, vol 74, no 1, pp 49–66.

Blackman, T., Elliott, E., Greene, A., Harrington, B.E., Hunter, D.J., Marks, L., McKee, L., Smith, K. and Williams, G. (2009) 'Tackling health inequalities in post-devolution Britain: do targets matter?', *Public Administration*, vol 87, no 4, pp 762–78.

Blackman, T., Hunter, D.J., Marks, L., Harrington, B., Elliott, E., Williams, G., Greene, A. and McKee, L. (2010) 'Wicked comparisons: reflections on cross-national research about health inequalities in the UK', *Evaluation*, vol 16, no 1, pp 43–57.

Brown, R.G.S. (1973) *The changing National Health Service*, London: Routledge and Kegan Paul.

Brown, R.G.S. (1979) *Reorganising the National Health Service: A case study of administrative change*, Oxford: Blackwell/Robertson.

Bulmer, M. (1986) *The Chicago school of sociology: Institutionalization, diversity, and the rise of sociological research*, Chicago: University of Chicago Press.

Checkland, K., Coleman, A., Harrison, S. and Hiroeh, U. (2009a) '"We can't get anything done because ...": Making sense of "barriers" to practice-based commissioning', *Journal of Health Services Research and Policy*, vol 14, no 1, pp 20–6.

Checkland, K., Harrison, S. and Coleman, A. (2009b) '"Structural interests" in health care: evidence from the contemporary National Health Service', *Journal of Social Policy*, vol 38, no 4, pp 607–25.

Coleman, A., Checkland, K., Harrison, S. and Dowswell, G. (2009) *Practice-based commissioning: Theory, implementation and outcome*, Final Report to Department of Health, Manchester: National Centre Primary Care Research.

Coleman, A., Checkland, K., Harrison, S. and Hiroeh, U. (2010) 'Local histories and local sensemaking: a case of policy implementation in the English National Health Service', *Policy & Politics*, vol 38, no 2, pp 289–306.

DHSS (Department of Health and Social Security) (1983) *NHS Management Inquiry Report* (The Griffiths Report), London: DHSS.

Draper, P. and Smart, T. (1974) 'Social science and health policy in the United Kingdom', *International Journal of Health Services*, vol 4, pp 453–70.

Exworthy, M., Frosini, F., Jones, L., Peckham, S., Powell, M., Greener, I., Anand, P. and Holloway, J. (2010) *Decentralisation and performance: Autonomy and incentives in local health economies*, Report for NIHR SDO programme, available online: www.sdo.nihr.ac.uk/files/project/125-final-report.pdf.

Ferlie, E. (1994) 'The creation and evolution of quasi markets in the public sector: early evidence from the National Health Service', *Policy & Politics*, vol 22, no 2, pp 105–12.

Fine, G.A. (ed) (1995) *A second Chicago school? The development of a postwar American sociology*, Chicago: University of Chicago Press.

Flynn, R., Williams, G. and Pickard, S. (1996) *Markets and networks: Contracting in community health services*, Buckingham: Open University Press.

Griffiths, L. (2003) 'Making connections: studies in the social organisation of health care', *Sociology of Health & Illness* (Silver Anniversary Issue), vol 25, pp 155–71.

Ham, C. (1981) *Policy making in the National Health Service*, London: Macmillan.

Harrison, S., Hunter, D.J. and Pollit, C. (1990) *The dynamics of British health policy*, London: Unwin Hyman.

Harrison, S., Hunter, D.J., Marnoch, G. and Pollitt, C. (1992) *Just managing: Power and culture in the National Health Service*, Basingstoke: Macmillan.

Haywood, S. and Alaszewski, A. (1980) *Crisis in the health service: The politics of management*, London: Routledge & Kegan Paul.

Heidenheimer, A.J., Heclo, H. and Adams, C.T. (1976) *Comparative public policy*, London: Macmillan.

Hughes, D. (2007) 'Participant observation and health research', in M. Saks and J. Allsop (eds) *Researching health*, London: Sage, pp 92–111.

Hughes, D., Allen, P., Doheny, S., Petsoulas, C., Roberts, J. and Vincent-Jones, P. (2011) *NHS contracting in England and Wales: Changing contexts and relationships*, final report, NIHR Service Delivery and Organisation Programme. Southampton: NIHR, available online at: www.sdo.nihr.ac.uk/projdetails.php?ref=08-1618-127.

Hunter D.J. (1979) 'Coping with uncertainty: decisions and resources within health authorities', *Sociology of Health & Illness*, vol 1, no 1, pp 40–68.

Hunter, D.J. (1980) *Coping with uncertainty: Policy and politics in the National Health Service*, Letchworth: Research Studies Press.

Illsley, R. (1975) 'Promotion to observer status', *Social Science & Medicine*, vol 5, pp 63–7.

Illsley, R. (1980a) *Professional or Public Health? Sociology in Health and Medicine*, Rock Carling Monograph, London: Nuffield Provincial Hospitals Trust.

Illsley, R. (1980b) Foreword in D.J. Hunter, *Coping with uncertainty: Policy and politics in the National Health Service*, Letchworth: Research Studies Press.

Klein, R. (1974) 'Policy making in the National Health Service', *Political Studies*, vol 22, pp 1–14.

Maddox, G.L. (1971) '"Muddling through": planning for health care in England', *Medical Care*, vol 9, no 5, pp 439–48.

Malinowski, B. (1922) *Argonauts of the Western Pacific*, London: Humphries and Co.

McDonald, R., Checkland, K., Harrison, S. and Coleman, A. (2009) 'Rethinking collegiality: restratification in English general medical practice', *Social Science & Medicine*, vol 68, pp 1199–205.

Payne, G., Dingwall, R., Payne, J. and Carter, M. (1981) *Sociology and social research*, London: Routledge & Kegan Paul.

Pettigrew, A., Ferlie, E. and McKee, L. (1992) *Shaping strategic change: Making change in large organizations: the case of the National Health Service*, London: Sage.

Platt, J. (1992) '"Case study" in American methodological thought', *Current Sociology*, vol 40, pp 17–48.

Pollitt, C., Harrison, S., Hunter, D.J. and Marnoch, G. (1988) 'The reluctant managers: clinicians and budgets in the NHS', *Financial Accountability & Management*, vol 4, no 3, pp 213–33.

Pollitt, C., Harrison, S., Hunter, D.J. and Marnoch, G. (1990) 'No hiding place: on the discomforts of researching the contemporary policy process', *Journal of Social Policy* 19, pp 169–90.

Pollitt, C., Harrison, S., Hunter, D.J. and Marnoch, G. (1991) 'General management in the NHS: the initial impact 1983–88', *Public Administration*, vol 69, pp 61–83.

Powell, E. (1967) *Medicine and politics*, London: Pitman Medical.

Ragin, C.C. and Becker, H.S. (1992) *What is a case? Exploring the foundations of social inquiry*, Cambridge: Cambridge University Press.

Roth, J.A. (1963) *Timetables: Structuring the passage of time in hospital treatment and other careers*, Indianapolis: Bobbs-Merrill.

Roth, J.A. and Douglas, D.J. (1983) *No appointment necessary: The hospital emergency service in the medical services world*, New York: Irvington.

Smith, K.E., Hunter, D.J., Blackman, T., Elliott, E., Greene, A., Harrington, B.E., Marks, L., McKee, L. and Williams, G.H. (2009) 'Divergence or convergence? Health inequalities and policy in a devolved Britain', *Critical Social Policy*, vol 29, pp 216–42.

Strauss, A.L., Schatzman, L., Bucher, R., Ehrlich, D. and Sabshin, M. (1964) *Psychiatric ideologies and institutions*, New York: Free Press.

Strong, P.M. and Robinson, J. (1990) *The NHS: Under new management*, Milton Keynes: Open University Press.

Taylor, R. (1977) 'The local health system: an ethnography of interest-groups and decision-making', *Social Science & Medicine*, vol 11, pp 583–92.

van Teijlingen, E. and Barbour, R. (1996) 'The MRC Medical Sociology Unit in Aberdeen: its development and legacy', in A. Adams, D. Smith and F. Watson (eds) *To the greit support and advancement of health. Papers on the history of medicine in Aberdeen, arising from a conference held during the quincentenary year of Aberdeen University*, Aberdeen: Aberdeen History of Medicine Publications, pp 54–63.

Vincent-Jones, P. (2006) *The new public contracting: Regulation, responsiveness, relationality*, Oxford: Oxford University Press.

thirteen

Shaping strategic change: changing the way organisational change was researched in the NHS

Louise Locock and Sue Dopson

Background: the policy and research context

Shaping strategic change by Andrew Pettigrew, Ewan Ferlie and Lorna McKee was published in 1992, a period when the combined effect of managerialist and marketising reforms was creating high turbulence in the history of the NHS. The Thatcher government's implementation of the Griffiths managerial reforms in the NHS had been under way for the past eight years (Macfarlane et al, Chapter Nine), and the introduction of quasi-markets heralded by the publication of the 1989 White Paper *Working for patients* (Secretary of State for Health, 1989) was starting to take effect (Allen, Chapter Eighteen). Both these reforming movements were born of the government's frustration with consensus management and professional power, which were perceived as obstacles to change. They epitomise the faith the government placed instead in the superiority of executive management control, market competition and consumer choice, and private sector practices (Osborne and McLaughlin, 2002).

At the same time, the government identified a management skills gap. Early attempts to import private sector managers and to encourage clinicians to take on the new management roles had not yielded the expected transformational results. As Pettigrew et al note, many private sector or clinical managers did not stay long, and by 1988, when they were conducting fieldwork, most managerial roles were filled by former administrators. This is not to say that they all continued to act as administrators – some took to managerialism with enthusiasm. However, a range of studies at the time were finding that the implementation of general management had been mixed, with evidence of some change but also of considerable continuity and the persistence of clinical autonomy relatively untouched by management action. Studies pointed to a trend towards greater centralisation of power, accompanied by increasing bureaucracy and a proliferation of policy objectives (Klein, 1983,

1984; Pollitt, 1990). Doctors did not flock to take up management posts, as had been expected (Stewart et al, 1987–8; Strong and Robinson, 1990).

The government therefore remained concerned about the ability of managers to overcome organisational inertia and traditional power relationships and to embed new patterns of thinking and behaviour. The commissioning by the then NHS Training Authority and a consortium of Regional Health Authorities of the research that led to *Shaping strategic change* was, in effect, part of the government's attempt to improve managerial control of the NHS.

In reviewing the literature of the time, from both healthcare and other organisations, Pettigrew et al identified a strong academic tradition of scepticism about the chances of success for top-down institutional reform. They noted that many classic policy studies, such as the 'garbage can' model proposed by Cohen et al (1972), had led to a consensus that

> top-down pressures were likely to be too weak to change locally negotiated rules of the game; 'policy' was constantly being renegotiated at the periphery; innovation was likely to be bottom-up and professionally driven; human service organisations were likely to be 'frontline' agencies where professionals exercised substantial discretion irrespective of formal 'policy'. (Pettigrew et al, 1992a, p 38)

On the other hand, 'new institutionalist' research was suggesting that political institutions might have a more autonomous role than previous studies had allowed, and that top-down state action might in some cases result in transformation. March and Olsen (1989) hypothesise that, while institutions are often change resistant, transformation could be brought about through processes of 'radical shock', and that Thatcherite public sector reforms could be an example of just such a process.

Shaping strategic change took issue with both sets of assumptions. On the one hand, it challenged the 'myths' of 'rational problem-solving processes and linear implementation' (p 7) that dominated NHS and government thinking about change and that were inherent in the assumptions of the Griffiths reforms. At the same time, it was critical of much health services research for the opposing sin: a continued presumption in favour of incrementalism as the best way to understand change in the public sector and a failure to look at a wider emerging literature that suggested that discontinuity and greater top-down influence were features of the 1980s.

Setting the scene for the empirical findings of *Shaping strategic change*, the authors paint three contrasting scenarios:

At one extreme (if bottom-up or 'garbage can' perspectives are correct) the impact of top-down reforms can be expected to be muted, as informal or chaotic organisational life reasserts itself. If a top-down 'radical shock' perspective holds, by contrast, we can expect to see similar significant processes of general managerial role creation and shifts in the balance of power across Districts and issues. A middle course might be one in which substantial variability was found, with general management making a big impact in certain sets of circumstances, but much less in others. (Pettigrew et al, 1992a, p 59)

This proposed middle course of 'substantial variability' is pivotal in two ways. First, it underpins the methodological approach adopted by Pettigrew et al, seeking a wide range of differing case studies and examining them over time. Second, understanding why and how 'substantial variability' occurs becomes a central theme in their analysis and theoretical contribution. We examine these in more detail below.

Methodological contribution

At the heart of the book is a series of 11 longitudinal case studies, illustrating different types of service (acute and priority group) as well as different types of change (growth versus retrenchment). Within acute services, case studies examined rationalisation of acute hospitals in two neighbouring London districts; the rapid expansion of HIV services in two London districts; and the creation of three new district general hospitals. The priority service case studies examined change in mental handicap and psychiatric services in four districts. Around 400 interviews were conducted, along with observation and documentary analysis. Not only was the study as a whole wide ranging and complex, but the individual cases were also of significant scope and scale (more so than usual micro cases) and examined strategic decisions that were of interest in their own right.

To detect the kind of 'substantial variability' anticipated from the theoretical review, a specific set of methods were needed. It required a *wide range of case studies*, to avoid misleading generalisation from one or two cases in favour of either the garbage can or the radical shock version of events. It required a *focus on impact* (in this case the degree of strategic change), not just on the implementation of general management structures. To assess how different sets of circumstances affected the outcome, a *focus on context* was needed, including local relationships, history, management style and environmental pressures. Finally, a *longitudinal approach* was essential so as to assess the spread and permanence of change.

The text led a surge of interest in the case study method as a strategy for research that was particularly suited to organisational studies (Yin, 1999). A number of facets of methodological design were highlighted:

- The study of organisation is embedded in complex contexts that need study and understanding, and which do not necessarily lend themselves to simple causal explanations.
- Cases lend themselves to a multi-stakeholder analysis, where competing interests and explanations can emerge among the different individuals and groups involved in change.
- A historical perspective on the 'case' is relevant – reflecting on how past events, relationships and power struggles continue to shape the present, rather than treating innovations as 'episodic ... as if they had a clear beginning and a clear end' (p 6).
- Case studies can be longitudinal and therefore more appropriate to the study of social processes over time, again not treating the innovation as purely episodic.
- The case needs to be holistic – requiring 'the continuous interplay between ideas about the context of change, the process of change and the content of change' (p 7) and 'a view of process which combines rational, political and cultural elements' (p 8).
- Within a case study, the elements of the design are flexible, but case studies must involve multimethods. Analysis of data should be multifactorial and should be triangulated.

The work placed case study method firmly as a rigorous design option in healthcare organisational studies. It was, and remains, one of the largest in-depth comparative case study research projects in the NHS. Until this point, case studies had often been small scale and localised, making it difficult to detect patterns and draw meaningful contrasts. In its time the book was also unusual in explicitly and transparently describing its methods and framework for analysis, enabling the reader to examine the evidence base for the claims made from the data. But more importantly, the authors go beyond the within-case analysis commonly found in this type of research. Rather they concentrate on cross-case analysis and continuous interplay between case studies, existing literature and theory building.

Pettigrew and colleagues make 'a plea for a more process-based and "contextual" mode of research where the organisation is seen as embedded in its social, cultural, political and historical context', noting that organisational studies have been 'preoccupied with the intricacies of narrow *changes* rather than the holistic and dynamic analysis of *changing*' (Pettigrew et al, 1992a, p 6; original italics).

At the heart of their approach is a determination to embrace complexity in their explanations, not simply to replace one set of theories (rational linear) with another (political process). As they argue in one compelling passage, their task is 'to identify the varied causes of change, to assess against the evidence alternative accounts such as rational, incremental, political and cultural views of process, quests for efficiency and power, the role of exceptional people and extreme circumstance, the untidiness of chance, unintended consequences and counterproductive actions' (p 8).

Theoretical contribution – receptive and non-receptive contexts

The authors argue that any analysis of change should focus not solely on the content of the change initiative but also on the process (including actions, reaction and interactions of key players) and on context (both local or 'inner' context and the 'outer' context of national and regional policies and events). They identify a lack of attention to the importance of context and receptivity in social science research in general, and in healthcare studies in particular.

The definition of 'context' in social science is contested and much debate remains (Dopson and Fitzgerald, 2005a). In organisational studies the term 'context' has been discussed in a number of different ways. In considering the social phenomena of 'context', those theorists preferring a more positivist outlook see context as a reality that can be observed and measured easily. At the other extreme there are those in the subjectivist camp, who argue that context is complex and not at all easily assessed and probably not quantifiable at all. Indeed an extreme example of this latter perspective would argue that context is a socially constructed phenomenon and can be understood only by exploring the power relationships that serve to shape what are perceived by organisational actors as relevant contexts. Context has also been considered within organisational studies in terms of the 'appropriate' levels of analysis that include the environment, the organisation, the individual and the group.

Pettigrew et al realised the danger of becoming trapped in unproductive arguments as to whether context is best considered as an objective entity or can be understood only in a more subjectivist fashion. We should not be surprised that the debates on context exist in such a form within organisational studies; after all, sociologists have for years been debating whether society or the individual is more real and which should come first as a point of departure in sociological investigation. Such polarity of debate is also found within discussions of research methodology where research is often described in such all-or-nothing terms, that is, as either totally 'objective' or, conversely, as completely lacking in objectivity, as being subjective in an absolute sense.

A number of important theoretical contributions have questioned the historical dualism of structure and agency. For example John Child's work on strategic choice (Child, 1972, 1997) combines an awareness of objective environment as well as the possibility of management action; and also Giddens' (1984) formulation of structuration theory. Structuration is a term that refers to the dynamic articulation between structure and action (what Giddens called 'agency'). Giddens argues that organisational theories have treated structure as an exogenous constraint on action and have viewed action as independent of structure. In organisational studies, the implicit gulf between structure and action is reflected in the distinction between micro- and macro-organisational behaviour. Giddens argues that action and structure are inextricably linked, that action both 'constitutes and is constituted by' structure. Actions may therefore replicate, but they may also alter existing structural patterns. Structuration is important in organisational studies because it provides a theoretical and empirical base for bridging the gulf between studies of organisational structure and studies of everyday action in organisations. The Pettigrew et al approach clearly draws upon on structuration theory.

In Pettigrew's terms, a contextualist analysis of a social process 'draws on phenomena at vertical and horizontal levels of analysis and the interconnections between those levels through time'. Here, the vertical level refers to the interdependencies between higher or lower levels of analysis upon phenomena, for example the impact of a changing socio-economic context on features of intra-organisational context and interest-group behaviour. The horizontal level refers to the sequential interconnectedness among phenomena in historical, present and future time. More specifically, in the book it is argued that 'contextualist' analysis would exhibit the following characteristics:

1. A clearly delineated but theoretically and empirically connectable set of levels of analysis.
2. Clear description of the processes under investigation at a system and action level.
3. A theory which specifies a view on human behaviour.
4. Linkage of the contextual variables in the vertical analysis to the processes under observation in the horizontal analysis.

In the book, the starting point for the analysis of change is that any new initiative inevitably involves managing both an outer and inner context and process. Outer context refers to the social, economic, political and competitive environment in which the organisation operates. Inner context refers to the structure, corporate culture, history and political context within the organisation within which ideas for change have to proceed.

This general approach has also been associated with the tradition of process research, itself described as the dynamic study of behaviour within organisations, focusing on the core themes of organisational context, activities and actions that unfold over time (Pettigrew, 1990). The handling of time distinguishes process research from other methods, which are more cross-sectional in nature. Process research seeks to identify trends or patterns of association rather than predictive laws (Pawson and Tilley, 1997) and stipulates that, because processes are embedded in outer or inner contexts, the interaction between context and human action should be the focus of study. As discussed earlier, Pettigrew and his colleagues point out that the existing NHS literature base is weakened because it is insufficiently processual (an emphasis on action as well as structure), comparative, pluralist (a description and analysis of the often competing versions of reality seen by actors in change processes), contextual (operating at a variety of different levels with specification of the linkages between them) and historical (taking into account the historical evolution of ideas and stimuli for change as well as the constraints within which decision makers operate) (Pettigrew et al, 1992a). This critique continues to be levelled at recent scholarship in this area (Ferlie et al, 2010; McGivern and Dopson, 2010).

Pettigrew et al's more analytical discussions of healthcare contexts are a welcome relief from discussions that see context as a layered and unidirectional set of influences where the outer layer involves influences from government health policy, which moves down to regional/local influences and finally to influences specific to a single organisation and individual practitioners. There are three difficulties in such a unidirectional view of context. First, organisations, groups and individuals are portrayed as passive recipients subject to aspects of healthcare context that shape behaviour, but with no leeway in choosing which aspects of context to bring into the organisation and with no influence by which they could reshape the context. Second, these contexts are somehow separated out rather than treated as an 'integrated configuration'. Third, such a view implies a static view of context, that is to say, context is seen as a particular setting at a particular point in time rather than as evolving and changing over time.

The authors draw on literature from the field of innovation in making their key proposition that 'receptive and non-receptive contexts for change' have a fundamental bearing on the outcome of change initiatives. They argue that receptivity and non-receptivity are not static, but rather that receptive contexts can be created – and equally that they may be destroyed, perhaps by the withdrawal of a key individual or by hasty, ill-considered actions. Through cross-case analysis of their NHS case studies, eight factors for a receptive context in healthcare are identified (pp 277–86):

- the quality and coherence of 'policy'
- availability of key people leading change
- long-term environmental pressure – intensity and scale
- a supportive organisational culture
- effective managerial–clinical relations
- cooperative inter-organisational networks
- simplicity and clarity of goals and priorities
- the fit between the District's[1] change agenda and its locale.

These factors can apply not just to the inner context, but also to the outer context of national policy. For example, the authors note that while the quality of policy generated at local level was important, financial difficulties at regional level could undermine policy goals. Long-term environmental pressure is particularly important for the outer context. The authors remind us of RAWP, the government's Resource Allocation Working Party, which aimed to redistribute funding from well-funded districts to more disadvantaged areas. The pressure for retrenchment that this caused helped to promote radical restructuring at local level.

The notion of a receptive context for change alerted those leading and managing health service change to the need to treat the context in which they were introducing change as an arena to be managed, in addition to the content of the change initiative. Pettigrew at al's eight features of a receptive context directed NHS leaders to elements of the local context to which they needed to attend and provoked them into considering other local contextual mediating factors for change.

Reflections on the influence of the text

In this section we will reflect on the research in this field and how it has been influenced by the debate about context and the process of change. Advances have undoubtedly been made and much of the research has become more nuanced and complex, as have calls for research from funding bodies such as the Service Delivery and Organisation programme. Indeed, the very existence of the SDO points to the recognition that change is a complex research area. *Shaping strategic change* fed into a developing body of work and policy interest that led to the formation of the SDO. The study had been funded by a regional NHS consortium, but at the time there was no national focus for such research.

Shaping strategic change – and studies influenced by it – featured prominently in two key reviews commissioned by the SDO (Iles and Sutherland, 2001; Greenhalgh et al, 2004). These two reviews have, in turn, been highly influential. The SDO's recent review of its own impact (NCCSDO, 2009) notes that the Iles and Sutherland report, a guide for managers, won the

British Academy Management Book of the Year Award and was downloaded 45,000 times during the first three months of 2006. The Greenhalgh et al review was awarded the Baxter Award in 2006 for the most outstanding publication contributing to excellence in healthcare management in Europe. *Shaping strategic change* was also a key text for the authors of the Walter et al (2003) cross-sector review of research impact. Nutley and Davies had previously used Pettigrew's (1985) original content, context and process model to structure articles in a special issue of *Public Money and Management* on evidence-based policy and practice in 1998, and their subsequent book (Davies et al, 1999). Since then, Huw Davies has gone on to become Director of Knowledge Mobilisation and Capacity Building for the SDO and has used the theoretical framework developed in *Shaping strategic change* to structure SDO calls for research proposals. He comments that the model is 'very widespread, I would have said: easy enough to understand; complex enough to reveal insights; and not too restrictive' (Huw Davies, personal communication). One feature of *Shaping strategic change* was that all the cases were fed back to the study sites through 'research in action' workshops. McKee has referred to this as 'an early experiment in knowledge transfer/ mobilisation' (personal communication). Again, the SDO has since been in the forefront of efforts to improve knowledge mobilisation.

While Andrew Pettigrew's work has remained largely within the wider field of management and organisational studies, both Ewan Ferlie and Lorna McKee have continued to focus their research largely in healthcare. At a personal level, they and their ideas have influenced not only the research field itself, but also research commissioning and health policy and practice. Ferlie, for example, was a speaker at the conference to launch the SDO and a member of the Expert Forum set up as part of the SDO's listening exercise in 1999 (Fulop and Allen, 2000). He is now a member of the SDO's national Commissioning Board. Lorna McKee was also involved in the creation of the SDO. She was a founder member of the SDO Commissioning Board, and has been its Vice-Chair. She has been on SDO commissioning sub-groups on change management and continuity of care. At the time of writing she continues as a member of the Commissioning Board, and is Panel Chair of the new responsive mode SDO Studies Panel. Both authors have continued to use *Shaping strategic change* to frame their own further studies, seeking to replicate and refine the model (for example, a study of managing crisis and change [Bennett and Ferlie, 1994] and a recent SDO study of organisational culture, patient safety and staff well-being, www.abdn.ac.uk/hsru/rsearch/ delivery/organisation/cultural-change/). Both have also continued to focus on knowledge transfer as a key aspect of their work. Our own work during the 1990s focused on the implementation of clinical-effectiveness initiatives and evidence-based medicine. Like Pettigrew and colleagues, we quickly encountered simplistic attitudes to an 'implementation gap', persistent beliefs in a rational linear model of change, and a failure to grasp why innovations that seemed self-evidently desirable in some quarters were resisted in others.

A first influence on our own work was the value of comparative case studies. We sought to compare results of qualitative research in which we had been involved, considering the topic of evidence-based healthcare innovation in 49 NHS case studies. This comparative exercise yielded a number of new themes beyond those that had emerged in the individual cases. It is of course no accident and no secret that one of our collaborators on this project was Ewan Ferlie. We were already influenced by *Shaping strategic change* and subsequent work, and were drawn to the work that he and others were conducting using similar methods and assumptions.

A second influence has been to consider the role of context in the career of innovation. In the book *Knowledge to action?* (Dopson and Fitzgerald, 2005b) we describe the contextual features that commonly interact to affect the diffusion of innovations in complex professional organisations. Our analysis, we believe, extends and develops contextual understanding of organisational 'context' as outlined in the work of Pettigrew and others (Pettigrew, 1987; Child and Smith, 1987). First, we can illustrate that context is a multi-dimensional and multi-faceted, configured phenomenon, with aspects that are largely external to the organisational boundaries, such as healthcare targets set by the Department of Health and aspects that are internal, such as labour turnover among senior managers in the organisation. Second, we demonstrate that context is not a set of static variables. We observe that the dimensions of context are not isolated, but that they interact in complex ways often leading to unintended consequences. Thus a change of chief executive officer will frequently lead to an altered perception and prioritisation of government targets. Third, the vignettes in the book that summarise our cases, and can thus be seen as case studies within case studies, illustrate the role of individual and group agency in innovation processes. Finally, we believe that we broaden the scope of structuration theory as used by Pettigrew et al by conceptualising the context as 'active', because the features of the context actively interact with and are influenced by the perceptions and behaviour of stakeholders during the process of adopting innovations. They do not simply form the 'backcloth' against which innovations diffuse.

In our work we identify a number of features of the context that we highlight as core contributory influences, which are thus factors for receptive contexts to support the implementation of evidence-based healthcare change:

- the availability and engagement of local, credible and skilled opinion leaders
- the foundation of prior relationships, particularly between different clinical professional groups and between clinicians and managers

- the historical development of the services, which influences current organisation
- the structural characteristics of the location
- the complexity, volume and configuration of the various organisational components
- the skills available
- the change management and project management capacity within the stakeholders' group(s)
- the support of senior management, though this may be at a distance.

These features of contextual receptivity mix indicators of structure and process (structural features included the degree of system complexity and level of volume of clinical work; more processual indicators included the historical development of services and a foundation of good relationships) with some features of action (credible opinion leaders; presence of change management and project management skills; support from senior management) (Dopson and Fitzgerald, 2005b).

The reader will see that we have found the idea of what makes a receptive context for innovation to become adopted a very useful question in analysing our case study data. This lens on our data led us to a more nuanced understanding of the influences on the career of the evidence-based innovation. A major influence on the progress of new knowledge is the way in which it is shaped by politicking, power struggles and debates, and the existence of the informal organisational structures within which these 'negotiations' took place. Where there had been a history of close working between doctors and other health professionals and managers who might be affected by the decision, the increased inter-professional trust and reduced barriers made it much more likely that the evidence would be quickly implemented, especially where it informed a widely agreed need for change. Good channels of communication among communities of practice within particular professions – for example, via unidisciplinary meetings or informal social networks – did much to make new knowledge less 'sticky' and to increase its flow. Similarly, cross-professional communities of practice and, to some extent, artificially created multi-disciplinary meetings and groups could reduce the stickiness of knowledge flow across the professional barriers. A good deal of the transfer and uptake of the knowledge into action therefore depended on the pre-existing structures, processes and cultures that either facilitated or hindered free and frank communication about the pros and cons of the proposed innovation. Interestingly, the theme of communities of practice is now a central explanatory concept in recent work on NHS change; however, at the time of the publication of Pettigrew et al's book, the concept rarely featured in discussions.

Entrenched views and resistance to uptake were much more likely to make knowledge 'sticky' where trusting communication was not already established. Access to the views of opinion leaders, their position in the hierarchy of decision-making power and the degree of cross-professional respect that they commanded were all at least as important to the uptake of new knowledge as was the source or strength of the evidence, its financial impact or the implications for organisational change.

Concluding thoughts

Within healthcare organisational studies there remains a tendency to conduct isolated case studies that fail to build on past research and fail to move beyond descriptive analysis, to a theoretical level (see Chapter Twenty). The challenge issued in *Shaping strategic change*, to avoid research that is 'ahistorical, aprocessual and acontextual in character' (p 6), has been only partially met. Nonetheless, there exists a cohort of context-sensitive and theoretically informed health service researchers who would trace their intellectual antecedents to this key text among others. They meet regularly in forums such as the Organisational Behaviour in Healthcare conference and SDO events. Many of them – including some of the original authors – have fanned out into national roles where they personally span the boundary between research, policy and practice, and feed their methodological and theoretical ideas into wider thinking. A recent manifestation of the book's lasting value for academics is an explicit consideration of its relevance for new Government policy on NHS commissioning (Allen and Currie, 2011).

In policy implementation, too, the impact has been mixed. There is no doubt that change management initiatives in the NHS have been directly and indirectly affected by the growing realisation that the rational linear model is an insufficient guide to practice and that local contexts must be worked with rather than against. In 2002, the recently retired chief executive of the NHS, Alan Langlands, explicitly cited *Shaping strategic change* as a key influence on his thinking. But political frustration with the endless variability of local change processes often resurfaces and the pendulum swings back to top-down diktat.

Recent health policies have created very complex contexts for NHS managers to influence. *Shaping strategic change* was written at a time when markets and networks were not pushed as policy levers. We now have contexts that are shaped by a complex combination of hierarchies, markets and networks, and in these circumstances the task of unpacking the context in which managers seek to influence becomes even more critical and difficult. Given this reality, it is timely that we are highlighting the importance of this book to those charged with managing and changing health services. Whatever the fads and fashions for change favoured by policy makers, the sound principles for the analysis of change laid out in *Shaping strategic change* are enduring.

The influence of *Shaping strategic change* has been substantial and lasting. We would argue that some of this influence has been wielded through Carol Weiss's (1977) enlightenment model, whereby research filters indirectly into the consciousness of policy makers and practitioners. Ideas from key texts are taken up, circulated and shared, and embedded into policy formulation at a general level, rather than directly used for specific problem solving. Policy makers and managers may have only a vague idea or none at all about the origin of these ideas. But a very direct influence is also discernible. A recent review for managers by the NHS Confederation (2009) on 'Leading Innovation' includes a box listing the features of a receptive context for change and the following direct quotation from the *Public Money and Management* article published by Pettigrew et al in the same year as their book:

> These features of receptivity should not be seen as a shopping list, but rather as a highly interrelated combination which, taken together, may raise energy levels around change that are highly [organisational] specific. However, even in relatively receptive settings, the process [is] full of complexity, indeterminacy and simultaneity. There [is] no simple recipe or quick fix in managing complex change. (Pettigrew et al, 1992b, p 31, adapted in NHS Confederation, 2009)

We could not put it better ourselves.

Note

[1.] In the context of the book, 'District' means District Health Authority or DHA. England was divided into approximately 190 DHAs, each of which managed and received a budget for hospital and community services within its boundary, and which could be geographically and historically quite varied.

References

Allen, B. and Currie, G. (2011) *Shaping strategic change: Making change in large organizations*. Online 14 June 2011 doi: 10.1258/jhsrp.2011.010184

Bennett, C. and Ferlie, E. (1994) *Managing crisis and change in healthcare: The organizational response to HIV/AIDS*, Buckingham: Open University Press.

Child, J. (1972) 'Organisational structure, environment and performance: the role of strategic choice', *Sociology*, vol 6, no 1, pp 1–22.

Child, J. (1997) 'Strategic choice in the analysis of action, structure, organizations and environment: retrospect and prospect', *Organization Studies*, vol 18, no 1, pp 43–76.

Child, J. and Smith, C. (1987) 'The context and process of organisational transformation – Cadbury Limited in its sector', *Journal of Management Studies*, vol 24, no 6, pp 565–93.

Cohen, M.D., March, J.G. and Olsen, J.P. (1972) 'A garbage can model of organisational choice', *Administrative Science Quarterly*, vol 17, no 1, pp 1–25.

Davies, H.T.O., Nutley, S. and Smith, P. (1999) *What works? Evidence-based policy and practice in public services*, Bristol: Policy Press.

Dopson, S. and Fitzgerald, L. (2005a) 'The active role of context', in S. Dopson and L. Fitzgerald (eds) *Knowledge to action? Evidence based health care in context*, Oxford: Oxford University Press.

Dopson, S. and Fitzgerald, L. (eds) (2005b) *Knowledge to action? Evidence based health care in context*, Oxford: Oxford University Press.

Ferlie, E., Dopson, S., Fitzgerald, L. and Locock, L. (2010) 'Reviewing policy to support evidence based health care', *Public Administration*, vol 187, p 4.

Fulop, N. and Allen, P. (2000) *National Listening Exercise: Report of the findings*, London: National Co-ordinating Centre for NHS Service Delivery and Organisation R&D.

Giddens, A. (1984). *The constitution of society; Outline of the theory of structuration*, Cambridge: Polity.

Greenhalgh, T., Robert, G., Bate, P., Kyriakidou, O., Macfarlane, F. and Peacock, R. (2004) *How to spread good ideas: A systematic review of the literature on diffusion, dissemination and sustainability of innovations in health service delivery and organisation*, London: National Co-ordinating Centre for NHS Service Delivery and Organisation R&D.

Iles, V. and Sutherland, K. (2001) *Organisational change: A review for health care managers, professionals and researchers*, London: National Co-ordinating Centre for NHS Service Delivery and Organisation R&D.

Klein, R. (1983) *Politics of the National Health Service*, London: Longman.

Klein, R. (1984) 'The politics of ideology vs the reality of politics', *Milbank Fund Quarterly*, Health and Society, pp 6211–17.

March, J.G. and Olsen, J.P. (1989) *Rediscovering institutions. The organizational basis of politics*, New York: Free Press.

McGivern, G. and Dopson, S. (2010) 'Inter epistemic power and object processes in a biomedical network', *Organisational Studies*, vol 31, no 12, pp 1667–86.

NCCSDO (National Co-ordinating Centre for NHS Service Delivery and Organisation) (2009) *The impact of the NHS Service Delivery and Organisation Research and Development Programme 2001–2006*, London: National Co-ordinating Centre for NHS Service Delivery and Organisation R&D.

NHS Confederation (2009) 'Future of leadership: leading innovation', Future of Leadership Paper 3, London: NHS Confederation.

Osborne, S. and McLaughlin, K. (2002) 'The new public management in context', in K. McLaughlin, S. Osborne and E. Ferlie (eds) *New public management: Current trends and future prospects*, London: Routledge.

Pawson, R. and Tilley, N. (1997) *Realistic evaluation*, London: Sage.

Pettigrew, A.M. (1985) *The awakening giant: Continuity and change in Imperial Chemical Industries*, Oxford: Basil Blackwell.

Pettigrew, A.M. (1987) 'Context and action in the transformation of the firm', *Journal of Management Studies*, vol 24, no 6, pp 649–70.

Pettigrew, A.M. (1990) 'Longitudinal field research on change: theory and practice', *Organization Science*, vol 1, no 3, pp 267–92.

Pettigrew, A.M., Ferlie, E. and McKee, L. (1992a) *Shaping strategic change: Making change in large organizations: the case of the National Health Service*, London: Sage.

Pettigrew, A.M., Ferlie, E. and McKee, L. (1992b) 'Shaping strategic change – the case of the NHS in the 1980s', *Public Money & Management*, vol 12, no 3, pp 27–31.

Pollitt, C. (1990) *Managerialsim and the public services. The Anglo-American experience*, Oxford: Blackwell.

Secretary of State for Health (1989) *Working for patients*, London: HSMO.

Stewart, R., Dopson, S., Gabbay, J., Smith, P. and Williams, D. (1987–8) The Templeton College Series on District General Management, April–January, London: National Health Service Training Authority (NHSTA) Publications.

Strong, P. and Robinson, J. (1990) *The NHS under new management*, Milton Keynes: Open University Press.

Walter I., Nutley, S.M. and Davies, H.T.O. (2003) 'Research impact: a cross sector review', St Andrews: Research Unit for Research Utilisation, University of St Andrews.

Weiss, C. (1977) 'Research for policy's sake: the enlightenment function of social research', *Policy Analysis*, vol 3, no 4, pp 531–45.

Yin, R. (1999) 'Enhancing the quality of case studies in health services research', *Health Services Research*, vol 34, no 5, pp 1209–24.

Part Four

The new NHS? The NHS since the 1990s

Ostensibly, the final section deals with the latest period of the NHS 'story'. It takes its title from the 1997 White Paper *The new NHS: Modern, dependable* (DH, 1997) and the moniker of the 'New' Labour government (1997–2010). Much of the institutional legacy of the health policies introduced by the Labour government is still apparent in the NHS, although the 2010 Coalition government plans offer a radical policy reform.

The five chapters in this section explore the health policy process in terms of major planks of policy (Patient Choice and the internal market) and associated developments (*viz*, the rise of clinical guidelines). Stephen Peckham and Marie Sanderson (Chapter Fourteen) delve into the problematic definitions of 'choice' and its ramifications for policy implementation. Likewise, Pauline Allen (Chapter Eighteen) also explores the implementation in terms of the NHS internal market. However, she selected Carolyn Tuohy's (1999) book to assess the constraints on implementation. Historical institutionalism is the theoretical perspective through which the 'dynamics of change' are viewed.

An alternative picture of implementation is offered by Calum Paton (Chapter Sixteen), a former chair of an NHS Trust. His first-hand account of NHS policy is a view of the NHS from the bottom up, charting the impact over time of (often contradictory) policy messages from central government. His case study echoes Pressman and Wildavsky (1973), who also note the implementation gap between centre and locality.

Arguably, this period of the NHS was one in which public health was more centrally addressed than at some other periods. This shaping of the health policy agenda is significant because it denotes the extent to which the 'centre of gravity' in health policy remains focused on healthcare (as opposed to improving health per se). Alison Hann (Chapter Fifteen) considers the shift in thinking about health itself, and its impact upon health systems, by drawing on Petr Skrabanek's (1994) book. Mark Exworthy and Adam Oliver (Chapter Nineteen) consider the ways in which evidence of health inequalities is translated into policy. By using the three major inquiries of health inequalities since 1980, they explore the template of each successive inquiry and the barriers that this establishes for 'new' policy developments.

Although it is too early to provide detailed assessment of the 2010 proposals for reform of the NHS, it is possible to discern aspects of both continuity and discontinuity with previous reforms. However, while the content of the reforms (published as a White Paper in July 2010) was initially rather cursory, their potential impact could be among the most far-reaching since the inception of the NHS. More detail has subsequently emerged (through working papers, and later the Health and Social Care Bill published in January 2011), yet we await their implementation in order to ascertain their impact.

References

DH (Department of Health) (1997) *The new NHS: Modern, dependable*, Cm 3807, London: Department of Health.

Pressman, J. and Wildavsky, A. (1973) *Implementation: How great expectations in Washington are dashed in Oakland*, Berkeley, CA: University of California Press.

Skrabanek, P. (1994) *The death of humane medicine and the rise of coercive healthism*, Bury St Edmunds: The Social Affairs Unit.

Tuohy, C. (1999) *Accidental logics: The dynamics of change in the health care arena in the United States, Britain and Canada*, Oxford: Oxford University Press.

fourteen

Patient choice: a contemporary policy story

Stephen Peckham and Marie Sanderson

This chapter aims to explore the use of a case study approach to a specific policy and how the use of narrative approaches to analysis provides both a way of understanding how policy evolves and also a framework for the analysis of policy. Drawing on the findings of a study that sought to examine the content and operationalisation of the different policies in respect of patient choice in the four countries of the UK, this chapter explores how (often ill-defined) policies can be examined in a case study approach. The chapter is divided into three sections. The first section discusses the nature of choice policy in the UK. The second draws on our own study of NHS choice policy (Peckham et al, 2010) to explore how policy can be defined as a 'case' for analytical purposes and what kinds of methods can be used to examine policy cases where the 'case' is indistinct and poorly defined. In the last section we discuss the relevance of such approaches to current policy analysis.

Background to patient choice policy in the UK

'Choice' is a ubiquitous concept that has multiple meanings, and this is a source of ambiguity in policy documents, in broader discussion about health choices, and in its application in health policy (Clarke et al, 2006). Choice has many 'common sense' meanings as well as specific meanings within policy.

Offering choice in public services can be associated with numerous concepts, including competition, contestability and consumer behaviour, and patient empowerment, agency and autonomy (Fotaki et al, 2005). Choice is not a new concept in the NHS. In principle, patients have always had a choice of GP and an option to decline to consent to (most of) the treatments that doctors offer them. Wider choice has tended to exist for those with resources and access, who could opt out of the NHS and obtain healthcare privately. However, many different types of choice can be provided to patients, including choice of what patients receive (choice of treatment), where they are treated (choice of hospital), whom they are treated by (choice of practitioner), when they are seen (choice of appointment time). In addition to the choices that may be available to the individual, public services also place an emphasis on engaging and involving patients and the public in healthcare decision making at a community level.

In contrast with the potential multiplicity of choice, choice in relation to recent public policy in the UK has come to be characterised in a particular way. In recent years, particularly during the time of the New Labour government post 1997, the development of UK policy across health, education and social care has been marked by a focus on consumerism as the route to modernisation of public services (Needham, 2003; Clarke et al, 2007). This is reflected in policy rhetoric in relation to health, which focuses on a new relationship between health services and the public in which the availability of consumer choices transforms the patient into an empowered and knowledgeable consumer who is a co-producer of their healthcare with responsibility for taking decisions relating to their own health (Newman and Vidler, 2006). Within health, a particular model of consumer choice has come to prominence in which choice is a means of public service delivery to increase quality, efficiency, responsiveness, accountability and equality. This model is perhaps best articulated by Le Grand, for whom consumer choice is a mechanism within a system of service delivery and improvement (Le Grand, 2007). Choice, in Le Grand's view, is not simply a good in its own right but has instrumental value. Specifically, when consumer choice operates within a competitive environment it incentivises providers to maximise patient numbers through improved quality of services and provision of efficient and effective choices. Le Grand's view of choice therefore relates to a very specific model: choice linked to competition mechanisms provides the right incentives, and the most effective mechanism, to secure continuous improvement in health services.

NHS choice policy has developed within the context of increasing devolution within the UK. The devolution of administrative decision making to the Scottish Parliament, Welsh Assembly and Northern Ireland Assembly from 1997 onwards has provided a context that allows explicit differences in policy rhetoric and objectives, giving each country the leeway to develop policies that suit their particular circumstances. It has been noted that devolution of responsibility for health policy has resulted in tension between the need for uniformity, particularly in relation to performance targets, and the increasing diversity in policy as countries take advantage of the opportunity to develop policy (Exworthy, 2001). It has also been noted that there is divergence in terms of the way in which choice is emphasised and the kinds of choices that are promoted for health service users in the four countries of the UK (Hughes et al, 2009). The political divergence has been particularly striking in relation to choice policy because policy makers in Scotland and Wales have regarded choice between healthcare providers as an issue on which they can fulfil a political commitment to policy difference with reference to England (Greer, 2007).

The opportunity for policy devolution has led to increasingly distinctive approaches to achieving choice for patients across the UK. NHS policy in England has focused on developing consumer choices, most notably through its choice-of-provider policy, which offers patients a choice of secondary care provider. Choice of provider, together with two other major government policies, payment by results and practice based commissioning, was aimed at introducing a market-type competitive environment in NHS healthcare provision so as to provide the context within which health service improvements would be achieved. Conversely, in the other countries the emphasis was on the need to engage patients and the public in order to help improve services and performance through voice mechanisms. In particular, the emphasis in Wales, and to a certain extent in Scotland, on collective approaches to achieving choice in healthcare contrasts starkly with policy in England, which focuses on individual choice in relation to choice of provider.

Constructing the case

This section of the chapter draws on our experience of researching patient choice to describe how policy can be defined as a 'case' for analytical purposes and the kind of methods that can be used to examine policy cases.

In 2007, the National Institute of Health Research Service Delivery and Organisation programme commissioned a research project to examine the content and operationalisation of the different policies in respect of patient choice in the four countries of the UK and to assess their impact on health system performance, including responsiveness to patients (Peckham et al, 2010). The focus of the study was consumer choices offered to individual patients as they are being referred into secondary care. Its aim was to determine the political and ideological origins of the policies on choice within each country in order to identify the essential elements and objectives of policies on choice and their relationship with other health policies in England, Wales, Scotland and Northern Ireland.

Setting the boundaries of the case

Examining choice policy involves a series of judgements about the nature of the case, constructing boundaries around policy that are both temporal and conceptual. In this instance the case was particularly complex. The area of interest covered all four countries of the UK and included not only how choice was conceptualised in the policy of each country, but also how choices were being delivered to patients in each country and what choices were available. Our methodology sought data that would examine the national policy and its implementation in each country. The intention was then to compare across countries so as to identify key policy differences and differences in the way choice was put into practice (if at all) in each country. Our approach was, essentially, to develop a comparative case study design exploring the contemporary phenomenon of specific choice policies (in this case, choice of elective referral) within real-life contexts – the national policy, service organisation and delivery contexts (Yin, 2003).

In recognition of this complexity, the investigation was designed as a multi-level study, with selected case studies within each of the four constituent countries of the UK. There were three levels corresponding to the overall policy formulation (macro), the implementation of policy through the managerial agencies and service providers of the NHS (meso) and the operationalisation of the policy with patients (micro). This policy study was essentially split into 12 separate but linked case studies, consisting of four countries each with three levels of interest, with comparison of countries across all three levels, and also allowed for analysis within each country of the provenance, development and implementation of choice policies. The cases comprise the policy documents and interviews at the macro level, interviews with selected NHS organisations and GP practices at the meso level and interviews with patients being referred for hospital treatment for orthopaedics or ear, nose and throat (ENT) surgery at the micro level. This research design allowed both a context-contingent understanding of how policy on this issue was constructed and put into practice in ways that reflect the varying politics and policy goals of each nation and an insight into how such policies impact on patients.

The definition of the case is often complex and unclear, and in practice the case or cases for analysis emerge during the research process (Yin, 2003). This study presented a number of challenges in terms of identification of the case. The potential cases include policy, countries, organisations (including local health economies and individual organisations) and individual patient experiences. In addition, we selected tracer conditions (orthopaedics and ENT) and these could also constitute cases. Comparison between cases is a normal approach in multiple case studies and the research team was faced with an array of potential comparisons that could be made within this study (Ragin, 2007). These included:

1. Between country – England, Northern Ireland, Scotland, Wales
2. Between levels – macro, meso, micro
3. Between areas – Primary Care Trust (PCT), Local Health Board, and Health Board areas – comparing healthcare purchasers and providers
4. Between practices
5. Between patients – categories of age, gender, ethnicity
6. Between conditions – orthopaedics, ENT at meso and micro level
7. Combinations of the above

Defining the case also involved constructing boundaries around what was to be included in each case. In order to identify official policy we undertook an analysis of policy and guidance documents and interviewed people involved in policy development in each country. As in other cases of policy research, the researcher is faced not with a clearly defined policy document that sets out the elements of choice policy but, rather, with an array of policy documents, guidance, ministerial statements and practice that all constitute 'choice policy'. In addition, different conceptualisations of choice are incorporated in political discourse – particularly within the devolved health systems of the UK. While consumer choice has emerged as a high-profile policy in England, the other three countries do not identify choice as a policy driver. The lack of specific policies on individual choice outside England does not necessarily imply that individual choice of some kind is not available elsewhere, but that it might take a different form or be located within other policies that prioritise other goals. Perception issues in relation to the definition of the case were also complex in relation to interviews. As specific 'choice policy' existed only in England it was difficult to frame questions in the other countries in relation to the concept of patient choice. In order to explore the extent of choices about decisions relating to elective surgery, interviewees were engaged in a discussion about referral pathways and where decisions about treatment, consultant, provider and so on are taken.

Further definition of the case to be studied came from a temporal definition of choice policy. As the research was clearly focused on the English model of patient choice, the frame of interest was selected from the year 2000 onwards because the NHS Plan for England (DH, 2000) is generally seen to mark the start of the conceptualisation of a particular version of choice policy that is strongly linked to health consumerism (Greener et al, 2006). However, the end point of the temporal boundaries of the case was less easy to define because policy concerning choice continued to develop throughout the period of the study (2007–09). For example, 'free choice' of secondary care provider for patients in England was introduced after policy interviews had been conducted, but before the patient interviews were conducted. Similarly, during the time of the study there were a number of key organisational changes, including a major reorganisation in Northern Ireland and the start of changes in the commissioning and provision structures in Wales.

Policy is not just the statement of policy as set out by policy makers – whether written or spoken. It is clearly recognised that the implementation of policy is an important element of policy in practice (Barrett and Fudge, 1981; Hill and Hupe, 2002). We aimed to capture organisational perspectives on patient choice and to explore how staff in organisations understood and operationalised choice policy, in order to determine the way choices were offered to patients within referral processes for elective surgery (orthopaedics and ENT). At the patient level we examined referral processes from primary to secondary care and, in particular, any choice offered within them, from patients' perspectives, in order to identify any qualitative differences in the effects of the four nations' different choice policies on patients' perceptions of access to care and on the responsiveness of services to their needs and preferences. The case studies were selected to explore how patient choice policy, in terms of referral for elective surgery, was being 'operationalised'. The sites were selected to provide illustrative examples of how choice was 'managed' by NHS and general practice services and experienced by patients. Case study sites were selected to reflect rural and urban differences because evidence on health services access and patient choice suggests that there are key differences in the availability of choice between such areas (Exworthy and Peckham, 2006). In each selected case study area there were one clearly identified NHS acute provider (including in England a Foundation Trust) and additional NHS and private providers within one hour's travelling time (Le Grand, 2004; Damiani et al, 2005).

Examining the case

Structuring the case in this way led to several findings that reflected the way choice was conceptualised and implemented. At a national policy level, there were clear political differences in emphasis on patient choice between England and the other countries. The main significant difference between the countries was the contrast between the dominance of consumer's choice of provider in England and the emphasis in Wales and Scotland, and to a certain extent Northern Ireland, on public and patient engagement and the importance of 'voice' as necessary for bringing about choice at the service level. For these countries, 'patient and public engagement' at a community level was seen as central to improving quality and meeting patients' needs in a more responsive way. A further difference was the need, particularly in Scotland and Wales, to develop policy that reflected national identity and therefore differed from that in England. However, our analysis of policy documents noted that the position/nature of choice within policy documents was not always unambiguous. This was markedly so in Scottish policy documents, which generally rejected the notion of choice, but also recognised the advantages of efficiency and waiting-time reduction that offering choice of provider could bring, and the need to establish a clear choice policy (NHS Scotland, 2005). In Wales, the policy position was described as oppositional to English choice policy, emphasising 'voice not choice' (Peckham et al, 2010). Yet there were some increasing similarities in the way choice became an accepted concept in each country – such as choice of time and date of appointment, choice of alternative provider.

The concept of patient choice in England emerged gradually, and over time there was a shift in how patient choice was conceptualised and what it covered. While the development of consumer choices for patients – and in particular, patient choice of secondary care provider – has emerged as the main focus of policy in England (Jones and Mays, 2009), our data suggests that the emergence of consumer choices and the development of the 'choice and competition' system in policy was a gradual process. The NHS Plan referred to a number of types of choice that should be developed in the NHS – choice of appointment time and date for patients, healthy eating choices, choice of access routes into the NHS and choice of GP (DH, 2000). Alongside choice-of-provider policy other types of choices have also been developed, such as choice of care for people suffering from long-term conditions (DH, 2007a) and the development of the Expert Patient Programme, which helps people to self-manage and to take a partnership approach to decisions about their care (DH, 2001). More recently, there has been increased emphasis on developing responsiveness via groups of patients rather than the individual, through the development of 'choice for long term conditions', which has emphasised participation of local patient groups in developing the 'choice sets' or 'service menus' (DH, 2007a).

There were objectives across all four countries that emerged in policy interviews. Most important was the central focus on tackling waiting lists. Allowing patients a choice of secondary care provider was a mechanism used across all four countries in initiatives to reducing waiting times for patients. In England, patient choice was introduced to provide a mechanism for patients to select another provider in order to reduce waiting times, while in the other countries the emphasis was on providing choices if waiting time guidelines were likely to be breached.

In contrast with the variation between the countries at a policy level, it appeared that choice had been operationalised in a much more uniform way across the countries. Despite misgivings and, in some cases, hostility to the English patient-choice policy in Wales, Scotland and Northern Ireland, at an operational level all systems aspired to offer as many choices as possible to patients, including offering a choice of provider where possible. In reality, similar choices of time and date of appointment and provider exist in all health systems. All countries identified a standard subset of referral choices that were potentially available within the referral pathway including:

- choice of provider
- choice of treatment
- choice of appointment date and time
- choice of location of appointment
- choice of consultant.

Apart from the fact that some NHS patients in England were offered a menu of specialist providers and/or could book appointments over the internet for a date and time of their choosing, the evidence from this study did not demonstrate any obvious systematic differences in patient experience across the four countries, with booking systems for arranging patient appointments operating in all health systems. However, there was a cultural difference between England and the other countries in the way in which choice was perceived by NHS staff. There was as much diversity of patient experience *within* countries as *between* countries, and patients raised similar issues in each of the four countries.

Constructing the case – the issues

Analysis of the empirical data collected in the study reveals that there are a number of key conceptual problems in defining patient choice and in the relevance of interpreting this within a specific policy case study approach. The lack of a common definition of choice remains a key problem for the analysis of policy. Our approach was to focus on a specific aspect of policy related to elective referrals, but this both helped to focus the study and caused problems in a comparative study because of the way in which this policy was closely associated with English policy by politicians and policy makers, despite the fact that operationally similar processes were being adopted in all four countries. During our research, we found that defining the boundaries and definition of choice policy was an active issue. While there was general support for offering options to patients in policy stakeholder interviews in all countries, we found that discussions about 'patient choice' with interviewees outside the English system were difficult, given the explicit rejection of the notion of choice as framed by English health policy in policy documents and by the interviewees themselves. Furthermore, studying the case of choice policy involved imposing boundaries and definitions upon a continuous and organic process of policy development in which choice was defined in a variety of ways by different parties and at different times. As in the case of English policy, where choice became part of a much wider reform programme, the boundaries between choice and other policies were often porous and unclear.

So what does this tell us about the nature of the case? While clearly a distinctive concept, choice, as articulated in policy, lacks any clarity. This is not untypical in policy, and many policies lack specificity. Key problems relate to selecting a time frame (for example, when did the policy 'start'?), identifying policy boundaries and the extent to which policies need to be seen as part of wider policy initiatives. In this case, in England choice policy has often been framed as part of wider market-orientated reforms, but our study suggests that choice policy is linked more to waiting-time initiatives and broader concepts of providing choice in order to be seen as responsive. As other studies have shown, research clearly demonstrated that policy is not always what is contained within policy documents, and in this case policy included wider debates about choice. The study also demonstrated the political context of policy making within a comparative context in the UK. This case comparison suggested that there are common forces that drive the way health policy is implemented, irrespective of rhetorical differences and emphases in policy at a national level.

Investigating choice policy: methodological approaches

As discussed earlier in this book, defining the case raises complex questions of definition. In policy this is particularly complex, given the often imprecise or fuzzy nature of policy. As described previously, identifying the temporal, substantive and specific nature of a policy is fraught with difficulties. In order to overcome this lack of specificity, policy analysts have often adopted a multiple-lens approach to exploring specific policies (see, for example, Cairney, 2007). Applying such an approach to patient choice illuminates different interpretations. For example, patient choice policy in England appears to be incremental in nature, as policy documents show gradual development of policy. But incremental policy is associated with a clear path or goal, and in our study we show that there was a substantial lack of clarity about the goals of patient choice, or at least there were competing goals (Lindblom, 1979). One alternative approach is that of policy streams. This highlights how the intersection of problems, solutions and political context need to be aligned to achieve successful policy formation (Kingdon, 1995). Adopting this approach starts to help understanding of why there are policy differences between England, Wales, Scotland and Northern Ireland, and also why there are similarities in implementation between different choice policies within the NHS in each country (Peckham et al, 2010). However, here again the evidence does not specifically support the idea that streams came together at a window of opportunity. Rather, policy developments and politics seem disjointed and mechanisms for implementing choice were not particularly well developed or used. One third approach could be to examine the development of choice policy from a punctuated equilibrium perspective. This would view choice policy within a shift in the *policy venue*, with New Labour in England providing a new political context that led to a shift in the way public services problems were conceptualised and thus a change in the way policy was viewed – a shift in the *policy image*. While perhaps useful in considering whether New Labour set a new policy context, it does not explain similarities and differences across the different countries. There is also a strong argument that the shift in policy venue was far more gradual in terms of changes in welfare perceptions than can be attributed to a change of government in 1997.

Approaches to policy analysis need to be able to uncover the 'emergent nature' of policy. While policy may shift over time it may not be incremental – rather, it may either 'unravel' or develop, contingent on wider factors. This can be distinguished from incremental policy, where policy makers have a policy goal and move gradually towards that goal in small steps, and contingent on factors that allow policy to develop. Therefore methods need to uncover the unobservable, and capture different perspectives.

Our methodological approach drew explicitly on developments in contemporary policy analysis that suggest that a narrative approach yields richer and more relevant insights into policy processes than do traditional approaches (Ball, 1993; Roe, 1994; Fischer, 2003; Kay, 2006). Narrative approaches 'situate new initiatives, drives or targets into a history, and that draws on images of societal change and/or institutional problems to legitimate … proposals' (Newman and Vidler, 2006, p 195). This approach has already been used to explore consumerism in healthcare (Newman and Vidler, 2006). It draws on a policy-as-discourse approach to identify the ideological underpinnings and institutional development of the different choice policies, as well as the roles of actors and relationships between key stakeholders (Shaw, 2010). The language of political discourse and policy texts provides insights into the ideological basis, policy content and the way in which policy narratives are negotiated and developed. Our analysis incorporated thematic content analysis of policy documents and interviews and data collection at national and local levels. The aim was to develop 'policy narratives' for each of the four countries within the UK. Our intention was to identify dominant discourses within the policy process that clearly identified the political and ideological basis of patient choice policies. These discourse analyses explored the policy variants described by policy makers and those implementing policy that emerged from the historical analytic narrative, and thus should not be interpreted as detailed discourse analysis of documents or interviews. Variation between respondents about the meaning and goals of policy were common, but it was also possible to identify specific narratives about the nature of choice policy, such as addressing waiting times, improving access, being more responsive to patients, offering choice. Such variations occurred within countries and between countries.

It was intended to combine this approach with more traditional methods of analysing the policy process that draw on policy process and institutional frameworks (Kingdon, 1995; Sabatier and Jenkins-Smith, 1999). However, it became clear in early interviews that concepts of policy networks or advocacy coalitions were not appropriate approaches to the analysis of policy development on patient choice, because in England there was no evidence of a network or policy community with very few key individuals involved.

In Northern Ireland, Scotland and Wales this approach to the analysis was not relevant because patient choice policy was not being developed and there was little if any political or policy discussion about choice. Political rhetoric about political difference emerged as the key factor in framing discussions of patient choice, as described earlier.

Marinetto (1999) argues that a multiple research strategy is needed for exploring policy. Policy–discourse approaches do offer an interpretive view of policy, looking at interconnections in the policy process and between policy and the social and political context (Fischer, 2003). Within a policy-as-discourse approach to analysis, 'Policy is thought of as a set of processes and actions (or inactions) that have some broad purpose (rather than a discrete decision or programme administered at one moment in time), and embraces both what is intended and what occurs as a result of that intention' (Shaw, 2010, p 201).

Shaw identifies a number of discourses to be explored in policy research, suggesting that discourses should be examined in texts, historical location, uncovering meanings and ways of speaking and power relations. Discourses also examine institutions and how they are reproduced and examine the ideological aspects of policy. Examining data in multiple ways allows a clear narrative to be developed. As Shaw argues, however, the policy-as-discourse approach continues to have a number of critics and remains highly contested as an approach to analysis. While, on the one hand, it brings a richness to the analysis that may not be uncovered in applying more traditional and 'rational' analytical approaches, it does have particular relevance to policy developments that are less defined and are perhaps evolving over time. Its use in case studies of policy may be of particular benefit because it provides a way of exploring the data from a number of different standpoints.

Methodological flexibility is a key aspect of case study research. Lack of definition of the case and problems of conceptual clarity are often key attributes of policy. Our analysis of patient choice demonstrated the importance of conceptualising policy in its broadest context and accepting that an examination of macro-level policy would not provide an adequate analysis of choice policy in healthcare in the UK. Empirical analysis of policy is still an important way of understanding policy itself. As Marinetto (1999) has pointed out, studying policy at different levels is important in order to fully understand the policy itself. If we had simply examined national policy documents and drawn on the interviews of policy makers in the four countries, we would have arrived at a very different interpretation of policy and concluded that there were distinct and fundamental differences in policy between the four countries. Adopting an approach that examined policy at different levels in different contexts through multiple case studies and by examining narratives at each level and in each health system, we arrive at a rather different conclusion. This suggests that national differences are rhetorical rather than real and that, in contrast to suggestions that patient choice in England is a response to market-driven agendas, choice policy reflects a wider consideration of changing relationships between the welfare state and those who use it. Thus, we would argue, the examination of narratives on policy and key discourses provides a useful way of analysing policy case studies. Two benefits are of immediate concern. The first is in helping to uncover and define the case and the second is to provide a much more nuanced analysis of policy as experienced by those involved in delivering and 'receiving' policy.

Conclusion

This chapter has highlighted both the difficulty of defining policy and the complexity of trying to examine the operationalisation, understanding and impact of policy. The multiple contexts of policy pose methodological challenges to the researcher, the policy analyst and the policy maker. What encompasses a case in this respect is, in itself, a problem. While focusing on a specific policy may have been possible in terms of documented choice policy, we found that choice policy unfolded over time – an issue of particular significance in Scotland, for example – and that to understand choice policy involved examining its application (and people's understanding of it) within the NHS as well. This was not an evaluation of choice policy, but set out to understand the nature of choice policy. While initially the intention, as in many case studies of policy, was to use multiple lenses or frameworks to analyse the policy, we found that choice unfolded as a story, and thus we focused on building narratives of policy in different countries and at different levels and in different locations. Through this approach, we were able to discover interpretations of policy and their application. In particular, the approach provided a way of examining the policy within context, that is, at the national (macro) policy level and at the organisational and operational (meso and micro) levels. The comparative nature of the project also highlighted the importance of thinking about health policy in the context of devolution.

Where policy is less or even non-specific, narrative approaches to case studies have considerable attraction. They provide a way of organising the analysis of policy, uncovering its internal context (actors, processes, implementation) and the context within which policy is enacted. The approach within this study was to become involved in redefining the unit of analysis as we drilled down into the different levels. However, each level clearly nested within higher levels (national, PCT, department, practice, GP–patient encounter). Essentially, we started from the generality of policy documents and interviews where we retrospectively examined a variety of policies under the broad banner of choice and how they changed over time.

In the end, we examined specific choices in the referral pathways being offered at a specific time. Combining multi-level case studies with narrative approaches to policy analysis provides a useful and robust way of examining policies which capture both the ideological or value base of policies and their application in practice.

Such an approach does not, however, solve other selection issues about the case. Narratives provide historical context, but selection of the temporal frame will be crucial. While our study explicitly focused on the period post the NHS Plan of 2000, we situated this within the broader political frame of the New Labour government – that is, from 1997. However, the study could have been set within a broader context of changes in welfare policy, which would have placed patient choice in a longer historical frame that took ideas about changes in the welfare state (emerging in the 1980s) as providing a framework for analysis. While this might influence the meta-narrative it would not (at least, to any great extent) change the specific findings of our study about the processes of choice, similarities between devolved health systems or how policy was conceptualised by our respondents. This highlights that case selection or construction still remains a complex task.

References

Ball, S.J. (1993) 'What is policy? Texts, trajectories, toolboxes', *Discourse*, vol 13, no 2, pp 110–17.

Barrett, S. and Fudge, C. (eds) (1981) *Policy and action*, London: Methuen.

Cairney, P. (2007) 'A "Multiple Lens" approach to policy change: the case of tobacco policy in the UK', *British Politics*, vol 2, pp 45-68.

Clarke, J., Smith, N. and Vidler, E. (2006) 'The indeterminacy of choice: political, policy and organisational implications', *Social Policy & Society*, vol 5, no 2, pp 327–36.

Clarke, J., Newman, J., Smith V., Vidler, E. and Westmarland, L. (2007) *Creating citizen-consumers: Changing publics, changing public services*, London: Sage.

Damiani, M., Propper, C. and Dixon, J. (2005) 'Mapping choice in the NHS: cross sectional study of routinely collected data', *British Medical Journal*, vol 330, no 7486, pp 284–7.

DH (Department of Health) (2000) *The NHS Plan: A plan for investment, a plan for reform*, London: DH.

DH (2001) *The expert patient: A new approach to chronic disease management for the 21st century*, London: DH.

Exworthy, M. (2001) 'Primary care in the UK: understanding the dynamics of devolution', *Health and Social Care in the Community*, vol 9, no 5, pp 266–78.

Exworthy, M. and Peckham, S. (2006) 'Access, choice and travel: implications for health policy', *Social Policy and Administration*, vol 40, no 3, pp 267–87.

Fischer, F. (2003) *Reframing public policy*, Oxford: Oxford University Press.

Fotaki, M., Boyd, A., Smith, L., McDonald, R., Roland, M., Sheaff, R., Edwards, A. and Elwyn, G. (2005) *Patient choice and the organisation and delivery of health services: Scoping review*, Manchester: University of Manchester.

Greener, I., Mills, N., Powell, M. and Doheny, S. (2006) 'How did consumerism get into the NHS? An empirical examination of choice and responsiveness in NHS policy documents', Cultures of Consumption Working Paper Series, ESRC–WHRC Research Programme, London: ESRC.

Greer, S. (ed) (2007) *Devolving policies, diverging values*, London: Nuffield Trust.

Hill, M.J. and Hupe, P.L. (2002) *Implementing public policy: Governance in theory and practice*, London: Sage.

Hughes, D., Mullen, C. and Vincent-Jones, P. (2009) 'Choice versus voice? PPI policies and the re-positioning of the state in England and Wales', *Health Expectations*, vol 12, no 3, pp 237–50.

Jones, L. and Mays, N. (2009) *Systematic review of the impact of patient choice of provider in the English NHS*, London: London School of Hygiene and Tropical Medicine.

Kay, A. (2006) *The dynamics of public policy*, Cheltenham: Edward Elgar.

Kingdon, J. (1995) *Agendas, alternatives and public policies*, New York: Harper Collins, King's Fund.

Le Grand, J. (2004) 'Choice and personalisation', presentation, Office of Public Service Reform, 21 July, available at: www.cabinetoffice.gov.uk/opsr.

Le Grand, J. (2007) *The other invisible hand: Delivering public services through choice and competition*, Princeton, NJ: Princeton University Press.

Lindblom, C.E. (1979) 'Still muddling, not yet through', *Public Administration Review*, vol 39, pp 517-25.

Marinetto, M. (1999) *Studies of the policy process: A case analysis*, London: Prentice Hall.

Needham, C. (2003) *Citizen-consumers: New Labour's marketplace democracy*, A Catalyst working paper, London: The Catalyst Forum.

Newman, J. and Vidler, E. (2006) 'Discriminating customers, responsible patients, empowered users: consumerism and the modernisation of health care', *Journal of Social Policy*, vol 35, no 2, pp 193–210.

NHS Scotland (2005) *Building a health service fit for the future: A national framework for service change in the NHS in Scotland*, Edinburgh: Scottish Executive.

Peckham, S., Sanderson, M., Entwistle, V., Thompson, A. et al (2010) *A comparative study of the construction and implementation of patient choice policies in the UK*, Final report, NIHR Service Delivery and Organisation programme.

Ragin, C. (2007) 'Comparative methods', in W. Outhwaite, and S.P. Turner (eds) *The Sage handbook of social science methodology*, London: Sage.

Roe, E. (1994) *Narrative policy analysis, theory and practice*, Durham, NC: Duke University Press.

Sabatier, P., and Jenkins-Smith, H. (1999) 'The advocacy coalition framework: an assessment', in P. Sabatier (ed) *Theories of the policy process*, Boulder, CO: Westview Press, pp 233–60.

Shaw, S. (2010) 'Reaching the parts that other theories and methods can't reach: how and why a policy-as-discourse approach can inform health-related policy', *Health*, vol 14, pp 196–212.

Yin, R.K. (2003) *Case study research: Design and methods*, Thousand Oaks, CA: Sage.

fifteen

The individualisation of health: health surveillance, lifestyle control and public health

Alison Hann

Of all tyrannies, a tyranny sincerely exercised for the good of its victim may be the most oppressive. It may be better to live under robber barons than under omnipotent moral busybodies. The robber baron's cruelty may sometimes sleep, his cupidity may at some point be satiated, but those who torment us for our own good will torment us without end for they do so with the approval of their own conscience. (C.S. Lewis)

When we consider the aims of 'health promotion' it would be difficult to argue against the apparent central premise, which is that it is a stated policy objective to, quite simply, promote health. Its assertions are presented as 'obvious', 'self-evident', 'common sense' or 'what observer could possibly deny?'. Or perhaps, 'what observer could possibly object?'. This case study looks at the work of Petr Skrabanek both in a broad context and also with particular reference to his book *The Death of Humane Medicine* (1994). He was highly critical of the aims and objectives of the 'new' public health and sought to 'question the question' at every opportunity. One of the ways he did this was by using theoretical concepts to interrogate not just the activity of health promotion but also the ideological premise on which it is built. He questioned what Jones-Devitt and Smith (2007) have called the 'assumption-inference process in public health', which I have reproduced in Figure 15.1.

The diagram captures nicely the way in which health promotion is underpinned by the assumption that 'everyone wants good health' – that is, if they are rational; the implication being that if they engage in health-detracting activities, then they must be either ignorant or irrational in some way. What is missing from Figure 15.1 is the role of the state and the medical profession, whose influence might form a layer between the lower two – that is, the medical profession and the state apparatus insist that the pursuit of health is almost a categorical imperative. This is a crucial link in the chain, as together they (the state and the medical profession) form what might be called (to borrow from Foucault) a kind of power/knowledge nexus. Thus,

Figure 15.1: Assumption inference process in public health

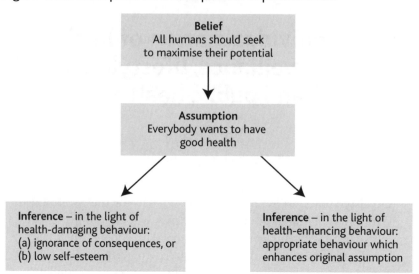

these taken-for-granted assumptions are articulated through health policy and medical practice. The last link here is that between evidence and policy/medical discourse. Skrabanek insisted that, in very important ways, the link between evidence and health promotion should be *stronger* than for other forms of medical intervention because health promotion deals with people who are not 'ill' and who have not approached a general practitioner (or any other health professional) asking for medical assistance. In the case of health promotion in general, and of screening in particular, Skrabanek points out that there should be conclusive evidence that the process causes no harm to those screened or counselled, and that also the activity should clearly be of benefit. He claims that

> Population interventions which have as their goal the prevention of heart disease and many cancers (among other things) should be regarded as population experiments and the same guidelines should be applied to them as clinical trials. That many such interventions are of an experimental nature and of uncertain benefit is made clear by the fact that they have been, and still are, tested by means of controlled trials. If a healthy volunteer, or a patient, has the right to be fully informed about the nature of trials and the benefits and risks which might be involved, then even more meticulous attention should be paid to the rights of whole populations of healthy people. (1994, p 110)

What Skrabanek did, then, was to subject the whole endeavour of health promotion and the 'new' public health to a critical analysis using the concept of 'healthism' – and this is, arguably, more relevant than ever before, given the expansion of policies aimed at making us more healthy.

The Death of Humane Medicine

The Death of Humane Medicine and the Rise of Coercive Healthism by Petr Skrabanek was published in 1994, shortly before the author's death from prostate cancer. It is an examination of the trend for the 'new' public health to use (as he would put it) various forms of coercion to ensure that individuals achieve a healthy body and lifestyle and, by extension, that the nation has a healthy population and workforce. His approach had two main strands: first, that health policy is devised by the government with a political agenda in mind. This is, of course, nothing new; health policy has always been deeply political. But he takes this one step further and suggests that, while claiming to have a firm evidence base, public health exists largely to 'operationalise' deeply embedded moral values that are given legitimacy by and through the authority of the medical profession. As such, public health interventions need not necessarily to rely on a firm evidence base; all that is needed is a strong political/medical advocacy coalition that drives policy towards a predetermined end point. An end point that is, in his words, the subtle (and sometimes not so subtle) coercion of the population into what he calls healthism. The second strand to Skrabanek's case is the false promise of longevity offered by 'healthism'. To put it crudely, this is the very familiar idea that if we do not smoke or drink too much alcohol, do not overeat, take regular exercise, attend for regular screenings and so on, then we will live longer and feel better. The other side to this coin is an obvious one: that failure to abide by these guidelines may result in your health being compromised, and this will in turn put a burden on the state in terms of costs to the NHS and days lost in productivity because of absence from work. Skrabanek agrees with Zola (1972) that the medical profession is a major institution of social control and the state has a great deal of interest in social control. The power invested in the medical profession is enormous: it makes decisions about employability, fitness to marry and to have children, the right to have an abortion, the time (and manner in which) a person is allowed to die, competence to enter into contracts, adopt children or rear one's own, access to certain types of welfare benefits and much more.

> [T]heir authoritarian judgement is sought on correct eating, sexual behaviour and the use of leisure time … [and] all this surveillance and control is expressed not it terms of power but in the language of 'science', it is implied that medical decisions are politically

neutral and scientifically objective. This makes their use by the state dangerous, as their real nature is concealed.' (Skrabanek, 1994, p 147)

Furthermore, the individual is invited to 'be in partnership' with the various health-promotion agencies to ensure their own (and others') compliance with the 'rules' of health promotion. Since Skrabanek's death, public health has blossomed. It is now a multi-dimensional business that has achieved a status that the public health physicians of the 1950s could only have dreamed about.

With the emergence of the Quality and Outcomes Framework (QOF) and the new GP contract, the connection between health policy and general practice is tighter than ever and, in addition to this, public health documents (such as *Healthy weight, healthy lives*) have paved the way for more individual approaches to health and lifestyle, while other approaches (such as the Black Report and, more recently, the Marmot Report) have been side-lined (see also Exworthy and Oliver, Chapter Nineteen).

In order to qualify for payments through the QOF, the general practitioner screens, tests, questions and measures patients on an opportunistic basis, in some cases whether the patient wants it or not. Advice is offered on a range of 'private' issues such as lifestyle choices, sexual practices, dietary habits, leisure activities, and detailed questions are likely to be asked concerning alcohol consumption, smoking habits and other 'risk factors' such as saturated fat intake. Few health professionals, politicians or members of the general public question the evidence base for these 'health promotion' activities, and little serious consideration is given to the right of GPs to penetrate so deeply into the private lives of their patients on behalf, arguably, of the state.

In *The death of humane medicine*, Skrabanek considers several areas that would now fall under what might loosely be called 'health promotion'. These include what he calls the 'unhealthy obsession with health', 'lifestylism' and 'coercive medicine'. In this chapter we will be examining obesity, diet and screening in the light of Skrabanek's observations.

Healthism, surveillance and childhood obesity

At the time of writing this, obesity is not a crime. This may seem an obvious and perhaps even a slightly silly statement. Yet, while it is not a crime, according to the legal definition, it is fast becoming a crime from the normative perspective, an act that contravenes a set of formal or informal norms or codes. Certainly, being obese attracts social (and medical) sanctions and stigma, and this is underpinned by medical 'evidence' that obesity is bad for your health and is 'caused' by people being lazy (slothful) or overindulgent (gluttons) or, of course, both. We are constantly bombarded with messages concerning what a 'healthy weight' should be (one commentator has referred to it as a tsunami of health-promotion literature); general practitioners are encouraged (through QOF) to ascertain a patient's Body Mass Index (BMI), and to give stern warnings to those whose BMI is over 25. Children are similarly subjected to scrutiny, and the rising concern with childhood obesity is becoming something of a national obsession. This has been fuelled by none other than Jamie Oliver (the TV chef), who, in campaigning for healthy school dinners, suggested that if something wasn't done (about unhealthy school dinners and overweight children – suggesting that these were linked), then today's children would die before their parents. This, coupled with a general medical/political obsession with childhood overweight and obesity has led to an unprecedented interference in children's eating habits and parental control. In the wake of Jamie Oliver, there have been drastic changes to school meals and inspection of children's lunchboxes in schools is apparently becoming routine, with strongly worded letters being sent to parents whose children's lunchboxes contain 'junk'. When New Labour became interested and brought Jamie Oliver on board, it turned a TV series into a national political campaign to encourage (force) schools to serve up healthy fare (O'Neill, 2009). As Andrew Lansley (then Shadow Health Minister, now Secretary of State for Health) pointed out, the campaign backfired. 'Hundreds of thousands of kids stopped eating school dinners altogether and instead brought in packed lunches. But then schools started rifling through children's lunchboxes – because headteachers now believed that "we've even got to determine what's in the packed lunches"', as Lansley (2010) put it. And so parents stopped giving their kids packed lunches, too, on the grounds that they didn't want to receive a letter from the school telling them off for giving their child a chocolate bar. As a result, many children were instead given money by their parents and encouraged to buy themselves snacks. Being children, they bought chips. Or sausages in batter. Or pork pies. Washed down with cans of Coke. As Lansley said of this healthy-eating debacle: 'If we are constantly lecturing people and trying to tell them what to do, we will actually find that we undermine and are counterproductive in the results that we achieve' (2010).

In addition to the obsession with children's diet, the focus on overweight and obesity in children has led to the weighing of children and measuring of their BMI becoming institutionalised in some schools (even though BMI is well recognised as being an unsuitable measure for children), and parents being sent letters concerning their child's weight and height ratio. Jennie Bristow, in 'Your child's body mass index is nobody's business but yours' (2009), describes a process in her daughter's school where parents are invited to consent to this process but warned that if they do not consent, 'your GP will be notified'. In some schools this 'weighing in' process is done in public – in front of classmates – and has been shown to lead to the stigmatisation and bullying of 'overweight' children (Fitzpatrick, 2006).

Indeed, even the government's own health advisers warned that mass 'weigh in' would stigmatise overweight children and provoke widespread anxiety and distress among both children and parents. Lyons (2008) points out that this campaign against childhood obesity simply makes parents feel guilty and 'chubby' children feel isolated and ashamed, and makes society an ever more-policed arena. He adds: 'New Labour, a government without any wider vision of how to lead or change society, has become obsessed with micro-managing our lives' (p 8). But while stigmatisation may be bad enough, worse is to follow. In 2004 in Albuquerque, New Mexico a three-year-old child was removed from the custody of her parents because she was 'overweight'. Anamarie weighed 130 lbs by the time she was three – but she was also twice as tall as other children her own age, had a full set of teeth (by the age of one year) and a full head of adult hair. Her parents had been concerned about her size and weight since she was eight months old, and she had been to see no less than 57 doctors by the time she was three, none of whom could explain her condition. At the time she was taken into state custody, the child was on a diet of 550 calories a day. Nonetheless, the child was placed in state custody and social services informed the courts that her parents were 'feeding her too much' and endangering her health (Campos, 2004). In the UK in 2008, all six of a Dundee family's children were taken into care because they were overweight. Later, child protection services removed the same family's new-born baby from the mother while she was recovering in hospital (The Dundee and Tayside Feed, 2009). In all, there have been 20 reported cases in the UK of obese children being removed from their parents on the basis of their being overweight (The Dundee and Tayside Feed, 2009).

In yet another case, Tom Halton took part in a scheme to measure children's weight. Barnsley Primary Care Trust, the local healthcare provider, wrote to Tom's parents to inform them that their son was overweight (he was 5 ft 1 in tall and weighed 108 lbs). The letter the parents received suggested that the boy was heading for a life of ill-health, with a high chance of getting cancer, heart disease and diabetes. Tom's father commented that he thought the letter was 'scaremongering', an assessment with which this author would agree. Both Tom and his parents found the whole incident distressing – the child because he felt guilty and stigmatised, and the parents because they felt their parenting was being undermined. Tom had been part of the National Child Measurement Programme, which is 'an annual programme to measure the height and weight of all children in reception and year six'(Lyons, 2008). The document *Healthy weight, healthy lives* (DH, 2008) states, without any apparent acknowledgement of the irony it carries, that 'many areas are *sharing* [my emphasis] each child's results with the parents' and that Primary Care Trusts (PCTs) are proactively inviting the parents of children identified as being overweight or obese to take up offers of 'support'. Such 'support' is also offered through the Healthy Child Programme, which 'offers every family a programme of screening tests, immunisations, developmental tests, reviews, and guidance to support parents and help them make healthy choices'. This 'support' even gives parents helpful advice on how to keep their babies and toddlers active and healthy. All of this is delivered via a partnership between schools, PCTs, general practitioners and, in some circumstances, as we have seen earlier, social services.

Healthism, surveillance and adult obesity

Overweight and obese adults are also subjected to social sanctions and stigmatisation. PCTs have commonly made some surgical procedures such as hip replacements contingent upon the weight of the patient – with some setting the bar at a BMI of 30 or over, but others setting it as low as a BMI of 25. It has also been well documented (Guard and Wright, 2005) that GPs regard their overweight and obese patients as 'lazy', less intelligent and weak willed. Alongside this, there has been a huge increase in bariatric surgery both within and outside the NHS, with some prospective candidates for 'weight loss surgery' actually being encouraged to put on weight in order to qualify for weight-reducing procedures. But the sanctions applied by the medical profession are underpinned by social stigmatisation because 'scientific' health information is incorporated into a pre-existing set of cultural beliefs that fat people are weak, lazy and greedy.

All of the above 'scaremongering', victim blaming and so-called health promotion might conceivably be justified if the evidence base supported the link between overweight (in both children and adults) and ill-health. But it does not. With regard to children, it seems to be clear that the whole idea of fat children is more a cultural construct than a scientific one. As Basham and Luik (2008) put it: 'the idea that children weighing over a certain amount are fat or obese has no scientific foundation, as the dividing line between fat and normal is pretty arbitrary ... furthermore, it is not at all clear that a fat child carries significant health risks or an increased risk of being a fat adult' (p 81). There is a similar position with regard to adult overweight and obesity. While it may be the case that the very overweight may have particular health problems related to their size, for most adults the link between weight and mortality and morbidity is extremely weak, apart from those at extreme ends of the scale. For Basham and Luik (2009), it would be a mistake to ignore the powerful moralistic slant in the discourse of obesity. For example, within the focus on 'junk food', such as the famous turkey twizzler debacle, and fast food outlets, there is 'a barely concealed contempt for the largely working class people who eat there, who are presumed to be lazy, unthinking and not sufficiently interested in healthy cooking and physical exercise' (p 48). They are seen as 'junk people' who –

for their sins – are being subjected to lectures, warnings, 'support', sanctions, stigmatisation and the ministrations of health-promotion zealots who have joined forces with schools, quangos and the medical profession to 'blame' overweight and obese adults and children for a whole variety of 'crimes', such as selfishly using up NHS resources and moral turpitude.

All this – and no one seems to notice the unprecedented intrusion into people's private lives. Quite the reverse; as the campaign gathers momentum, few question its wisdom. While the overweight are being subjected to specific torment, the population at large is being told that it must take responsibility for its own health, while the government 'has a responsibility for making it easier for people to make healthy choices' (Hewitt, 2009). These policies end up shifting the burden of 'ill health' onto the public. As one NHS manager put it, 'encouraging people to make healthier lifestyle choices plays a crucial role in tackling the increased costs to the health system'(Lyons, 2010b). A UK government report published in March 2010, *Mindspace: Influencing behaviour through public policy* (Dolan, 2010), made clear the future direction of healthcare. The report's authors argue that problems such as the increase of chronic conditions like obesity (*sic*) or diabetes can be resolved only if 'we are successful in persuading people to change their behaviour, their lifestyle or their existing habits' (Perks, 2010); and we must not forget, as Basham and Luik (2009) point out, that 'the existence of an obesity epidemic offers enormous commercial, financial and power maximising opportunities for ... the medical profession, academic researchers, the public health community, the government health bureaucracy, the pharmaceutical industry, the fitness industry and the weight loss industry' (p 44). Part of this particular 'mission' is to coerce people into particular dietary choices, and it is founded on the assumption that it will make them more healthy and they will live longer.

Healthism and dietary choice

The dietary choices are well known. We are, first and foremost, to eschew saturated fats, we must eat five pieces of fruit or vegetables a day and we must restrict our intake of salt. In this endeavour we are 'helped' by the food industry, who produce low-fat, low-calorie, low-salt foodstuffs to the point where it becomes difficult to find salted butter and full-fat cream cheeses on supermarket shelves. Consumers are told that certain products (for example, shredded wheat, skimmed milk and polyunsaturated fats) may protect their heart, and that these are 'healthy choices'. The important thing to note here is that the evidence base for all of the above claims is extremely thin or even non-existent. Energetic campaigns have been waged to stop us eating salt, in order to avoid cardiovascular disease. Yet, while there may be some benefit in reducing salt intake for those already being medicated for high blood pressure, or for those who suffer from kidney disease, for most people salt intake is clinically irrelevant. So strong is the anti-salt message that, in one worrying instance, Heinz has decided to change its long-standing recipe for tomato ketchup and lower the salt content. This change was not demanded by consumers. A spokesperson from Heinz told the *New York Post* that the decision came from 'the changing needs of our consumers and our commitment to health and wellness' (Lyons, 2008). Lyons reports of one New York mother who was worried about the reformulation, that she said: 'My son only eats two vegetables. And Heinz ketchup is one of them. Actually the other one was smothered in ketchup so I'm not sure it counts … I'm not exaggerating when I say this could be the end of vegetables for him.' However, and joking aside, Lyons suggests that Heinz's decision was taken under pressure, with the 'authorities' forcing food manufacturers to change their recipes. In a similar manner, McVities changed the formulation of digestive biscuits to reduce the amount of saturated fat. Saturated fats, in particular, have become known as being 'bad for you' because of the link between fat and both obesity and heart disease. Neither of these links is scientifically proven (Hann and Peckham, 2010).

Lyons (2008) comments, after outlining the weakness of the evidence against salt, saturated fat and other 'junk' foods, that:

> regardless of the evidence, there is a more principled basis on which we should object to these kind of policy proposals – namely, that we, and not NICE or anybody else, should have control over our own lives and our own, sometimes bad habits. Let us eat junk, slob out on our sofas, smoke our fags and drink our booze. If these things turn out to shorten our lives, so be it … That's surely a better way to live than to be endlessly subjected to the high fibre, low-fat, salt free dictatorship of Those Who Know What's Good For Us. (p 2)

Healthism and screening for cholesterol

What has also become firmly embedded in health promotion and public health policy is the link between saturated fat and cholesterol, and between cholesterol and heart disease. Screening for cholesterol is something that is part of the proposed health 'MOT'. Speaking on the 60th anniversary of the founding of the NHS, then Prime Minister Gordon Brown said that his government would be launching a whole raft of screening tests to detect the risk of heart disease, stroke, diabetes and kidney disease. Screening for risk factors has long been recognised as problematic. As Skrabanek noted in 1994:

> The search for risk factors on a mass scale divides the populations into the normal responsible group, and those who are irresponsible people. [...] Technically speaking, risk factors have nothing to do

with causes of diseases, and their introduction was an example of trickery to provide an 'explanation' for causative mechanisms, which in fact are not known. For example, possession of a driving license is a risk factor for car accidents. Being Japanese is a risk factor for dying by hara-kiri. In general, the study of risk factors and their detection in individuals does not bring us nearer to an understanding of causal mechanisms. (p 163)

The relationship, between dietary fat, cholesterol and heart disease is complicated and contains three independent propositions, which contain a number of assumptions: first, that lowering cholesterol prevents heart disease; second, that eating less fat (or less saturated fat) not only lowers cholesterol but also prevents heart disease; and third, that lowering cholesterol prolongs life. In simple terms, therefore, it is assumed that screening for cholesterol (and controlling cholesterol levels) prevents cardiovascular disease and will prolong life. This orthodoxy has had important consequences for clinical practice because GPs are encouraged to screen 'healthy' patients on an opportunistic basis and to meet their targets in order to meet quality thresholds for screening – and, as a result, trigger financial payments. The upshot of this is that cholesterol and saturated fat have both become linked with an increased risk of developing coronary heart disease, and as a result, people are encouraged to cut down on their consumption of saturated fat and to have their cholesterol levels regularly tested. But the usefulness of cholesterol testing as a screening test has been contested right from the start (see for example Texon, 1989; Davey Smith et al, 1993; Ravnskov, 2000). As Wald et al (1999) explain, the link between cholesterol and heart disease is far from proven and, despite the apparent popular consensus, remains controversial. In addition, the idea that consumption of saturated fat is 'bad' is also contested. Taubes (2001) comments: 'mainstream nutritional science has demonised dietary fat, yet 50 years and hundreds of millions of dollars of research has failed to prove that eating a low-fat diet will help you live longer' (p 1). Taubes also points out the influence of the food industry in promoting the 'healthy eating' message that has become synonymous with avoiding fat in the diet. He says: 'The low fat gospel spreads farther by a kind of osmosis, continually reinforced by physicians, nutritionists, journalists, health organisations and consumer advocacy groups such as (in the USA) the Centre for Science in the Public Interest, which refers to fat as the "greasy killer". In America, we no longer fear God or the Communists, but we fear fat' (p 2). We in the UK too, it seems, fear it. In the US people can buy cholesterol-lowering drugs over the counter; in the UK statins are not (yet) available over the counter, but many food 'supplements' and foodstuffs (such as Flora margarine) are sold specifically on the claim that they help to lower cholesterol. Being responsible for your own health is all very well, but there is plenty of evidence that lowering cholesterol, by whatever method, will not prevent heart disease (Hann and Peckham, 2010). Because of this steadfast belief in saturated fat as a demon and cholesterol as a risk factor, people are screened, tested, put on diets, put on drugs – sometimes for life – and yet they will actually have no significant health gain. Or as Oliver (1985, p 8) put it: 'In fact, no clinical trial on reducing saturated fat intake has ever shown a reduction in heart disease.' Some have shown the exact opposite:

> As multiple interventions against risk factors for coronary heart disease in middle aged men at only moderate risk seem to have failed to reduce both morbidity and mortality such interventions become increasingly difficult to justify. This runs counter to the recommendations of many national and international advisory bodies which must now take the recent findings from Finland into consideration. Not to do so may be ethically unacceptable. (Hargreaves et al, 1991)

Instead, what we find is that the case of cholesterol is similar in some respects to the cases outlined above: not only is the information we are given wrong, it is actually damaging. Kendrick (2007) remarks: 'Before looking at the connection between blood cholesterol levels and heart disease, it is worth highlighting a critically important – remarkably unheralded – fact: After the age of 50, the lower your cholesterol level is, the lower your life expectancy' (p 92).

Healthism and screening for cancer

A similar 'war' is being waged against various other conditions, with cancer being top of the list. This 'war' has led to a huge increase in screening. The enthusiasm for screening for breast and cervical cancer has continued unabated for decades. In the UK, women are invited for cancer screening on a regular basis (every three years for cervical cancer and either every three or five years for breast cancer, depending on a woman's age). In the case of cervical cancer, GPs are encouraged under QOF to gain 80% coverage of their eligible patients (cervical cancer screening is predominantly carried out as part of primary care). It has been suggested that, in order to secure the necessary percentage, GPs' surgeries have been generating an inordinate quantity of 'information leaflets', invitations to screening and other 'promotional' material to encourage women to come forward. Invitations to 'non-attenders' are followed up with 'reminder' letters and phone calls from the GP's surgery, and women are opportunistically reminded of their screening test by GPs and other surgery staff, such as the practice nurse or receptionist. The nature of the information has been described by some commentators as highly misleading, and in other cases just plain wrong. In many instances, women are informed that the screening will 'prevent cervical cancer' or that it could save their lives. This has, to some extent been fuelled by the 'Goody effect'[1] (Fitzpatrick, 2009; Hann and Peckham, 2010). However, there is a considerable body of evidence that, despite the claims for the cervical cancer screening programme, it is not as good as it might seem, and that perhaps not only does it not save as many lives as is claimed, but it is the cause of considerable iatrogenic harm. For example, it has been estimated that for every 10,000 women who are screened, 10 deaths may have been avoided (Pettigrew et al, 2001), but to prevent these 10 deaths, 1,564 women are referred for 'further investigations', which could range from a simple retest to colposcopy or biopsy. Thus, many women who were not destined to get cervical cancer are treated and investigated unnecessarily. Furthermore, this obvious physical harm does not take into account the stress and anxiety caused to the women concerned, who have been told that they have an 'abnormal' smear. However, deaths avoided and iatrogenisis are not the only consideration; the rate of false negatives is also an important consideration, one study finding that the rate might be as high as 30% (Pettigrew et al, 2001).

A similar case can be made for breast screening. Women are told by most leaflets and other health-promotion campaigns that they have a 'one in twelve' chance of developing breast cancer (in some information, this has now been increased to a one in seven chance), which is highly misleading. This is a cumulative risk for women who live to the age of 85, not an individual risk. To put it simply, and individual has a 100% or a 0% chance of developing cancer. Or to put it yet another way, for women between the ages of 30 and 50 the risk is about 1 per 1,000 per year (or 1% on aggregate), between the ages of 50 and 70 the risk rises to about 2 per 1,000 per year (2% on aggregate). In addition to this, the benefits of breast screening are consistently overestimated, a risk reduction of 30–50% being claimed for it (Slaytor and Ward, 1998). But this is also misleading. A hypothetical woman of 50 who is screened three times between the ages of 50 and 59 has, during that time period a 2% chance of developing breast cancer and, at worst, a 1% chance of dying from it. The risk reduction from screening is actually 25% of 1% – in other words, 0.25% (Hann and Peckham, 2010). The other side of this coin is that 99.75% of women who go for breast screening derive no benefit from it whatsoever and that, in addition, the breast screening programme also suffers from the problems associated with high rates of false positive and iatrogenic harm done through women's being subjected to unnecessary breast surgery. Yet, despite all the problems associated with both the breast and the cervical cancer screening programmes, both have been a resounding success, at least in terms of compliance rates and political support. As Skrabenek pointed out in 1994, 'anyone who questions the wisdom of screening for cancer is regarded as a kind of heretic, or a misanthrope or a fool' (p 98). Women are thus being recruited into a screening programme without being given full information; indeed, we might go as far as to say that they are being misinformed about the benefits and that the repeated invitations, media campaigns and other activities (such as the Pink Ribbon campaign) promote the idea that the risks of cervical and breast cancer are much higher than they actually are. The benefits are overplayed and the harms not discussed at all.

Healthism and current policy

In the foreword to his book, Skrabanek comments:'The roads to unfreedom are many. Signposts on one of them bear the inscription *Health For All*' (1994, p 11). He goes on:

> The pursuit of health is a symptom of the unhealthy. When this pursuit is no longer a personal yearning but part of state ideology, *healthism* for short, it becomes a symptom of political sickness ... in the weak version of healthism ... [t]he state goes beyond education and information on matters of health and uses propaganda and various forms of coercion to establish norms ... all human activities are divided into approved and disapproved, healthy and unhealthy, prescribed and proscribed, responsible and irresponsible. (p 15)

From this perspective, health promotion, or healthism, represents a huge potential for harm, either physical or social, and those sections of the population that find themselves in the 'irresponsible' half of the equation are subjected to the full force of the health-promotion mission, to the point where the norms of healthy eating, a healthy weight and a healthy lifestyle become internalised and the individual 'polices' herself, and chastises herself for 'moral' lapses from the health-promotion doctrine. This governance of the individual is something addressed by Foucault, who draws a clear distinction between sovereign rule and the 'art of government'. The latter is concerned with the 'protection' of individuals to ensure their health, wealth, happiness and so on, and he makes the point that this requires the cooperation of the individuals themselves, who engage in practices of 'self-government'. As he puts it: 'the subject constitutes himself [*sic*] in an active fashion, by the practices of self, these practices are nevertheless not something that the individual invents himself. They are patterns that he finds in his culture, his society and his cultural group' (Foucault, 1998, p 11). Foucault identifies this as a type of 'pastoral power', which is connected with the 'pastoral' role of the church in days gone by. This ensured 'salvation' for the individual, but to attain this she must make sacrifices; but so must the 'pastor' who undertakes the lifelong task of 'looking after' the individual. To do this, the pastor needs to know people's minds, souls, secrets and all the details of their actions.

> Pastoral power no longer implies, of course, that individuals be led to salvation, but rather that they be assured of other worldly goods such as health, wellbeing and security. In tandem with this change, the officials of pastoral power, who were previously members of religious institutions 'spread into a whole social body' and 'found support in a multitude of institutions' such as those of family, medicine, psychiatry, education and employers. (Nettleton, 1997)

Thus, the individual is 'recruited' and required to participate in the 'policing' of themselves and of others around them in order to conform and comply to the requirements of (in this case) health promotion.

The case study in question here is two-fold – first, Skrabanek's idea of healthism, and second, the whole endeavour of health promotion. Both, he says should be subjected to critical analysis. In particular, the 'partnership' between the medical profession and the state needs to be treated with healthy scepticism, especially when the concern for a healthy population morphs into coercive policy which subjects people to victim blaming, guilt, stigmatisation and which accuses those who are ill of moral weakness. There is a world of difference between legislation in the case of a well-established link between harm and a given practice – seatbelt legislation might be an example here – and the enforcement of healthism. There is nothing wrong, Skrabanek might say, with informing and educating the general public concerning what might be called 'healthy choices', but these should be based on very sound (scientific) evidence and not on assumptions, morals or guesswork. While it may be possible and even acceptable to be paternalistic, this need not necessarily involve being coercive. That is to say, individual rights and freedoms must not be compromised in the name of health promotion.

What is clear from the earlier discussion is that healthism is stronger than it ever was in 1994, when Skrabenek published his book. In the intervening years, the discourse of health promotion has become so embedded in politics and medical practice that it is no longer questioned or subjected to scrutiny. The most recent government White Paper on health, *Equity and excellence* (DH, 2010), does not concern itself too much with public health because this was going to be the subject of a separate report, published separately in December 2010, but what is clear from *Equity and excellence* is the much stronger positioning of the National Institute for Health and Clinical Excellence and the central position of health promotion in future policy. It would seem unlikely that this will involve a reduced role for health promotion or healthism in the future.

Note

[1] The Goody effect – used to describe increased awareness of cervical cancer, and cervical cancer screening, especially in young women as a result of the death from the disease of Jade Goody, TV celebrity.

References

Basham, P. and Luik, J. (2008) 'Is the obesity epidemic exaggerated? – Yes', *British Medical Journal*, vol 336, p 244.

Basham, P. and Luik, J. (2009) *Diet nation: Exposing the obesity crusade*, London: Social Affairs Unit.

Bristow, J. (2009) 'Your child's body mass index is nobody's business but yours', *Spiked*, available at: www.spiked-online.com/index.php/site/printable/6752/.

Campos, P. (2004) *The obesity myth: Why America's obsession with weight is hazardous to your health*, New York: Gotham Books.

Davey Smith, G., Song, F. and Sheldon, T.A. (1993) 'Cholesterol lowering and mortality: the importance of considering initial level of risk', *British Medical Journal*, vol 306, pp 1367–73.

DH (Department of Health) (2008) *Healthy weight, healthy lives: A cross government strategy*, London: DH.

DH (2010) *Equity and excellence: Liberating the NHS*, London: The Stationery Office.

DHSS (1980) *The Black Report: Inequalities in health – report of Working Group*, London: DHSS.

Dolan, P. (2010) *Mindspace: Influencing behaviour through public policy*, Institute for Government, Cabinet Office, available at www.instituteforgovernment.org.uk.

Dundee and Tayside Feed, The (2009) 'Social workers remove Dundee children for being too fat', available at: http://news.stv.tv/scotland/tayside/124368-social-workers-remove-dundee-children-for-being-too-fat/.

Fitzpatrick, M. (2006) 'Stop bullying fat kids', *Spiked*, available at: http://spiked-online.com/index.php/site/printable/315.

Fitzpatrick, M. (2009) 'Jade and the dangers of smear testing', *Spiked*, available at: http://spiked-online.com/index.php/site/printable/6384.

Foucault, M. (1998) 'The ethic of care for the self as a practice of freedom', in J. Brenaur and D. Rasmussen (eds) *The final Foucault*, Cambridge, MA: MIT Press.

Guard, M. and Wright, J. (2005) *The obesity epidemic: Science, morality and ideology*, London: Routledge.

Hann, A. and Peckham, S. (2010) 'The gold effect and screening for cholesterol', *Health Risk and Society*, vol 12, no 1, pp 33–50.

Hargreaves, A.D., Logan, R.L., Thompson, N., Elton, R.A., Oliver, M.F., Riemerson, R. (1991) 'Total cholesterol, low density lipoprotein cholesterol, and high density lipoprotein cholesterol and coronary heart disease in Scotland', *British Medical Journal*, vol 303, pp 378-81.

Jones-Devitt, S. and Smith, L. (2007) *Critical thinking in health and social care*, London: Sage Publications.

Kendrick, M. (2007) *The great cholesterol con*, London: John Blake Books.

Lansley, A. (2010) 'Minister rejects "Jamie Oliver approach" on health', *Guardian*, 30 June.

Lyons, R. (2008) 'Let's call a ceasefire in the war on obesity', *Spiked*, available at: www.spiked-online.com/index.php/site/printable/4303/.

Lyons, R. (2010a) 'Squeezing the joy out of ketchup', *Spiked*, available at: www.spiked-online.com/index.php/site/printable/8898/.

Lyons, R. (2010b) 'The tyranny of the anti-junk crusade', *Spiked*, available at: www.spiked-online.com/index.php/site/printable/9073/.

Marmot, M. (2010) *Fair society, healthy lives. Strategic review of health inequalities in England post-2010: The Marmot Review final report*, London: The Marmot Review.

Nettleton, S. (1997) 'Governing the risky self', in A. Petersen and R. Bunton (eds) *Foucault health and medicine*, London: Routledge.

O'Neill, B. (2009) 'Putting St Jamie in the dock, at last', *Spiked*, available at: www.spiked-online.com/index.php/site/article/9102/.

Oliver, M.F. (1985) 'Consensus or nonsensus conferences on coronary heart disease', *The Lancet*, vol 2, pp 1087–9.

Perks, M. (2010) 'We have ways of making you healthy', *Spiked*, available at: www.spiked-online.com/index.php/site/printable/8660/.

Pettigrew, M., Snowden, A. and Lister-Sharp, D. (2001) 'False negative results in screening programmes, medical, psychological and other implications', *International Journal of Technology Assessment in Health Care*, vol 17, no 2, pp 164–70.

Ravnskov, U. (2000) *The cholesterol myths: Exposing the fallacy that cholesterol and saturated fat cause heart disease*, Washington, DC: New Trends Publishing.

Skrabanek, P. (1994) *The death of humane medicine and the rise of coercive healthism*, Bury St Edmunds: The Social Affairs Unit.

Slaytor, E. and Ward, J. (1998) 'How the risks of breast cancer and the benefits of screening are communicated to women: analysis of 58 pamphlets', *British Medical Journal*, vol 317, no 7153, pp 263–74.

Taubes, G. (2001) 'The soft science of dietary fat', *Science*, vol 291, pp 2536–45.

Texon, M. (1989) 'The cholesterol–heart disease hypothesis critique – time to change course?', *Bulletin of the New York Academy of Medicine*, no 658, pp 836–41.

Wald, N.J., Hackshaw, A.K. and Frost, C.D. (1999) 'When can a risk factor be used as a worthwhile screening test?', *British Medical Journal*, vol 319, pp 1562–5.

Zola, D.W. (1972) 'Medicine as an institution of social control', *The Sociological Review*, vol 20, pp 487–504.

sixteen

NHS confidential: Implementation, or ... how great expectations in Whitehall are dashed in Stoke-on-Trent

Calum Paton

Brief description of the case study and the political context

The subtitle of this study borrows from Pressman and Wildavsky's (1973) *Implementation*, moving Washington to Whitehall, and Oakland to Stoke. The title genuflects to Sir Christopher Meyer's (2005) memoirs *DC confidential* – for the separate, longer version of this case study (available from the author) 'spills the beans'. This study is one of failed policy as well as of failed implementation. But an endemic 'implementation deficit' is one reason why the lessons extend beyond both the NHS and (arguably) New Labour.

There is merit in the late (Speaker of the US House of Representatives) Tip O'Neill's dictum that 'all politics is local'. Yet paradoxically, although that may be true of the vast US, it may be less true of the politics of the 'nationalised' NHS in England. This study is about how national policy missiles fired from discreet silos nested in central government have the potential to create local infernos when they land in localities. Phrases like 'local voices' (Conservative) in 1992 and 'devolving power to the frontline' (New Labour) in 2002 create expectations locally that are at odds with the national government's 'great expectations' – which generally involve compliant local agencies delivering good news and good 'stats' to national politicians. This culture, in the NHS, has produced (in the phrase of our transatlantic cousins) the politics of 'kiss up, kick down'. In the NHS, this primarily operates through meso-level apparatchiks (eg in Strategic Health Authorities) transmitting kisses up to politicians and kicks down to NHS Trusts – monitoring performance rather than managing it. And in the era of the 'new market' in the English NHS, the 'new regulators' (Monitor; the Care Quality Commission; the Audit Commission; Strategic Health Authorities) are frequently at sixes and sevens with each other, exacerbating serious quality concerns.

On one interpretation, the study is of über-localism – the antithesis of central control. Yet my argument is that the local disintegration depicted is the bastard child of *uncoordinated national policy*: man makes his own localism, but not in circumstances of his choosing.

The method and type of case study

Like all narrative case studies (as opposed to multi-method, triangulated studies), this one suggests rather than proves. (The longer version suggests more strongly than space here allows – that the local dysfunction depicted is chronologically, structurally and behaviourally linked to the wider political and policy environment.) Part of the point of doing case studies is to shed light on whether it is 'policies or personalities' that explain events. Many of the Harvard Kennedy School's narrative case studies of public decision-making seek to show how effective leaders, 'product champions' and facilitators (ie individuals) achieve things (Moore, 1995) (see Marinetto, Chapter Two).

In most of these cases, key aspects of the external environment (such as the US political structure, and the dominant political decision-making culture) are taken as a 'given'. Thus the heuristic or pedagogical intention is that the cases inform more effective action 'within the status quo'. But in general they do not explore broader or deeper issues such as how individuals' actions are conditioned by external circumstances – configurations of power, political or administrative structures or other 'structural' factors which affect (and are affected by) agency. Indeed the 'agency'-dominated and incrementalist bias of such cases set me on the road of seeking to combine case studies of policy with theoretical concerns such as the theory of the state (Paton, 1990).

Yet in structure, this is a 'Harvard' study, telling a punctuated, chronological story. I was Chairman of the University Hospital of North Staffordshire NHS Trust from 1 November 2000 to 1 January 2006 and therefore a participant: the study may be considered a hybrid. It seeks to tell a rounded story, rather than just being one view of one episode – but it is written by a former protagonist.

Contemporary relevance: learning from poor policy and poorer implementation

Matthew Taylor, former 'think-tanker' and adviser to former Prime Minister Tony Blair, confessed that, as a young policy-maker, 'I knew little or nothing about systems and was uninterested in implementation … Policy may provide the recipe for successful change, but systems provide the ingredients (the materials on which the recipe must operate), implementation does the cooking and, however enticing the dish, without clear communication no one will come to dinner' (2008, p 119). Unfortunately, the Blair government collectively did not learn in time what was later encapsulated by Taylor (or Peter Hyman; see Hyman, 2005). For the duration of the Blair regnum – from 1997 to 2007 – implementation was ignored and undervalued (Hyman, 2005), as was understanding of 'systems' (which were imposed on top of each other without much regard for compatibility) and of communication (which was seen as announcement, re-announcement and spin, rather than undistorted communication or even the establishment of hegemony for a New Labour-friendly 'narrative' (Humphries, 2004). The implosion of New Labour under Blair's successor Gordon Brown is some testimony to the latter claim – the breadth of New Labour's dominance disguised, in its heyday, its lack of depth, which is to say shallowness, in terms of political support but arguably also in terms of innovative political impact. According to Simon Jenkins (2006), John Major, Blair and Brown are, to a man, Margaret Thatcher's sons.

Introduction: national policy

In 2000, the NHS Plan was launched, against the backdrop of Prime Minister Blair's ad hoc promise on television in January of significant extra money for the NHS (which in the event continued up to 2008). Part of the 'reform agenda' was a three-year budgetary cycle instead of the annual bear-garden, although this remains an aspiration rather than a reality at the 'coalface'. What controversy there was in the early days came from targets – which were geared ad hoc to 'pull the NHS up by the scruff of the neck'. In the heyday of targets from 2000 to (at least) 2006, and in reality now, much of the NHS cultural metaphor was military – not least the 'sitreps' (situation reports) which saw Chief Executives reporting even solitary 'breaches' of targets or directives on a weekly basis to Regional Offices (ROs) and even the national Department of Health (especially when the ROs were abolished at the end of 2001) and then to the smaller Strategic Health Authorities (SHAs) from 2002 to 2006, at which point Regions were restored in all but name.

Two remarks_illustrate the culture, the first made to me by the Chief Executive of a large acute hospital NHS Trust (winter 2001):

> ... it would have been nice if, before I embarked on a train journey to London in the January snow which took four hours each way instead of the usual two, the Minister had checked with her own Regional Office as to why we only had four new intensive beds in our special care baby unit, as opposed to eight, instead of summoning me to tell her personally – it was because the Regional Office had turned down the funding for more!

The second was made by a retired army general talking to a private NHS leadership seminar (2002):

> "the thing about describing the NHS as like the army in its command and control misses the point. In the army, we really do devolve, to companies ... leadership really means making decisions which may concern life and death, and carrying the can; in the NHS things really are centralised – by leadership, they really mean followership ..."

Of own goals and too many balls

New Labour, despite its NHS achievements, scored a spectacular own goal. Itchy fingers when it came to announcements of new policy, new structures and new institutions of governance for the NHS (I distinguish between institutions and structures in a manner similar to Tuohy, 1999) led to a plethora of contradictory policies hatched in a plethora of initiatives from the 'garbage can' of ideas and structural options (Paton, 2006). These policies, as well as having a large collective opportunity cost, also had high collective administrative and transactions costs (Paton, 2007). The need to save 33% of Primary Care Trusts' costs, following the fiscal freeze from 2010 onwards, can be read as a subconscious plea of guilty by Ministers.

By 2009, the English NHS had five balls in play on one policy pitch, confusing the players charged with winning on behalf of Ministers – at least four, arguably five, contradictory policies in force for steering the NHS. These were: the old market (based on the purchaser/provider split, with the purchaser now called the 'commissioner'), inherited and never abolished; collaboration; central targets; the new market based on 'patient choice' and the accompanying 'payment by results'; and yet also the 'new planning' – based on the 'need' for regional 'reconfiguration' of hospital services and enhanced primary and community services, the so-called 'Darzi' agenda, based on the *NHS next stage review* led by clinician and former junior Health Minister Lord Ara Darzi (2008).

The case study

This story records the change 'overnight' of one of the country's most-improved Trusts from 'hero to zero' – in the context of local health economy dis-integration and then disintegration. Politicians are good at creating new policies, and new structures and institutions to go with them, and less good at removing the institutional traces of previous policies, partly out of inertia and partly because such institutions have created new interests along the way which politicians are loath to challenge except at 'critical' times. Thus the new system of local Primary Care Trusts created in 2001/02 saw all sorts of local actors and activists seeking advantage from new institutions with new decision-points, from local politicians through newly created local bureaucrats to 'local voices' always looking for a megaphone. For those who like the whiff of 'small is beautiful' and 'local pluralism', the tableau may be an appealing one; the reality (Newton, 1980) in terms of policy output – and public interest – may be somewhat different.

Key agencies in the local health economy

The hospital

In 2001, the University Hospital of North Staffordshire (then the North Staffordshire Hospital Trust) entered a period of expansion, becoming one of the largest acute Trusts in the country. The poor health of the local population and the poor quality of community services (especially 'out of hours') was, and is, the source of severe pressure upon the hospital. Between 2001 and 2005, the hospital broke even in financial terms, and moved – in the star system which operated up to 2005 – from lower mid-table status to narrowly missing 3-star status in both 2004 and 2005, resulting in it being put into the Foundation Trust 'diagnostic process' in 2005. Ironically in the light of later events, it was the Board's refusal to 'spend their way' to 3-star status which kept it, in footballing terms, at the top of the Championship rather than in the Premier League.

For two years up to 2005, it was the only acute hospital within the SHA's territory which was in financial balance; and it brokered money via the SHA to other Trusts over that period. The Trust Board had to resist understandable frustration on the part of some clinicians and managers that other Trusts were 'spending their way to 3 stars' whereas we refused to give up on 'prudence'. In 2004 for example, we missed 3 stars by a whisker – had we scored higher on one element of one indicator (had we spent more on food), we would have made it.

The 'commissioners'

In 2001, Alan Milburn, the Health Secretary, 'abolished health authorities'. Locally, this meant that the five Primary Care Groups (Stoke-on-Trent North; Stoke Central; Stoke South; Newcastle-under-Lyme; and Staffordshire Moorlands) which had evolved up to 2001 became four Primary Care Trusts, taking over the purchasing from one health authority. Most other strategic actors had argued that this was a dysfunctionally large number for a local area, but they were overruled by the Secretary of State, no doubt influenced by local politicians and local MPs with local fiefdoms. It was a decision –

taken in the heyday of 'devolving to the frontline' – which his successors would come to regret. In 2002, the new PCTs brought into public life hosts of non-executive directors who were unaware of recent history, and entering a brave new world of 'local voices'. The dilemmas of the 1990s were a foreign country, and they were condemned to repeat history as a result.

Reaction at the hospital to the new PCTs in North Staffordshire was sceptical. This is a typical remark, from a hospital Executive Director:

> "people are getting appointed as PCT Chief Executives who wouldn't get appointed as divisional managers in this hospital ..."

In return, of course, the hospital was seen as "that wretched hospital" (one PCT Chair, July 2006), swallowing so much money.

The problem of collective action

A major structural problem was as follows: if each small PCT sought to make its own decisions on each type of service (ie electives; emergencies; what would have been 'regional' (ie specialist) services; mental health, and so on), then 'the left hand would not know what the right hand was doing': that is, individual PCT decisions would be likely to be collectively incoherent. For example, one PCT's decision to 'buy' specialist cancer services from Hospital A might depend upon a 'critical mass' of demand for that hospital's cancer services from other PCTs – otherwise, the hospital might not have the finance and scale for a viable service (especially in the light of what was then the EU Working Time Directive [WTD], now the Working Time Regulations [WTR]). This is essentially similar to a problem encountered with the 1990s 'internal market'.

Yet if the PCTs came together and created a division of labour in commissioning/purchasing – eg one local PCT in the 'health economy' leads on electives, another on emergencies, another on specialised services and so on – then the question arises – why have local purchasers in the first place? More significantly, this would remove the PCTs' 'global' role in local purchasing: that is, each PCT would not be able even to think of 'rationally' trading off investment in one type of service (eg electives) against another.

The consequence was that, where collectively PCT made verbal agreements (say, at the health economy-wide Executive of joint executive–non-executive meetings), individual PCTs were always likely to renege when the going got tough or when their own local stakeholders were unhappy. And sometimes, inversely, when individual PCTs agreed to something with the hospital or other NHS Trusts, the collectivity of PCTs might later reverse that.

Differing targets, differing ambition

In North Staffordshire, by 2003, the hospital saw 3-star status as being well within its grasp, ie combining both financial excellence and clinical excellence (at least as defined by the government's own yardstick, later to be that of the Health Care Commission). Yet none of the PCTs could envisage getting more than one star, for various reasons. As a result, the PCTs sought only to satisfice on those targets where they were struggling. Since overall star status reflected achievement of a list of core targets plus high achievement in nine further additional targets, this could put hospital strategy at odds with PCT strategy (if indeed strategy was developed to this extent).

A category mistake

With PCTs, there was from the outset a confusion between localism in commissioning and localism in provision. Confusing the two localisms in one reform (*Shifting the balance of power*, DH, 2001) led to the need for quick reversal of one expensive reform through another expensive reform. As well as creating commissioning that was "not fit for purpose" (Patricia Hewitt, September 2005, NHS Chairs' Conference, Westminster), the question of conflict of interest arose. To wit: PCTs that were providers as well as purchasers could go easy on their own providers while 'putting the screws on' the hospital (a reversal of the orthodoxy depicted by the 'anti-hospital' brigade).

In North Staffordshire in 2004 and 2005, we suffered from these confusions, with PCTs seeking to highlight hospital costs but less willing to draw attention to their own primary care reference costs – in one notorious case scoring higher than 150 (ie 50% above the national average). Additionally, the PCTs lived the dream of their local causes, which meant that, in the words of warning of the hospital Chief Executive (Letter to SHA CE, 27 May 2004), "PCTs in this patch have made 'laudable' but 'non-priority' investments and reserves that we simply cannot afford. (I feel we are not party to understanding the investments that are proposed)".

The 'internal regulator' – strategic manager or performance monitor?

The SHA between 2001/02 and 2006, when Regional Offices were recreated in all but name, was like Monty Python's Flying Circus, recalling that Python was so named because 'there's no one called Monty Python; it doesn't involve flight; and it's not a circus'. Likewise, the SHA was not strategic; it was in poor health; and had no authority. In North Staffordshire, the only thing the NHS Trusts and PCTs could agree on was a version of this wry half-joke. The only thing the hospital and SHA could agree on was the 'uselessness' of the PCTs. The only thing the PCTs and the SHA could agree on was the 'truculence' of the hospital. The following quote comes from University Hospital of North Staffordshire (UHNS) Chief Executive (personal communication, 2004):

> "they talk of performance management; all they do is performance monitoring. There are three levels we need to address to make things add up – within the hospital; within the North Staffs health economy; and within the wider SASHA [the Shropshire and Staffordshire SHA]. We're trying to do our bit, but nothing's happening at the other levels."

This view was shared by many in the PCTs, covertly (interviews, former PCT Chief Executive Officers, 2006/07). The SHA Chairman talked of an "escalating response strategy" (July 2004) to health economy problems.

The PFI

Underlying the development strategy for the UHNS and the local health economy was the private finance initiative (PFI) project to replace 'antediluvian' buildings ('21st-century healthcare in Victorian buildings') and build a new 'superhospital', as the famous local newspaper, *The Sentinel*, called it; and the wider 'Fit for the Future' health strategy to reconfigure care across the whole North Staffordshire health economy, emphasising 'post-acute intermediate care' as well as 'pre-acute' provision to obviate the need for admission to hospital where possible.

Each agency of the local health economy had to approve each stage of the project, from the Strategic Outline Case through the Outline Business Case through the Full Business Case in 2005. By July of that year, the SHA approved the Full Business Case, following the meeting on 28 July at which the UHNS's key officers were congratulated on the soundness of the case:

> MB (SHA Chair) reiterated that the development is important, iconic for North Staffs and the political impact ... BC (SHA Chief Executive) confirmed his support – that the project was well negotiated and fundamentally sound. To be put on record that the SHA were extremely impressed with the approach taken by ... [UHNS]. (Minutes of the meeting, 'Fit for the Future Financial Recovery Plan presentation to SHA Board', 28 July 2005)

Yet only three months later, the same SHA governors were calling into question the affordability of the PFI/Fit for the Future project, and condemning all and sundry for widespread financial deficits across its patch.

What had happened? The immediate story, part 1

The outgoing Shropshire and Staffordshire SHA yielded on 1 August 2005 to a 'division' of the larger West Midlands SHA-designate (pending parliamentary approval) under the 're-re-organisation' intended to reverse the damage of the 2001 re-organisation known as 'Shifting the balance'. The new SHA Chief Executive (later national NHS Chief Executive Officer), David Nicholson, put in a Managing Director for the Shropshire and Staffordshire 'patch' of the larger SHA.

The latter catapulted the hospital to national prominence in April 2006 by announcing 1,000 redundancies (a figure which was later both reduced by two thirds and then reversed). This was the era of the expensive 'turnaround teams', sent scuttling around the NHS to save Health Secretary Hewitt's blushes when confronted by deficits. On 4 April 2006, accompanied by Acting NHS Chief Executive Iain Carruthers, Health Secretary Hewitt toured the University Hospital. Interviewed on Radio Stoke, Hewitt stated, "the problem is that this hospital was treating too many patients …".

Carruthers was later quoted in *Health Service Journal*:

> "we couldn't understand how a situation like that had gone on for such a length of time." (HSJ, 2006, p 7)

An official rewrite of history was under way, and the 'one-club golfer' NHS had moved from using only the driver (service targets) to solely the iron (fist to drive though temporary cuts).

What had happened? The underlying story

Storm clouds were beginning to form by May 2004. The PCTs were worried about hospital 'over-performance'.

As just one example among many, the PCT Chair was keen to show me (as UHNS Chair), a graph demonstrating the PCT's perspective on how UHNS should manage waiting times, that is to keep waiting times, condition by condition, to as near as possible the maximum permissible, to deflate costs in-year. (Incidentally, behaviour such as this replicated nationally would nicely explain the King's Fund's findings in 2006 that 'outlier' waiting times were tackled fairly successfully but that average waiting times were not much affected – at that time.)

My response to this was: 'Yes, but that ignores how clinicians organise their sessions' (eg they 'squeeze in' shorter operations after a longer one); also, 'it stores up trouble for the following year or two', that is a greater caseload is carried forward, which – with targets becoming more ambitious year-on-year (at that time) – would prevent target achievement the following year (by clogging up the first part of the year with historic cases); and, further, 'it ignores the fact that the lion's share of over-performance is not elective-related, ie it is emergency admission driven'.

The underlying problem was that the PCTs had generally not invested in effective primary care of the sort that could keep chronically ill people out of hospital (the so-called 'repeat patients': the hard core of genuinely needy people who formed a large part of hospital attendances and admissions). The cost of keeping or treating them in hospital was, annually, more than the PCT was prepared to budget for; yet they could not obviate the admissions – on this, they were at odds with the majority of 'their' GPs.

Over time, it produced a vicious circle – they had to pay the hospital more than they wished as a result (not hospital 'over-performance', in that Orwellian phrase, but inevitable admission and treatment), which left less (a negative amount!) for belatedly investing in primary and community services. By the time Patricia Hewitt's gratingly titled document advocating extra-hospital care, *Our health, our care, our say* (DH, 2006) was produced, the commissioners of North Staffordshire found themselves a million miles from the aspiration. In this case, Whitehall's great expectations really did founder in the sticks.

And of course there was less money with which to be ambitious as regards 'electives targets', putting the PCTs and the UHNS at odds over how ambitious to be. On this issue, the hospital's approach – up to summer 2005 – was to assume a rising PCT income available for hospital expenditure, in line with national allocations which were increasing in so-called 'three-year settlements'.

The budgetary process

One must distinguish between the technical budgetary process and the politics of the budgetary process. Technically NHS contractors were supposed to sign up to the Local Delivery Plan (LDP), the successor to the Service and Financial Framework (SAFF) between the SHA and its providers.

Example

The North Staffordshire 2004/05 budget had only been agreed late in financial year 2004/05; and later still the PCTs sought to reduce the amounts paid to the hospital, necessitating arbitration by the SHA – which it sought to avoid at all costs. In the end, the SHA ruled that UHNS should not be reimbursed for some services delivered on behalf of some PCTs, on the grounds that the latter could meet more of their targets, and have a better financial out-turn, while UHNS could still meet its targets (principally the percentage of patients seen or treated in target times) through its 100%

performance for non-local PCTs that actually paid up! Arcane, messy but in line with the incentives of the different PCT/hospital targets.

In 2005/06, the situation was even worse. The PCTs offered us a reduction in inpatient activity – which bore no relation to reality, but had much to do with their financial position. The UHNS Board felt unable to sign up to what it saw as fantasy figures in which available finance drove clinical assumptions rather than the other way around. It was not a case of empire-building, as our incentive was to treat fewer people given the difficulty, growing over time, of securing appropriate reimbursement: our concern was treating unavoidable emergencies and clinically necessary admissions, of people who had nowhere else to go – reflecting GP referral patterns that were at odds with PCT assumptions.

The first quarter of the financial year 2005/06 showed a growth in inpatient activity in all categories, with emergencies and urgent/major cases dominating the financial implications (ie activity necessitated on clinical/quality grounds). On that basis, the provisional budget agreed by the Trust's finance team assumed that later settlement or arbitration would occur as before.

As late as September 2005, the UHNS was given a clean bill of health as regards governance and control by District Audit (the local arm of the Audit Commission), which had produced positive 'Audit Letters' to the Board at the end of each financial year, including 2004/05. But what triggered a change was the Acting Chief Executive's (ACE's) request to the Board, at the beginning of October 2005, that he call in District Audit to investigate finance. With hindsight, we should have carefully specified the remit of any such investigation. For, as we later discovered, the request suited the 'cunning plan' of the SHA suits.

District Audit, for its part, was usually retrospective in its assessments, a problem with audit and inspection in general. In this case, when it issued its retrospective criticisms, it failed to take account of the political reality of the budgetary process, and was indeed unable to explain how it was unaware of problems only a couple of months before. (Other external auditors also, commissioned by the SHA as it faced criticism for tardiness in apprising itself of problems, had ironically suggested that the former Chief Executive of UHNS and myself were over-egging the pudding in our warnings about the storm clouds blackening the whole health economy.) Audit's 'story', therefore, was arguably structured by the preoccupations of those engaged in rewriting history from inside the Trust, as they were its primary informants.

What had happened? The immediate story, part 2

In late September 2005 the ACE had told me that he had worries about Trust finances. We also needed to appoint a new Director of Finance (DF).

The ACE told me that our Associate Finance Director (who had successfully been Acting DF in the recent past) did not wish to apply for the vacancy. I was disappointed, as she had done a good job since I had chaired the Trust. With hindsight I wish I had been of more suspicious mindset. The SHA 'found' an Interim DF for us, and she made accusations that led to the Associate's departure on sickness leave. These accusations were later unequivocally withdrawn.

The Public Interest Report issued surreptitiously by District Audit in May 2006 noted that, as in many good organisations, an assumption that things would continue to go well had been made by the Board. If this refers to the financial situation, it is false. But if it applies to trust in a continuing culture – of frank talking, Chief Executive to Chair; frank talking at private Board; collegiate relations among the Executives; cooperation sought with health economy partners but not at any price – then the suggestion may be justified in part. Meanwhile, returning to late 2005, the Interim DF lost little time in rewriting the budget. With hindsight, she and the ACE were the main source of 'intelligence' for Audit's inquiries. Her main conclusions as to the Finance Department were: the budget overestimated income, as a result of 'mistakes' within Finance, principally concerning the move to Payment by Results and income from PCTs (not unconnected, but two separate points); various personal issues (later found to be misleading at least); and the Cost Improvement Programme was not on time or on target.

District Audit produced a draft report by 27 October 2005, which claimed that there had been a partial breakdown in financial governance. Given the fact that the Interim DF now posted the most likely scenario for the deficit to be £18 million and not the £9 million the Board had posted, the Board considered its position. We (myself and the non executive directors) were loath to resign, but decided to offer to do so, not least at the urging of the SHA Chair after a December meeting – ironically the Foundation Trust Diagnostic 'Board-to-Board' meeting (of the SHA Board with the UHNS Board), a consequence of our good performance leading to us being a candidate Foundation Trust. We were no quitters, and our offer to resign was on the basis of going only when a new Board was ready. *The Sentinel* quoted the SHA Chair to the effect that a 'new Board was waiting in the wings', as we had been told. So our resignation was accepted for 1 January 2006. By September 2006, a new external Chair could not be found; and the SHA Chair from 2001 to 2006 was confirmed as Trust Chair by the Appointments Commission later in 2006.

On 21 December 2005, the applicant Foundation Trust Diagnostic Board-to-Board Challenge held under the auspices of Monitor, the Foundation Trust 'regulator', took place in the UHNS boardroom. This concentrated mostly upon the Trust's financial position in the short term, rather than following its remit.

This meeting could be described surreal. At NHS governance level, two snippets pieced together from my notes give the tenor:

David Nicholson (West Midlands SHA, later national CEO): "How do you think you are seen by the PCTs?"

Chairman (present author): "… as filling spaces where necessary, given the absence of services elsewhere."

Nicholson (later, aware that the ACE was displaying contrition to the point of choking on humble pie): "But there are some things you're proud of … for example, being a teaching hospital now …?"

ACE: "Well, even that … it hasn't been popular with all the staff; … perhaps we should concentrate on being a DGH [District General Hospital] for the local population …"

Thus ambition as well as reputation had gone from hero to zero – to my disbelief, given our resolve earlier that day to be resolute.

What had happened? The financial story

The rewritten budget was partly based on replacing the June 2005 'reasonable estimate' of net income with a lower sum. The Interim DF restored between £1 million and £2 million at a later date, based on a negotiation with the PCTs.

The other main part of the rewritten budget concerned Payment by Results (PBR). The Interim DF claimed that the budget she had inherited overestimated income in this realm. Change in the PBR income was based on the SHA policy on 'local' (non-elective) PBR, resulting in reduced income that was not known to the hospital earlier in the year. Before the Trust's regime change, the shortfall was estimated at £30 million, reduced to £25 million on assumption of 'reasonable' reimbursement by the PCTs. (Financial shortfall is the amount estimated before cost improvement is made in-year.) The financial shortfall after the Interim DF's work in October 2005 was £34.5 million, reduced to £32 million after reimbursement assumptions from PCTs.

Of the two main factors (PCT/PBR, totalling £5.2 million), the first – PCT income – was the result of a changed approach 'behind our backs' rather than technical mistakes; the second was an in-year change rather than a mistake.

The implication by 'the centre' was that the Trust had been complacent. Yet it was the Trust alone in the health economy that had 'cried wolf' up to summer 2005. That summer, a management consultant hinted to me that a 'posted' deficit of £9 million for 2005/06 was alarmist – and this from a body that was reviewing the PCTs as well as the UHNS. Even in September 2005, the new SHA regime was demanding a £5 million contribution from the UHNS to its 'control total' (ie to ameliorate the Staffordshire and Shropshire deficit, now about £50 million), despite a break-even having been posted at the Department of Health. This would have necessitated reducing the deficit to £4 million in year, not increasing it – hardly suggestive that the SHA, old or new, was on top of the situation.

The other side of the coin to income is, of course, cost improvement. It may be that the Financial Recovery Task Group was required to sharpen its approach. If so, with hindsight, my instruction to the ACE in September 2005 should have been 'well, do it!' rather than agreeing to call in District Audit on a broad as opposed to a specific remit. After all, the ACE had been a core member of the Financial Recovery Task Group since it was set up, and we had been reassured (orally) that it was operating as intended.

Post-Board resignation

The UHNS eventually posted a deficit of £15 million in 2005/06. In the end most of our projected £16 million cost savings were made. Regarding the PCT income: "They were just giving it all away, the family silver ... it'd never have happened with [the former Chief Executive, 2001–05 and DF, 1998–2001)" (interview with a Trust Divisional General Manager, 2006).

The PFI commercial close was renegotiated, with the 'unitary payment' (the total annual payment from the Trust to the private partner, comprising the cost of building, equipping, running and partly staffing the new hospital – ie staffing outsourced services under the PFI contract, plus the cost of finance to the partner, plus their profit) reduced from around £53 million to around £43 million.

'Financial turnaround' reduced the Trust's bed stock (both present and future, ie in the new PFI hospital and related community support, beds would be reduced by 250, but see section below, '2009 in Staffordshire') on the grounds that more would be done outside the hospital and that shorter lengths of stay would ensue; plus a variety of cost-saving measures were proposed at great cost by management consultants (primarily, fewer follow-up outpatient appointments, different procurement, and better theatre use – all of which had been in the Trust's strategy prepared as part of the Cost Improvement Programme and for moving to a new clinical model associated with Fit for the Future/PFI, but to operate before that if and where possible). But the PCT's own financial turnaround up to 2007 actually reduced expenditure in the areas where expansion was needed (including mental health), that is, there was no 'joined up' health economy turnaround, despite in some cases the same management consultants having assessed and advised across the health economy!

The UHNS's deficit crisis spearheaded the national deficit crisis of 2005/06, and it was useful to Ministers and their managerial advisers to 'make an example' of the hospital. Yet analysis later of the 40-odd worst financial performers did not include the UHNS.

The hospital's PFI was subsidised by the grant of £60 million of public capital, in June 2006, the largest public capital allocation of the year. But, £18 million requested by the Interim Chief Executive for community places – to compensate for the cuts he was making in the hospital – was turned down. As a result, it was 'Groundhog Day' (see Exworthy and Peckham, Chapter Twenty) in the local NHS, every year up to 2009, in terms of inadequate community care.

Four PCTs were replaced with two ('all-Stoke' and 'North Staffordshire'). Combined Health Care, the mental health Trust, had to withdraw its successful application to be a Foundation Trust when the PCTs withdrew from financial agreements, seemingly as part of their own 'financial turnaround'.

In 2006, the hospital's Medical Assessment Unit was moved from one part of the split site to join up with A&E – ignoring the fact that the new unified Urgent Care Unit was part of the site due to be abandoned when the new hospital was built in three years' time (see below).

2009 in Staffordshire

If the NHS were being interviewed and asked the time-dishonoured question 'Where do you see yourself in five years' time?', it would not fare well. For it is a repeat offender in failing to learn from the past. One of the reasons is that short-termism suits politicians and managers, respectively, alike – they can 'take initiatives' and 'take action', respectively....and often be long gone when the proverbial hits the fan. Consider the following in the Staffordshire health economy as a whole.

By 2008, it was clear that the Stafford General Hospital (the Mid Staffordshire NHS Foundation Trust, a smaller but still substantial hospital to the south of the UHNS) was in trouble. Excessive death rates in 'emergency care', although the data were disputed, brought the spotlight of regulators and the Department of Health squarely onto the Trust. The rest is history: its emergency care was proclaimed the 'biggest scandal ever', and by July 2009 the same 'turnaround' Chief Executive who had stayed seven months at the UHNS had been appointed as Chief Executive.

So how had Monitor recommended that the Trust become a Foundation Trust, advice taken by the Secretary of State only a year before the crisis began to hit – with the then Chief Executive receiving the letter of congratulation only days before the Health Care Commission (HCC) (as it then was) announced its special investigation into the Trust's quality problems? How had the HCC missed things hitherto? Or District Audit? It seemed that the regulatory regime of the NHS was rotten to the core – perhaps not surprising, given that the NHS's version of the 'new regulation' was based *inter alia* on the philosophy underpinning the financial sector (Paton, guardian.co.uk, Comment, 19 April 2009).

The hasty creation, abolition and recreation of regulators, to mirror New Labour's careless haste and hyper-activism in policy-making, has left the public confused as to which hospitals are even safe – a point illustrated by the divergent stories as to whether the Mid Staffordshire Hospital had improved significantly by the end of 2009, and by the fact that a significant number of the Trusts 'failing' on clinical quality (according to the reputable Dr Foster) had been given Foundation (ie top) status by Monitor.

The Hollywood blockbuster 'Groundhog Day' tells the story of the reporter condemned to relive the same day over and over again, learning to cope with it better each time. The NHS both local (Staffordshire and Shropshire) and national is still living its own Groundhog Day, but without the learning.

In 2009, it was 'leaked' that the reduced bed stock in the new PFI hospital was unsustainable and would have to be reversed.

How national policy and local 'unravelling' interacted in detail

I have explored elsewhere (Paton, 2006, 2007, 2008, 2009) the story of how national policy's contradictions vitiated New Labour's health strategy and wasted money. Blairite 'sofa government' was responsible for much 'making it up as we go along' on the NHS.

A longer version of this case study (available from the author) explores in detail how national policy and both regional and local reactions affected the North Staffordshire health economy from 2001 to 2009. That version provides full references to documents, meetings, quotes and notes.

Some key factors of national interest, directly or indirectly related to the North Staffordshire story, are as follows.

- The policy of attracting private sector providers has adversely affected public budgets, with PCTs in North Staffordshire, for example, forced by central diktat to worsen the public health economy's budgetary deficit through subsidising a private treatment centre in South East Staffordshire. Thus a self-fulfilling vicious circle: the public sector is financially lax, so we need more private sector involvement …;
- Double, triple or quadruple counting: the UHNS's deficit was occasioned and worsened by the fact that different cost pressures were to be accounted for by recounting the same 'efficiency savings'. These pressures included:

the new hospital/PFI; university status, gained in 2001; the costs of the Agenda for Change (a government initiative on staff grading and pay); the costs of the new consultant contract from 2003 (Ministers later argued that savings should have been gained by employing fewer doctors, ignoring their own 'target culture' of the time, as well as a key lesson from Kaiser Permanente and the Veterans Administration hospitals in the US: having many *more* senior specialists per capita can dramatically *reduce* lengths of stay). To this list can be added the local costs of the ill-fated national information strategy; and the annual 'efficiency savings' (often an oxymoron born of NHS-speak).

- Rapid turnover of NHS executives is functional for Ministers who see institutional memory as productive of 'cynicism' or 'whingeing': fresh-faced marketeers who do not recall the mid 1990s (see Paton et al, 1997) are preferable. Embarrassingly, there seems to be a shortage of 'turnaround' short-timers also.

- The market NHS will arguably worsen the phenomenon noted in North Staffordshire whereby individual organisations seek financial balance, or surplus, at the expense of others. Monitor's latest 'scorecard' to measure Foundation Trust viability overtly ignores the external effects (on other Trusts; on patients) of disinvestment by Trusts in 'unprofitable business'. 'Commissioning' may be improved incrementally, but the dysfunctional commissioner/provider split remains, causing havoc in practice in inverse proportion to the theoretical benefits it possesses if one subscribes to neoliberal or public choice economics.

- The Resource Accounting and Budgeting (RAB) scheme devised by the Treasury has been removed (see Harper, 2005). This imposed a draconian 'recovery' regime on the hospital, which was neither fair nor sustainable – nor compatible with a 'market NHS' in which there are annual winners and losers

- The spirit of *Shifting the balance of power* was replaced with the spirit of *Commissioning a patient-led NHS*, with fewer PCTs and a tougher approach to PCT competencies … on paper, but 'world-class commissioning' has fast become a standing joke, hoisted by the grandiosity of its own petard (and its failure to diagnose the real problem – an absence of integrated service planning).

Key readings

Cohen, M., March, J. and Olsen, J. (1972) 'A garbage can model of rational choice', *Administrative Science Quarterly*, vol 1, pp 1–25.

DH (Department of Health) (2001) *Shifting the balance of power in the NHS*, London: DH.

DH (2005) *Commissioning a patient-led NHS*, London: DH.

Paton, C. (2006) *New Labour's state of health: Political economy, public policy and the NHS,* Aldershot: Ashgate.

Paton, C. (2009) 'Resistible force meets moveable object', in T. Casey (ed) *The Blair legacy,* London and New York: Palgrave Macmillan.

(Other) References

Darzi, A. (2008) *NHS next stage review: Final report,* London: Department of Health

DH (Department of Health) (2006) *Our health, our care, our say,* London: DH.

Farrell, J. (2001) *Tip O'Neill and the democratic century,* Boston, MA: Little Brown.

Harper, K (2005) *NHS reform: Getting back on track,* London: The King's Fund.

HSJ (*Health Service Journal*) (2006), 26 April.

Humphries, J. (2004) *Lost for words,* London: Hodder and Stoughton.

Hyman, P. (2005) *1 out of 10,* London: Vintage.

Jenkins, S. (2006) *Thatcher and sons,* London: Allen Lane.

Meyer, C. (2005) *DC confidential,* London: Weidenfeld and Nicholson.

Moore, M. (1995) *Creating public value.* Cambridge, MA: Harvard.

Newton, K. (1980) 'Is small really so beautiful; is big really so ugly', *Political Studies,* vol XXX, no 2, pp 190-206.

Paton, C. (1990) *US health politics,* Aldershot: Avebury.

Paton, C. (2006) *New Labour's state of health.* Aldershot: Ashgate.

Paton C. (2007) '"He who rides a tiger can never dismount": six myths about NHS "reform" in England', *International Journal of Health Planning Management,* vol 22, no 2, pp 97-111.

Paton, C. (2008) 'The NHS after 10 years of New Labour', in M. Powell (ed) *Modernising the welfare state: The Blair years,* Bristol: The Policy Press.

Paton, C., Birch, K., Hunt, K., Jordan, K. and Durose, J. (1997) 'NHS reforms. Counting the costs', *Health Service Journal,* vol 107, no 5567, 24-27.

Pressman, J. and Wildavsky, A. (1973) *Implementation: How great expectations in Washington are dashed in Oakland,* Berkeley, CA: California University Press.

Taylor, M. (2008) 'Speaking truth to power', in N. Timmins (ed) *Rejuvenate or retire? Views of the NHS at 60,* London: Nuffield Trust, p 119.

Tuohy, C. (1999) *Accidental logics,* Oxford and New York: Oxford University Press.

seventeen

Implementing clinical guidelines: a case study of research in context

George Dowswell and Stephen Harrison

The case described here is a research study in which the authors were participants between 1998 and 2002. The study sought to evaluate the effect of a particular approach to implementing clinical guidelines in primary care in the English NHS. Although an account of the aims, methods and findings of the study must necessarily be given, the aim of this chapter is somewhat broader. We attempt to use this research as a vehicle for understanding something about the policy, organisational and academic context in which it took place, and the manner in which this subsequently developed. The chapter is divided into five sections. The first provides the context for our study, while the second describes the study itself. The third and fourth sections examine evidence and experience from the study as a means of illuminating subsequent changes in two related aspects of the NHS, the conceptualisation of 'evidence-based medicine' and its implementation in general medical practice. We conclude with brief reflections.

Context: evidence-based medicine in the National Health Service

'Evidence-based medicine' (EBM) is the doctrine that daily clinical practice should be based on sound and systematically assembled research evidence about the effectiveness of each therapeutic intervention employed. It has been a formal component of UK health policy since the early 1990s (for a summary history, see Harrison and Checkland, 2009), and parallel doctrines have developed in clinical professions other than medicine, including nursing, midwifery, dentistry and physiotherapy, as well as in sectors other than health, especially education, criminal justice and social work (Davies et al, 2000) and to aspirations for 'evidence-based policy' more generally (for example, Black, 2001). EBM is usually conceived in the language of science, especially in relation to the so-called 'hierarchy of evidence' (Sackett et al, 2000, pp 173–7), widely cited as an authoritative definition of the soundness of scientific research purporting to demonstrate the effectiveness of clinical interventions. Randomised controlled trials (RCTs) and systematic reviews of RCTs occupy the pinnacle of this hierarchy, with other methods ranked lower. Non-randomised controlled studies rank second to the RCT, and uncontrolled methods a poor third. However, EBM is not simply a question of how medical knowledge is generated, but also raises questions how it should be *implemented*. It has become the orthodoxy that the application of EBM is not primarily a matter of the internal motivation of professionals, but that managerial and/or organisational effort is required in order to implement it (Harrison, 2002). Such efforts are typically manifest in algorithmically structured rules such as 'clinical guidelines' or 'protocols' (Berg, 1997) that guide their users to courses of clinical action. Thus EBM is a political as well as a scientific phenomenon, in at least two senses (for a more extensive discussion, see Harrison, 1998). First, as we recount below, it has become institutionalised in UK public policy. Second, EBM is a *normative* doctrine that seeks to prescribe how clinicians should behave.

The adoption of EBM as UK policy can be seen in two phases: first under the Conservative governments of the early and mid-1990s, and subsequently after the election of the Labour government of 1997. Following recommendations from a parliamentary committee (House of Lords, 1988), the then Conservative government created a national research and development strategy for the NHS in 1991, involving the appointment of national and regional research directors, the establishment of national and local research budgets to be the object of competitive bidding, and reorganisation of the flow of research funds through NHS hospitals (Baker and Kirk, 1996). The central objective of this programme became the assessment of the effectiveness of both new and previously unevaluated healthcare interventions. A range of specialist institutions were publicly funded as the means of reviewing, collating and disseminating the findings of effectiveness research to the NHS, perhaps most notably the Cochrane Collaboration (www.cochrane.org), established in 1997 to produce and disseminate systematic reviews of healthcare interventions and to promote the search for evidence of effectiveness in the form of clinical trials. It duly became the conventional academic and policy wisdom that valid evidence of the effectiveness of clinical interventions should be defined by the 'hierarchy of evidence' (Centre for Reviews and Dissemination, 1996) and that clinical guidelines were the appropriate medium for its dissemination (NHS Executive, 1996). These developments coincided with the so-called 'internal market' in the NHS, under which its institutions were divided into 'providers' of care (such as hospitals) and 'purchasers' whose role was to commission services from providers and pay for the care for defined geographical populations (Robinson and Le Grand, 1993). The consequent need for purchasers to develop criteria for their commissioning priorities and decisions led to increasing interest in health economics, specifically the analysis of the cost-effectiveness of clinical interventions. Such analyses required research data about the effectiveness of interventions and generally adopted the 'hierarchy of evidence' as their criterion of validity.

1However, the Conservative governments seem largely to have assumed that clinical guidelines would simply be adopted by clinicians, an assumption that became increasingly questioned on both theoretical (Harrison, 1994) and empirical (Grimshaw and Russell, 1993) grounds; in short, clinical guidelines proved not to be 'self-implementing'. In due course, the New Labour government elected in 1997 went on to institutionalise EBM and clinical guidelines through the establishment in 1999 of the (then) National Institute of Clinical Excellence (NICE) to make recommendations (based on the results of health technology assessment and associated microeconomic analysis) about what interventions should be made available to patients by the NHS, and to commission the production of evidence-based guidelines on specific topics by groups of experts (for overviews of NICE, see Syrett, 2003; Rawlins and Culyer, 2004). This was accompanied by the central specification of *service* models defined in 'National Service Frameworks' for such topics as coronary heart disease, mental health and cancer, and the inclusion of compliance with evidence and guidelines as a dimension of NHS performance management administered by the NHS quality regulators of the moment, from 1999 the Commission for Health Improvement and from 2004 its successor, the Healthcare Commission. Somewhat later, the 2004 general practice contract and its associated Quality and Outcomes Framework (QOF) offered general medical practices substantial additional financial rewards in return for meeting specified 'evidence-based' performance requirements in relation to the management of chronic diseases in their patients (for an overview, see Roland, 2004).

However, when our study was conceived in the mid-1990s, the institutions had only just begun work, so that the initial response of the EBM community to the discovery that clinical guidelines might not simply be put into automatic practice by clinicians was to posit and evaluate a series of organisational and educational interventions that might be expected to improve the rate of uptake of such guidelines. The term 'interventions' is used advisedly here; researchers working within this frame of reference evidently saw the measures that might be taken to improve guideline implementation by doctors as analogous to clinical interventions with patients. Thus, evaluations of such interventions naturally enough took the form of RCTs in which guideline uptake was compared between groups of doctors who had been exposed to various educational and other organisational interventions and 'control' groups who had not. Moreover, such researchers tended to conceive and publish their studies with little (if any) attention to theories of behaviour change or to organisational context, and to focus only on differences between the groups and obscuring any changes over time common to both (Cohen et al, 1982; Grimshaw and Russell, 1993). Our study sought to address these *lacunae* in the course of evaluating an intervention aimed at increasing the uptake of two evidence-based guidelines in English general medical practice.

Case study analysis

Our study, designed and undertaken by a multi-disciplinary group of researchers from the universities of York and Leeds and Bradford Royal Infirmary, comprised two elements, given the acronyms BACKING ('Bradford, Airedale, Calderdale and Kirklees Implementing National Guidelines', after the research locations) and EGUS ('Explaining Guideline Uptake Study'). It was conceived in the late 1990s, at a time when the EBM movement was gathering momentum, but when it had also become evident that the clinical guidelines which had become the movement's preferred vehicle for translation of research evidence into clinical practice could not be assumed to be self-implementing. The study (which was designed and largely completed before NICE had become operational) was focused on the only three clinical guidelines that had in 1999 been officially endorsed by the Department of Health as appropriate for NHS-wide implementation. These related to the treatment of back pain, asthma and stable angina, all in the context of general medical practice. The back pain guideline was used only to design and test the feasibility of various aspects of the study, so that the substantive study and published results (and the remainder of this chapter) concerned the asthma and angina guidelines. (For a full account of our research methods, both quantitative and qualitative, see Harrison et al, 2003; Wright et al, 2003.)

The study employed a relatively sophisticated design, featuring a 'Latin square' in which each guideline was allocated for implementation in one of two (then) Primary Care Group (PCG) areas, with the other PCG serving as a control. (PCGs, introduced in 1999, can be seen as an early attempt to exert NHS hierarchical influence over GPs: see Peckham and Exworthy, 2003, pp 151ff.)

Each PCG was therefore the intervention site for one guideline and the control site for the other. The aims of this choice of design included: equalisation of any 'Hawthorn effects', since both PCGs were observed; avoidance of 'resentment' effects in which control groups try to compete with intervention groups; and a consistent macro-environment. It transpired that it was not feasible to allocate guidelines to PCGs randomly, so that the study was a quasi-experiment. The organisational intervention aimed at increasing guideline uptake by GPs was based on earlier studies. It included the minor modification of guidelines by local consensus groups to fit local contexts, a series of educational meetings on the relevant topic, educational outreach visits to some general practices, and reminders such as mouse mats and posters. (For a detailed account of the intervention, see Wright et al, 2003.) Finally, the study employed mixed methods. In addition to the quantitative analysis of guideline uptake and data drawn from patient casenotes (the BACKING component), semi-structured interviews (the EGUS component) were conducted with a stratified random sample of GPs in some 49 practices, each being interviewed three times over a period of 15 months. The aim of the interviews was to explore explanations for the quantitative findings, though the timing of interviews was such that the latter were not then known to either participants or the research team. Practice nurses were also interviewed where possible.

The quantitative (BACKING) results showed a significant difference between intervention and control groups in respect of only one of the six elements of guideline implementation for which data were collected (recording of smoking status for asthma patients). Otherwise, no significant differences were found, leading to the overall conclusion that the organisational intervention had little effect on guideline uptake. However, the quantitative data also showed a marked increase in uptake of both asthma and angina guidelines *by both control and intervention groups* over the period of the study (Wright et al, 2003). Conventionally, the published results of such trials would be expressed as odds ratios, so that our study would have simply appeared as 'no effect'. Only by taking an interest in comparisons of the real data was it possible to see that guideline uptake had increased markedly in both intervention groups and both control groups, and thereby to adduce an 'environmental' explanation of a type that medical health service researchers typically do not seek. The qualitative (EGUS) component of the study found that almost all GPs welcomed clinical guidelines in principle, believing that they would improve quality of care and not objecting to guidelines that 'save money without reducing quality'. The study's main overall conclusion was that external factors, in particular the expectation that government regulation of clinical practice was in the ascendant, were likely to have been responsible for the increasing adoption of guidelines (Harrison et al, 2003). A subsequent longitudinal cohort study (1998–2003) found dramatic improvements, particularly in coronary heart disease care, which it attributed to 'systematic quality improvements in the NHS' (Campbell et al, 2005).

Our research was undertaken during a period when two important transitions were occurring in health services research and in general medical practice, and some of our qualitative findings and experiences with the study can be used to illustrate these.

Transitions in health services research

The research was conceived, and much of the fieldwork undertaken, at a time when health service researchers saw little or no need to adapt the methods typically employed to evaluate clinical interventions when researching other phenomena, including the social (Greenhalgh et al, 2005). As noted above, it was assumed that educational and related efforts to implement clinical guidelines should be regarded as analogous to clinical interventions and thus investigated in randomised controlled trials designed solely to establish the presence or absence of an effect. Although the most advanced clinical trialists were already experimenting with post-trial evaluative methods (Dowswell et al, 1997, 2000), and medical journals had carried some discussion of the value of qualitative methods (Pope and Mays, 1995), the Medical Research Council (MRC) was still issuing guidelines to researchers based on the assumption that the randomised controlled trial was the basic research approach to be adopted (Campbell et al, 2000). Yet, within eight years, this narrow view had broadened to an astonishing extent in the subsequent revision of MRC guidance, a document which does little more than acknowledge RCTs as one element of many methods, each having equal status, depending on the research question and the circumstances (Craig et al, 2008). More than 10 years after the BACKING and EGUS studies were designed, mixed research methods have become utterly orthodox.

In parallel, consumers of 'evidence-based medicine' have shifted their perspectives on what is to count as valid evidence. Appropriate evidence is no longer restricted to 'the best available external clinical evidence' (Sackett et al, 1996), for a variety of reasons (Miles, 2009). There may be no RCTs (in surgery, for example) (Hoppe et al, 2009); existing measures (QALYs in pharmacoeconomics, for example) may have been judged to be imperfect or inadequate (Ferner et al, 2010); disputes about dealing with either absent or conflicting clinical perspectives may have arisen (Schilling et al, 2010); and it is unclear how population-based evidence should be applied to individual patients (Byrne, 2004). Taking NICE as an example of a body rooted in the original EBM ethos, it is apparent from revisions to its guidance on technology appraisal that a number of non-traditional perspectives must now be considered. Acceptability to patients, carers and clinicians, perceived appropriateness, preferences, feasibility and impact from organisational perspectives, equity and equality have all been added to NICE's criteria (NICE, 2008). More recently, NICE has begun to consider population health topics, for which research methods aimed at evaluating clinical interventions are poorly suited. According to one leading participant in the field, EBM had by 2002 effectively become 'Certain Types of High Quality and Clinically Relevant Evidence from Healthcare Research in Support of Healthcare Decision Making-based Medicine' (Haynes, 2002). Yet, perhaps paradoxically, the earlier medical approaches had already spread to fields of study outside healthcare; the Campbell Collaboration was established in 2000 and explicitly modelled on the approach developed by the Cochrane Collaboration in the health field (www.campbellcollaboration.

org/background/index.php), focusing especially on experimental methods and the aggregation of research findings through systematic reviews (see Davies et al, 2000).

Despite these apparent epistemological convergences, the academic worlds of health services research and the older social sciences (such as medical sociology) remained somewhat separated from each other, as our own experiences with publications from our study illustrate. The studies gave rise to six papers in peer-reviewed journals, plus a letter to the *British Medical Journal*. The main empirical reports of the quantitative and qualitative data and overall findings were published in two papers in the same issue of the *Journal of Health Services Research and Policy* (Harrison et al, 2003; Wright et al, 2003). Despite forming the main output of a highly topical study conducted in a somewhat novel manner, these have been cited relatively rarely. Other papers used aspects of the empirical data for conceptual analysis, notably a publication in the *Journal of Advanced Nursing* (Harrison et al, 2002) and another in *Sociology of Health and Illness* (Harrison and Dowswell, 2002). In contrast, these 'spin-off' papers have been much more widely cited, and indeed the latter was reprinted as a chapter in a major international compendium on the sociology of work (Beynon and Nichols, 2006).

Transitions in general practice organisation

Our research was conducted before general medical practices had been 'corporatised' in the manner that has since become common. The GPs whom we interviewed seemed very much to operate as individuals, generally claiming to have little knowledge about colleagues' clinical practices and preferences, and stating that GP partners did not generally develop collective clinical policies for the practice (Dowswell et al, 2001; see also Exworthy et al, 2003). It was common for GPs to express the view that guidelines were sometimes helpful for GPs in terms of making work easier, but that they were much more appropriate as guidance for nurses. Older GPs often saw the routinisation implied by guidelines as the end of autonomous medicine based on craft skills and long experience. Most GPs felt that it was appropriate to document the reasons for deliberate deviations from guidelines in individuals' casenotes, and felt that the guidelines studied were more likely to have changed their casenote *recording* behaviour than their actual clinical practices (Harrison and Dowswell, 2002). Practice nurses were generally committed to guidelines and there was some evidence that they sought to persuade GPs (their employers) to make use of them (Harrison et al, 2002). GPs were much more likely to report familiarity with the guideline for which their PCG was the intervention site than with that for which it was the control site, but (as implied earlier) this was not related to changes in guideline uptake and PCGs were not regarded as influential

(Dowswell et al, 2002). Taken together with the observation that guideline uptake had increased sharply in all study groups, this led the researchers to conclude that an external factor was likely to have been responsible, suggesting that GPs' knowledge of the increasing policy importance of evidence-based medicine and clinical guidelines (as represented, for instance, in high-profile statements about the role of NICE and the development of National Service Frameworks) had led them to conclude that a new era of 'bureaucratic accountability' in medicine was being ushered in (Harrison and Dowswell, 2002; Harrison et al, 2003).

In summary, early attempts to diffuse research-based knowledge did not seem to stimulate substantive discussion or action within general practices. Following the introduction in 2004 of 'pay-for-performance' for GPs through QOF, practices began to behave much more like corporate organisations in an apparent (and often successful) attempt to secure high levels of financial reward. These organisational changes can be summarised as follows.

First, standardised forms of patient data recording via templates may have become the norm. Crucially, such templates do not simply record data, but also define the nature of the clinical work to be performed by acting as 'prompts' and discouraging the recording of information that is not important for QOF (Checkland et al, 2007). The result seems to be a more 'biomedical' rather than holistic style of practice in which, for example, reminder systems are created so that when patients attend for unrelated problems, clinicians are reminded to fulfil QOF requirements, establishing an additional QOF-related agenda running alongside the patient's own agenda (Checkland et al, 2008). Second, practices have developed new staffing arrangements to pursue QOF requirements. In particular, there has been increased employment of information technology and associated specialist staff, and greater use of practice nurses and/or healthcare assistants to deliver the requirements of QOF. Practice managers' roles gained in importance as they assumed responsibility for delivering the QOF points devoted to 'managerial' domains and for overseeing the achievement in the clinical domains. Third, new distinctions had grown up within practices between those practice staff who carried responsibility for QOF targets and those who did not, 'chasers' and 'chased' respectively (McDonald et al, 2007). The former had developed a number of strategies for influencing the behaviour of the latter, ranging from sending electronic reminders and setting computer systems to generate 'pop up boxes', to public 'naming and shaming'.

In general medical practice, QOF has generated a new form of stratification within UK general practice, with some clinicians (both doctors and nurses) involved in surveillance of their colleagues (McDonald et al, 2009). The originator of the notion of 'stratification' within the medical profession (Freidson, 1985) suggested that such changes would threaten the solidarity of the professional group as a whole. However, this does not seem to have occurred. Some older GPs in the EGUS study were well aware of themselves as anachronisms, and quick to acknowledge the inevitability of change. They attributed this to many factors, including the activities of the GP and serial murderer Harold Shipman, the triumph of accountants and bureaucrats, declining public respect for institutions and even to young doctors having their heads filled with 'rubbish' by medical schools. Many acknowledged that novel ideas like work–life balance and the emergence of new contracts of employment directly with Primary Care Trusts (rather than the traditional independent contractor status of family doctors) were beginning to undermine the vocational aspects of medicine and accelerating the slide towards proletarianisation, at worst, or corporatisation, at best. In contrast, although GPs in more recent studies have expressed reservations about being 'chased' and about the substantive content of some QOF targets, there is little apparent contemporary dissent in relation to such matters (Checkland et al, 2008; see also Jones and Green, 2006). Indeed, they often maintained the stance that there had been 'no real change' in practice in response to QOF; they claimed to be 'doing it already' or that the additional work had easily been 'fitted in' alongside their usual work, and that the holistic philosophy of general medical practice was still in place. QOF has evidently been construed by UK general practices as a technical problem, which has been efficiently solved.

Concluding reflections

EBM in the 1990s was the brash 'new kid on the block', its participants often self-identified with science, progress and the sweeping away of perceived old fallacies. The apparent undermining of the EBM discourse by a consistent political rhetoric in favour of consumer choice and 'patient centred' healthcare (Miles et al, 2008) has in fact been somewhat less pervasive than our account in the third section of this chapter implies when taken on its own. Once our account of transitions in general practice organisation (our fourth section) is added, it becomes evident that, despite the pluralisation of abstract discourses about the nature of 'evidence', guideline-driven EBM has to an important extent been institutionalised by QOF and its bureaucratic requirements, perhaps pointing to the contemporary pervasiveness of discourses of management and 'performativity' (Harrison, 2002).

Looking across our two topics, it is striking that considerable substantive change has occurred with relatively little comment having been passed by those affected. Indeed, as we noted earlier, some GPs thought that nothing of any great significance had changed. The main intent of our case study is to serve as a metaphorical vantage point from which to note that a good deal has in fact changed in relation to the central matters that the

BACKING and EGUS studies were designed to investigate. The narrow case of our research is in effect 'nested' within a wider case of the recent history of general practice organisation and the manner in which it deals with evidence and guidelines about clinical interventions.

References

Baker, M.R. and Kirk, S. (eds) (1996) *Research and development for the NHS: Evidence, evaluation and effectiveness*, Oxford: Radcliffe Medical Press.

Berg, M. (1997) 'Problems and promises of the protocol', *Social Science and Medicine*, vol 44, no 8, pp 1081–8.

Beynon, H. and Nichols, T. (eds) (2006) *Patterns of work in the postfordist era*, Cheltenham: Edward Elgar.

Black, N. (2001) 'Evidence-based policy: proceed with care', *British Medical Journal*, vol 323, pp 275–8.

Byrne, D.S. (2004) 'Evidence-based: what constitutes valid evidence?', in A.G. Gray and S. Harrison (eds) *Governing medicine: Theory and practice*, Buckingham: Open University Press, pp 81–92.

Campbell, M., Fitzpatrick, R., Haines, A., Kinmonth, A.L., Sandercock, P., Spiegelhalter, D. and Tyrer, P. (2000) 'Framework for design and evaluation of complex interventions to improve health', *British Medical Journal*, vol 321, no 7262, pp 694–6.

Campbell, S.M., Roland, M.O., Middleton, E. and Reeves, D. (2005) 'Improvements in quality of care in English general practice 1998–2003: longitudinal observational study', *British Medical Journal*, vol 331, no 7525, p 1121.

Centre for Reviews and Dissemination (1996) *Undertaking systematic reviews on effectiveness*, Report no 4, York: University of York.

Checkland, K., Harrison, S., McDonald, R., Grant, S., Campbell, S. and Guthrie, B. (2008) 'Biomedicine, holism and general medical practice: responses to the 2004 General Practitioner contract', *Sociology of Health and Illness*, vol 30, no 5, pp 788–803.

Checkland, K., McDonald, R. and Harrison, S. (2007) 'Ticking boxes and changing the social world: data collection and the new UK general practice contract', *Social Policy and Administration*, vol 41, no 7, pp 693–710.

Cohen, D.I., Littenberg, B., Wetzel, C. and Neuhauser, D.B. (1982) 'Improving physician compliance with preventive medicine guidelines', *Medical Care*, vol 20, pp 1040–5.

Craig, P., Dieppe, P., Macintyre, S., Michie, S., Nazareth, I., and Petticrew, M. (2008) 'Developing and evaluating complex interventions: the new Medical Research Council guidance', *British Medical Journal*, vol 337, p 1655.

Davies, H.T.O., Nutley, S. and Smith, P.C. (eds) (2000) *What works? Evidence-based policy and practice in public services*, Bristol: Policy Press.

Dowswell, G., Lawler, J., Young, J., Forster, A. and Hearn, J. (1997) 'A qualitative study of specialist nurse support for stroke patients and care-givers at home', *Clinical Rehabilitation*, vol 11, no 4, pp 293–301.

Dowswell, G., Harrison, S. and Wright, J. (2001) 'Clinical guidelines: attitudes, information processes and culture in English primary care', *International Journal of Health Planning and Management*, vol 16, no 2, pp 107–24.

Dowswell, G., Harrison, S. and Wright, J. (2002) 'The early days of primary care groups: general practitioners' perceptions', *Health and Social Care in the Community*, vol 10, no 1, pp 46–54.

Dowswell, G., Lawler, J. and Young, J. (2000) 'Unpacking the "black box" of a nurse-led stroke support service', *Clinical Rehabilitation*, vol 14, no 2, pp 160–71.

Exworthy, M., Wilkinson, E.K., McColl, A., Moore, M., Roderick, P., Smith, H. and Gabbay, J. (2003) 'The role of performance indicators in changing the autonomy of the general practice profession in the UK', *Social Science and Medicine*, vol 56, no 7, pp 1493–504.

Ferner, R.E., Hughes, D.A. and Aronson, J.K. (2010) 'NICE and new: appraising innovation', *British Medical Journal*, vol 340, p b5493.

Freidson, E. (1985) 'The reorganisation of the medical profession', *Medical Care Review*, vol 42, no 1, pp 11–35.

Greenhalgh, T., Robert, G., Bate, P., Macfarlane, F. and Kyriakidou, O. (2005) *Diffusion of innovations in health service organisations*, Oxford: Blackwell.

Grimshaw, J.M. and Russell, I.T. (1993) 'Effect of clinical guidelines on medical practice: a systematic review of rigorous evaluations', *Lancet*, vol 342, pp 1317–22.

Harrison, S. (1994) 'Knowledge into practice: what's the problem?', *Journal of Management in Medicine*, vol 8, no 2, pp 9–16.

Harrison, S. (1998) 'The politics of evidence-based medicine in the UK', *Policy and Politics*, vol 26, no 1, pp 15–31.

Harrison, S. (2002) 'New Labour, modernisation and the medical labour process', *Journal of Social Policy*, vol 31, no 3, pp 465–85.

Harrison, S. and Checkland, K. (2009) 'Evidence-based practice in UK health policy', in J. Gabe and M.W. Calnan (eds) *The new sociology of the health service*, London: Routledge, pp 121–42.

Harrison, S. and Dowswell, G. (2002) 'Autonomy and bureaucratic accountability in primary care: what English general practitioners say', *Sociology of Health and Illness*, vol 24, no 2, pp 208–26.

Harrison, S., Dowswell, G. and Wright, J. (2002) 'Practice nurses and clinical guidelines in a changing primary care context: an empirical study', *Journal of Advanced Nursing*, vol 39, no 3, pp 1–10.

Harrison, S., Dowswell, G., Wright, J. and Russell, I.T. (2003) 'General practitioners' uptake of clinical practice guidelines: a qualitative study', *Journal of Health Services Research and Policy*, vol 8, no 3, pp 149–52.

Haynes, R.B. (2002) 'What kind of evidence is it that evidence-based medicine advocates want health care providers and consumers to pay attention to?', *BMC Health Services Research*, vol 2, no 1, p 3.

Hoppe, D.J., Schemitsch, E.H., Morshed, S., Tornetta, P. (III); Bhandari, M. (2009) 'Hierarchy of evidence: where observational studies fit in and why we need them', *Journal of Bone and Joint Surgery: American Volume*, vol 91, Supplement 3, pp 2–9.

House of Lords (House of Lords Select Committee on Science and Technology) (1988) *Third report: Priorities in medical research*, HL Paper 54-1, London: HMSO.

Jones, L. and Green, J. (2006) 'Shifting discourses of professionalism: a case study of general practitioners in the United Kingdom', *Sociology of Health and Illness*, vol 28, no 7, pp 927–50.

McDonald, R., Checkland, K., Harrison, S. and Coleman, A. (2009) 'Rethinking collegiality: restratification in English general medical practice', *Social Science and Medicine*, vol 68, pp 1199–205.

McDonald, R., Harrison, S., Checkland, K., Campbell, S.M. and Roland, M. (2007) 'Impact of financial incentives on clinical autonomy and internal motivation in primary care: an ethnographic study', *British Medical Journal*, vol 334, pp 1357–9 (full electronic version at doi: 10.1136/bmj.39238.890810.BE).

Miles, A. (2009) 'Evidence-based medicine: requiescat in pace? A commentary on Djulbegovic, B., Guyatt, G.H. and Ashcroft, R.E. (2009) "Cancer Control", 16, 158–168', *Journal of Evaluation in Clinical Practice*, vol 15, no 6, pp 924–9.

Miles, A., Loughlin, M. and Polychronis, A. (2008) 'Evidence-based healthcare, clinical knowledge and the rise of personalised medicine', *Journal of Evaluation in Clinical Practice*, vol 14, no 5, pp 621–49.

NHS Executive (1996) *Clinical guidelines: Using clinical guidelines to improve patient care within the NHS*, London: Department of Health.

NICE (National Institute for Health and Clinical Excellence) (2008) *Guide to the methods of technology appraisal*, available at: www.nice.org.uk/media/B52/A7/TAMethodsGuideUpdatedJune2008.pdf.

Peckham, S. and Exworthy, M. (2003) *Primary care in the UK: Policy, organisation and management*, Basingstoke: Palgrave.

Pope, C. and Mays, N. (1995) 'Reaching the parts other methods cannot reach: an introduction to qualitative methods in health and health services research', *British Medical Journal*, vol 311, no 6996, pp 42–5.

Rawlins, M.D. and Culyer, A.J. (2004) 'National Institute for Clinical Excellence and its value judgements', *British Medical Journal*, vol 329, pp 224–7.

Robinson, R. and Le Grand, J. (eds) (1993) *Evaluating the NHS reforms*, London: King's Fund.

Roland, M. (2004) 'Linking physician pay to quality of care: a major experiment in the UK', *New England Journal of Medicine*, vol 351, pp 1488–54.

Sackett, D.L., Rosenberg, W.M. et al (1996) 'Evidence based medicine: what it is and what it isn't', *British Medical Journal*, vol 312, no 7023, pp 71–2.

Sackett, D.L., Straus, S., Richardson, W.S., Rosenberg, W. and Haynes, R.B. (2000) *Evidence-based medicine: How to practise and teach EBM,* 2nd edn, Edinburgh: Churchill Livingstone.

Schilling, R.J., Sporton, S.C. et al (2010) 'The NICE guidelines for percutaneous epicardial catheter ablation of ventricular tachycardia: symptomatic of a guideline-obsessed health service?', *Heart*, vol 96, no 3, pp 229–30.

Syrett, K. (2003) 'A technocratic fix to the "legitimacy" problem? The Blair government and health care rationing in the United Kingdom', *Journal of Health Politics, Policy and Law*, vol 28, no 4, pp 715–46.

Wright, J., Reeves, J., Warren, E., Bibby, J., Harrison, S., Dowswell, G., Russell, I.T. and Russell, D. (2003) 'Effectiveness of multifaceted implementation of guidelines in primary care', *Journal of Health Services Research and Policy*, vol 8, no 3, pp 142–8.

eighteen

Accidental logics, Carolyn Hughes Tuohy's analysis of the English National Health Service internal market of the 1990s

Pauline Allen

Background to the introduction and form of the NHS internal market in the 1990s

Since 1948, the British NHS had been a tax-financed healthcare system that is free at the point of delivery to all patients (Webster, 2002). On the establishment of the NHS in 1948, virtually all hospitals had become state owned and all clinical staff (except for general practitioners [GPs]) had become employees of the state. General practitioners remained independent contractors, with a complex system of payment involving a mixture of capitation and incentive payments for carrying out certain health-screening tasks. The contract for paying GPs was negotiated at national level between the government and GP representatives.

In order to understand why the NHS internal market was introduced in the 1990s, it is necessary to explain the broad structure of the NHS prior to that time. One of the important themes in analysing that structure is the degree to which the NHS was a centralised, hierarchical, as opposed to a decentralised and/or market-based system (Allen, 2006). Since its inception, the British NHS has seemed very centralised, compared with other European health systems, such as Germany's (Allen and Riemer Hommel, 2005). When the NHS was set up, it was conceptualised as a national service, replacing the existing local health services. There was central parliamentary accountability, as characterised in the often-quoted remark of Aneurin Bevan (the Minister of Health who was a key political participant in the introduction of the NHS): 'When a bedpan is dropped on a hospital floor its noise should resound in the Palace of Westminster' (Jenkins, 1995, p 65). Funding was also centralised through the use of national insurance payments, distributed to regions by central government, and the aim was to provide a uniform standard of service for all (Klein, 2001). It could certainly be understood as a hierarchical system, as opposed to a market-based one (Allen, 2006), and was characterised as an 'example of a command and control healthcare system' by Moran (1994). Nevertheless, even at this time, there was a clear policy strand, also emanating from Bevan, advocating local decision-making autonomy (Webster, 2002). Furthermore, when it came to the implementation of policies, the command structure became a negotiated order, with power at the periphery (Peckham et al, 2005). The reorganisation of the NHS in 1974 was an attempt to transform it into a national service with national standards (Allsopp, 1995), demonstrating that this degree of centralisation had not in fact been achieved in the period from 1948. The introduction of performance management by the Conservative government under the 'Griffiths reforms' of 1983 can be seen as a further attempt to centralise the NHS (Klein, 2001) (Macfarlane et al, Chapter Nine). However, the concept of 'general management' was introduced at the same time, and this is more equivocal: the new breed of general managers was meant to be responsive to consumers, and to have the autonomy to achieve centrally set goals in the manner they saw fit (Baggott, 2004).

Despite all these organisational changes in the broad structure of the NHS, by the late 1980s there was a general political consensus that there were serious problems in the NHS, mainly concerning the underfunding of the service. There was a groundswell of discontent about the funding of the NHS, as is evidenced by a House of Commons Social Services Select Committee report in 1987 that expressed concern about the funding shortfall. In addition, the three Royal Colleges (interest groups training, regulating and representing medical specialities, such as surgery) made public calls for an increase in funding to the NHS in 1987 (Webster, 2002). Moreover, stories were circulating in the press about cut-backs to services and their adverse effects on patients (Webster, 2002), and there was a nurses' strike in 1988 to protest about this (Butler, 1992). Matters were made worse for the NHS when the then Secretary of State, John Moore, was forced publicly to accept a poor financial settlement from the Treasury for the year 1988/89.

At the same time, in the late 1980s there were political ideas circulating which claimed that decentralised market structures for the NHS would be more effective than retaining centralised hierarchical control. These were in tune with prevailing political opinion under which nationalised industries such as the supply of gas and electricity were being privatised. Initially, proponents suggested that the whole funding basis of the NHS should be changed from national insurance (in effect, general taxation) to a range of private insurers (Webster, 2002). However, the Prime Minister, Margaret Thatcher, realised that this was politically unacceptable and, moreover, the Treasury did not accept the idea of using tax concessions to help fund private insurance contributions. Nevertheless, Mrs Thatcher announced a review of the NHS in 1988. This ruled out funding changes and concentrated on the structure of health services provision instead. The main idea to come out of the review was an internal market for the NHS, which would at least introduce part of the market ideology that Conservative politicians were keen to implement across Britain.

The new organisational policy for the NHS in England was set out in the White Paper *Working for patients* (DH, 1989). The principal reform consisted of the introduction of an internal market for community, secondary and tertiary healthcare by means of a split between the purchasers of care and its providers. There were two categories of purchaser: district health authorities and certain 'fundholding' GPs (fundholders) (Wainwright and Calnan, Chapter Eleven). The remit of the health authorities was to purchase healthcare for their resident population with money that was allocated by central government. No change was made in the source of such money, which was from general taxation, and healthcare continued to be free to all at the point of delivery. Fundholders were given part of the budget for the district health authority in which their practice was located. The providers of healthcare were constituted into entities which were not directly managed by the health authorities. Instead, they were 'self governing trusts' who had a special legal status within the NHS. The trusts had to compete with each other to obtain funds from the purchasers. Thus, a degree of economic incentive was introduced on the provider side, as there was an expectation that if trusts could not obtain sufficient funds from purchasers, they would be forced to cease operation.

The government's reasons for the introduction of the internal market into the NHS were made explicit in *Working for patients* (DH, 1989, pp 4–6). First was the desire to achieve better 'value for money' (DH, 1989, p 5). Proponents of the internal market ideology (such as Enthoven, 1985) contended that technical efficiency was more likely to be achieved in a situation of competition between providers than in a structure (such as a hierarchy) that effectively contained monopoly providers. This was because purchasers in a market could use the threat of exit from their contractual relationships with providers to enforce improvements in performance. Thus, it was thought that competition on the supply side would improve efficiency. Hierarchies, on the other hand, were seen as less likely to promote technical efficiency because of the lack of possibility of exit. In other words, the incentive structures on providers were thought to be weaker in hierarchies (Allen, 2002a).

A second reason given for the introduction of the internal market was that it would stimulate staff and professionals to behave in a more responsive manner in relation to the needs and desires of patients (DH, 1989). A third reason was that patients should be given a greater choice of the services available (DH, 1989). A series of 'key measures' was proposed in *Working for patients* to achieve the preceding objectives. The first of these was the decentralisation of decision making and delegation of authority to the local level.

In order for the internal market to work, it was necessary for purchasers and providers to agree with each other what healthcare should be provided and at what price. It has been argued that, in the context of the delivery of public services, the contractual approach could create a structural bias in favour of the delegation of decision-making authority to accountable and effective units (Harden, 1992). In this way the contract could help the implementation of the 'key measure' of delegating responsibility to local levels. Local knowledge could be used to make explicit and clear choices about local services. It was intended that purchasers of healthcare would undertake strategic planning of services by assessing the needs of their local populations and by translating their aims for individual services and quality standards into contractual specifications. It was argued in *Working for patients* (DH, 1989) that such delegation of contracting power to local organisations would lead to the NHS being more responsive to the needs of patients.

Discussion of the case study of the NHS internal market by Carolyn Hughes Tuohy

Tuohy's book sets out to provide a comparison of the 'dynamics of change in the healthcare arena in USA, Britain and Canada'. This chapter will discuss only her analysis of the British NHS in the 1990s. Tuohy uses a political science approach to look at the structural issues affecting the NHS internal market introduced by Margaret Thatcher in the 1990s. Political science is mainly interested in the wielding of power. Tuohy uses two particular strains of analysis in political science to do this. The first is historical institutionalism and the second is rational choice. The book

> explores the distinctive logics of decision making systems, within which actors respond rationally, to the incentives facing them given the resources they can bring to bear. But it also recognises that the dynamics of change in decision making systems cannot be understood entirely in terms of 'rational choice' of the actors within them. Periodic episodes of policy change establish the parameters of the systems within which the actors make their choices. And those episodes are best understood as products of particular historical contexts. (Tuohy, 1999, p 6)

Thus, rational choice is based on economic theory of how people respond to incentives. Historical institutionalism is concerned with the previous history and experience of a system, and the notion of path dependency. 'Path dependency' is the view that 'specific patterns of timing and sequence matter, ... that particular courses of action, once introduced, can be virtually impossible to reverse; and that consequently political development is punctuated by critical moments or junctures which shape the basic contours of social life' (Pierson, 1997, p 1, quoted in Tuohy, 1999, p 6). Tuohy argues that key features of healthcare systems are 'accidental' in the sense that they were shaped by ideas and agendas in place at the time a window of opportunity was opened by factors in the broader political system.

Tuohy then uses two analytical concepts to look at national health systems. The first is structural dimension. This relates to the balance of influence across key categories of actors. In the case of healthcare, these are the state, private finance and the medical profession. The second is the institutional dimension. This refers to the mix of instruments of social control, namely: hierarchy, market and what she calls collegiality. These two sets of concepts tend to map onto each other in the way set out in Figure 18.1.

Figure 18.1: Mapping of structural and institutional dimensions

Structural dimension	State	Private finance	Professions
Institutional dimensions	Hierarchy	Market	Collegiality

Tuohy argues that change in the policy parameters establishing the structural balance and the institutional mix of a healthcare system requires an extraordinary mobilisation of political authority. This political will is likely to come from outside the healthcare system, from broader political arenas, and is rare. Once the institutional mix and structural balance of the individual healthcare system is established, they 'intersect to generate a distinctive logic that governs the behaviour of participants and the ongoing dynamic of change' (Tuohy, 1999, p 7).

Important elements of the healthcare system to consider when analysing the particular logic of a system are information flows and lines of accountability. In respect of information, the issue is that, although the incentives to use information are greater in markets than in hierarchies or collegiate arrangements, the costs of collecting information are greater too. This is because in markets, the number, variety and independence of sites at which information is held are all greater. But, on the other hand, hierarchical and collegiate systems run the risk of excluding certain information that can be overlooked by normal forms of transmission.

Similarly, Tuohy argues that channels of accountability vary, depending on the institutions. State actors need political support, which leads them to seek to accommodate a range of interests, which gives them an affinity with authority. Private finance must respond to demands of private capital for a rate of return, which leads them to have an affinity with the deployment of wealth. Professionals must maintain standing in their groups, which leads them to have an affinity with skill, as they need to continue to meet the group's standards and norms.

Tuohy considers the origins and challenges to institutional mix and structural balance. She notes that policy episodes where the fundamental institutional mix and structural balance are altered are rare. Mobilisation of political authority is required to upset the balance of forces inside the healthcare arena, and success depends on the durability of forces and the fit between the change proposed and internal logic of the system. System logics depend on the legacy of past episodes of change. Moreover, institutional mixes vary in how they shape actors' behaviour. These derive from how they handle actors' needs for information. Drawing on the transactions costs work of Williamson (1975), Tuohy argues that in healthcare, markets are too costly in information so hierarchies work better. Hierarchies allow for adaptive behaviour and contain stable relationships between actors. She also argues that collegial relationships are important, and implicitly draws on the extensive work about networks and clans exemplified by such authors as Ouchi (1991) and Powell (1991). Unlike the broad reach of hierarchies, collegial arrangements between medical professionals are seen by Tuohy as being suitable only for small groups of professionals who are carrying out forms of peer assessment. The other important theoretical point to note from Tuohy's work is that she sees state hierarchies as more capable of introducing big change than either markets or collegial arrangements. This change is carried out through the chain of command and established channels of communication inherent in hierarchies. But she also notes that delay in implementation is likely.

Now we will turn to Tuohy's analysis of the NHS internal market using the concepts set out earlier. In order to gather data about the NHS internal market, Tuohy drew on both previously published material analysing the NHS and also elite interviews she carried out herself on visits to Britain. The first thing to note is that she sees the introduction of the internal market in the NHS in the 1990s as a rare policy episode involving mobilisation of political authority. In this way, she likens it to the introduction of the NHS itself in 1948. The 1990s were a time in which broader political forces outside the NHS were at work and were able to make significant changes to the NHS system.

What she sees pervading the NHS prior to the introduction of the internal market is the logic of 'hierarchical corporatism' (Tuohy, 1999, p 28). This consisted of strong state control, but with the following additional feature: there was also a strong dimension of collegiality and a strong role for the medical profession. Spheres of authority were based on functional expertise, creating a set of parallel authority structures – some hierarchical and some collegial. These spheres were brought together in hierarchical structures of 'consensus management' which gave effective powers of veto to key functional groups. This gave doctors an effective veto at each level of the organisation. Hospital consultants were not employed by the hospitals where they worked, but instead their contracts were held at regional level.

So they did not report to local managers at all. GPs were self-employed, and their referrals to specialists were determined by professional networks, not administrative rules. Although budgets were set at the top, and then resources allocated downwards, the clinical autonomy of doctors to determine patterns of care was preserved. Thus, although there was heavy influence of state actors and hierarchical control, the doctors were also important players. Mechanisms of control *within* the structures relied on hierarchical lines of accountability on budgetary matters; and upon collegial networks among professionals concerning quality and appropriateness of care. In this way, transaction costs were kept relatively low by the use of mutual understandings. What was not important was the logic of the market.

Tuohy notes that in the late 1980s a rare window of opportunity for institutional and structural change opened when the Conservatives won their third successive electoral victory. There was an ideological tide in broader political society which made it possible to introduce ideas of markets into public services in Britain. Nevertheless, Tuohy argues that the implementation of the details of the Conservatives' reform was very much shaped by and incorporated into the characteristics of the existing system. In other words, the hierarchical aspects of the NHS were still very important. What she sees happening is that the logic of the market clashed with the existing hierarchical corporatism of the NHS. The political intervention from outside the healthcare arena did not go with the flow of the corporatist system. She observes that formal modes of relationships changed with the purchaser–provider split, as contracts were introduced and a degree of competition encouraged on the supply side. Nevertheless, she sees that informal networks and modes of relations persisted, as the internal market was socially embedded in relationships. Faced with the high information and other transaction costs of writing and enforcing contracts for healthcare, purchasers and providers were drawn to stable forms of relationships that reduced the need for specificity in contracting. (These contracts can be seen as relational, using Macneil's terminology – Macneil, 1978.) She sees that the market incentives introduced were weak. The contracts were for 'blocks' of care, akin to passing over a budget to the provider, rather than operating as an incentive for providers to produce more care to be paid more. (One advantage of these block contracts was to substantially reduce transactions costs, however.) Tuohy notes that there was, in fact, only a limited degree of competition between providers, so that this did not produce any serious incentives. Although the hierarchical relationship between health authorities and provider units was tempered by market elements, the low levels of competition between providers meant that the internal market did not transform authority relationships into relationships of voluntary exchange.

Tuohy also sees that the clinical arena was preserved as 'a zone of collegial decision making' (1999, p 197). One aspect of this was the introduction of clinical audit, to be carried out by clinical, not managerial staff. Managers did not make great incursions into medical spheres. They instead consolidated their authority over budgetary processes and financial management. But she notes that one aspect of collegial relationships between doctors was affected by the internal market. This was because of the introduction of fundholding. This produced a cash nexus between consultants and GP fundholders, because fundholders, being smaller purchasers, could actually switch their patients to different hospital providers. Tuohy points out that the introduction of the internal market did not lead to significant gains for the private sector, in terms of either finance or provision. Finally, she notes that managerial behaviour was in fact still regulated through the hierarchy, and not decentralised to any large degree as the market had promised. The numbers of central directives and 'guidances' are evidence of this. The balance of centralisation and decentralisation may have changed in a different way, however: Tuohy argues that, at local level, district managers lost some authority upwards to the centre, as regional health authorities were replaced by regional offices of the NHS itself; and downwards to the NHS trusts, which were accountable through a separate bureaucratic line to other parts of the NHS hierarchy.

Thus, an institutional mix in which hierarchy and collegiality were dominant survived the introduction of what should have been a market logic. The market was institutionally embedded in a hierarchical system. The end result was that there was little change in the structural balance between state, medical profession and private finance. It should be noted that the considerable power of politicians within the system had changed little, despite the rhetoric of decentralised market decision making. Tuohy points out that the establishment of the internal market was 'above all an act of public policy ... for which politicians were accountable, and in whose consequences they continued to intervene' (1999, p 199).

Tuohy's explanation for this lack of change in the balance of the actors in the British NHS lies in the logic of agency. The introduction of the internal market was an attempt to make the responsibility of the actors (both medical and managerial) clearer, by requiring them to bargain with each other and monitor compliance, using the contracts made. But in practice, old patterns of relationships proved resilient. Tuohy asserts that this resilience was derived from the centrality of trust-based relationships in the functioning of the system. The obvious forms of these relationships were the collegial networks between professionals and the agency relationships between doctors and managers that had developed in the NHS. But stability was also provided by hierarchical forms, which allowed trust to develop between managers too. Thus, Tuohy analyses the British NHS internal market as being institutionally embedded in a hierarchical regulatory system and also socially embedded in networks of relationships. She points out that persistence of pre-internal market forms is due to not only habitual ties: they may also be rational. Where there were budgetary uncertainty and deep reservations about the adequacy of data, modes of relationship which avoided the need for costly information were attractive.

Reflections on contemporary relevance of the case study

Tuohy provides a very useful analytical framework to deal with analysis of policy change and continuity. She makes good use of both institutional analysis and rational choice concepts. The mixture of understanding the importance of path dependency in policy change, at the same time as understanding economic theory concerning incentives and the importance of minimising costs is very useful. Other studies broadly confirm her analysis. Although the government did not fund any large-scale evaluations of the internal market, there is evidence to indicate that it was not entirely successful (Allen, 2009). Research concerning efficiency in the internal market does not provide any convincing evidence that efficiency was, in fact, improved by the introduction of the new structures (Le Grand et al, 1998). Responsiveness and choice for patients were not significantly improved. Institutions (health authorities and fundholders) were the purchasers, acting as agents for patients. Studies find that incentives operating on purchasers did not have the effect of aligning purchasers' goals with those of patients (Propper, 1995; Flood, 1997; Fotaki, 1998; Le Grand et al, 1998; Enthoven, 1999; Allen, 2002a). One of the reasons researchers have identified for this lack of success was that the incentives to behave in market-like ways were not strong enough and the hierarchical elements of the NHS continued to exercise control (Enthoven, 1999; Allen, 2002b). The lessons learned from this type of analysis vary. Rather than understanding the institutional issues, the more common political and academic view has been that markets *must* work, and that the lack of strong incentives was the problem.

Following the Tories' NHS internal market, since 1997 New Labour has had two main policy phases (see also Paton, Chapter Sixteen). First, an initial re-emphasis on hierarchy (using targets). This, arguably, follows the logics of existing NHS structures, although there is some evidence of encroachment into collegiality. The latter was precipitated by a series of scandals about the weakness of medical self-regulation, such as the excess number of deaths of infant cardiac surgery patients in Bristol (Smith, 1998). The early indications following New Labour's election victory in May 1997 were that, despite a softening of the rhetoric about competition and markets, there would be a continuing commitment to the purchaser–provider split (Allen, 2002b). After an initial period when the New Labour government emphasised the need for purchasers and providers to cooperate within a re-integrated public service, a series of new policy initiatives started moving towards a more overtly marketised system. Attempts to focus on standards and modernisation coupled with the use of centrally defined targets and performance management were tried, but, especially after the general election in 2001, an increased emphasis on markets and choice appeared (Hughes and Vincent-Jones, 2008). This second phase of structural reforms in the NHS can be seen as a response to what is perceived as the failure of the hierarchical model in the early New Labour years, combined with a particular form of learning from the deficiencies of the Conservatives' internal market of the 1990s. The notion of markets as a core mechanism for improving public services, and health services in particular, has not been abandoned. Indeed, the objectives of the internal market of the 1990s started to be re-articulated through a set of more radical restructuring reforms under New Labour. The New Labour government tried to take account of the failures of the internal market structures, particularly in relation to motivation and incentives on the supply side. The re-emphasis on markets as a motor for improvement was encapsulated in 'four inter-related pillars of reform' which 'are designed to embed incentives for continuous and self sustaining improvement' and produce 'better quality, better patient experience, better value for money and reduced inequality' (DH, 2005). These were:

1. Demand side reform – more choice and a stronger voice for patients;
2. Transactional reform – money following patients, rewarding the best and most efficient providers, giving others the incentive to improve;
3. System management and regulation – a framework of system management, regulation and decision making which guarantees safety and quality, fairness and equity; and
4. Supply side reform – more diverse providers, with more freedom to innovate and improve services. (DH, 2005)

(For details of these mechanisms, and how they interrelate, see Allen, 2009.)

Arguably, these policies were 'going against the grain' in Tuohy's conception of the NHS, as they were pushing the role of markets further, and trying to lessen the effect of hierarchy. But, these policies also sat side by side with other pre-existing elements. Despite the increase in market-like elements in the NHS, under New Labour there were still many hierarchical corporatist elements coexisting with them. The targets introduced in the early New Labour period from 1997 continued. The most salient of these hierarchical policies was the fact that each year an operating framework was issued to the NHS by the Department of Health setting out annual priorities for the whole system to follow (for example, DH, 2004). All NHS hospitals were required to return data to the centre about the extent to which they met national targets. Further examples of central control included the introduction of a standard form of contract to be used in the market regime (thus somewhat undermining the notion of a market as involving the devolution of power from the centre) and actual direct planning of services, such as the reconfiguration of health services in London (Healthcare for London, 2007). Thus, Tuohy's conceptual model and empirical analysis may well still be valid for the second internal market of the new millennium. (Since this chapter was written, a new Coalition government has taken power and increased the emphasis on markets in the NHS [see Health and Social Care Bill 2011].)

Summary points

- The structure of any particular healthcare system is context and path dependent.
- The interrelationships between different interest groups (such as the state, private finance and the medical profession) and between different institutions (such as the market, hierarchy and professional networks) are vital to understanding a healthcare system.
- The NHS in England is strongly influenced by the state and its hierarchical structures, despite the attempt to introduce market elements in the 1990s and again in the 2000s.

References

Allen, P. (2002a) 'A socio-legal and economic analysis of contracting in the NHS internal market using a case study of contracting for district nursing', *Social Science and Medicine*, vol 54, no 2, pp 255–66.

Allen, P. (2002b) 'Plus ça change, plus c'est la même chose: to the internal market and back in the British National Health Service', *Applied Health Economics and Health Policy*, vol 1, no 4, pp 171–8.

Allen, P. (2006) 'New localism in the English NHS: what is it for?', *Health Policy*, vol 79, pp 244–52.

Allen, P. (2009) 'Restructuring the NHS again: supply side reform in recent English Healthcare policy', *Financial Accountability and Management*, vol 25, no 4, pp 343–89.

Allen, P. and Riemer Hommel, P. (2005) 'What are third way governments learning? Health care consumers and quality in England and Germany', *Health Policy*, vol 76, no 2, pp 202–12.

Allsopp, J. (1995) *Health policy and the NHS*, 2nd edn, Harlow: Longman.

Baggott, R. (2004) *Health and health care in Britain*, 3rd edn, Basingstoke: Palgrave Macmillan.

Butler, J. (1992) *Patients, policies and politics*, Buckingham: Open University Press.

DH (Department of Health) (1989) *Working for patients; the health service in the 1990s*, Cm 555, London: HMSO.

DH (2004) *Planning and priorities framework: National standards local action*, London: DH.

DH (2005) *Creating a patient led NHS: Delivering the NHS Improvement Plan*, London: DH.

Enthoven, A. (1985) *Reflections on the management of the National Health Service*, Occasional Paper 5, London: Nuffield Provincial Hospitals Trust.

Enthoven, A. (1999) *In pursuit of an improving National Health Service*, London: Nuffield Trust.

Flood, C. (1997) 'Accountability of health service purchasers: comparing internal markets and managed competition reform models', *Dalhousie Law Journal*, vol 20, no 2, pp 470–531.

Fotaki, M. (1998) 'The impact of market orientated reforms on choice and information: a case study of cataract surgery in outer London and Stockholm', *Social Science and Medicine*, vol 48, pp 1415–32.

Harden, I. (1992) *The contracting state*, Buckingham: Open University Press.

Health and Social Care Bill (2011) www.publications.parliament.uk/pa/bills/cbill/2010-2012/0221/cbill_2010-20120221_en_1.htm.

Healthcare for London (2007) *A framework for action*, London: Healthcare for London.

Hughes, D. and Vincent-Jones, P. (2008) 'Schisms in the church: NHS systems and institutional divergence in England and Wales', *Journal of Health and Social Behavior*, vol 49, pp 400–16.

Jenkins, S. (1995) *Accountable to none: The Tory nationalization of Britain*, London: Hamilton.

Klein, R. (2001) *The new politics of the NHS*, 4th edn, Harlow: Pearson.

Le Grand, J., Mays, N. and Mulligan, J. (eds) (1998) *Learning from the NHS internal market: A review of the evidence*, London: King's Fund.

Macneil, I. (1978) 'Contracts: adjustment of long-term economic relations under classical, neoclassical and relational contract law', *Northwestern University Law Review*, vol 72, no 6, pp 854–905.

Moran, M. (1994) 'Reshaping the healthcare state', *Government and Opposition*, vol 29, no 1, pp 48–62.

Ouchi, W. (1991) 'Markets, bureaucracies and clans', in G. Thompson, J. Frances, R. Levacic and J. Mitchell (eds) *Markets, hierarchies and networks: The co-ordination of social life*, London: Open University Press and SAGE Publications.

Peckham, S., Exworthy, M., Powell, M. and Greener, I. (2005) *Decentralisation, centralisation and devolution in publicly funded health services*, London: NHS Service Delivery and Organisation R&D Programme.

Pierson, P. (1997) *Path dependence, increasing returns, and the study of politics*, Cambridge, MA: Harvard University Center for European Studies.

Powell, W. (1991) 'Neither market nor hierarchy', in G. Thompson, J. Frances, R. Levacic and J. Mitchell (eds) *Markets, hierarchies and networks*, London: Open University Press and SAGE.

Propper, C. (1995), 'Agency and incentives in the NHS internal market', *Social Science and Medicine*, vol 40, no 12, pp 1683–90.

Smith, R. (1998) 'All changed, utterly changed', *British Medical Journal*, vol 316, pp 1917–18.

Tuohy, C. (1999) *Accidental logics. The dynamics of change in the health care arena in the United States, Britain and Canada*, Oxford: Oxford University Press.

Webster, C. (2002) *The National Health Service: A political history*, 2nd edn, Oxford: Oxford University Press.

Williamson, O. (1975) *Markets and hierarchies: Analysis and anti trust implications*, New York: The Free Press.

nineteen

Evidence and health inequalities: the Black, Acheson and Marmot Reports

Mark Exworthy and Adam Oliver

Introduction

Health inequalities have long been totemic of the way in which public policy has addressed complex, 'wicked' issues (Graham, 2009; Exworthy and Hunter, 2011). These inequalities reflect the persistent and systemic variations in the social determinants of health, access to care, service provision and health status. Such inequalities are stratified by socio-economic status, education, gender, ethnicity, *inter alia*. Health inequalities have long been recognised as a 'policy problem', dating beyond the inception of the NHS in Britain to the work of, among others, Edwin Chadwick in the 19th century (Lewis, 1952).

At periodic moments in the NHS, inquiries have been held to synthesise extant evidence about health inequalities and to make recommendations for their alleviation (cf Higgins, Chapter Six). The focus of health inequalities in this chapter also gives an insight into the dramatic rise in the volume and extent of studies examining the translation of evidence into policy. The emphasis on evidence-based policy reflects a belief in a progressive approach to policy making (Oliver and Exworthy, 2003; Exworthy et al, 2006). Ensuring that policy is rooted in evidence about 'what works' is increasingly important for the 'effective governance of complex social systems', a crucial component of which, Sanderson (2002) argues, is 'reflexive social learning' (p 1). However, as Macintyre and colleagues (2001) note, there is often little or no evidence to guide policy development regarding health inequalities. Thus, we do not always know what works or why (Asthana and Halliday, 2006); policy making remains shrouded by uncertainty (Klein, 2002).

Policy learning often takes place through the medium of reports and documents. This is especially relevant in the case of public health, where research communities have invariably sought to influence policy objectives and processes. The interface between research and policy illustrates the ways in which research evidence is (or is not) translated into policy, and documents are one way of exercising the 'politics of health equity' (Freeman,

2006, p 51). These inquiry reports are important not simply because they gather and synthesise evidence but also because of the ways in which they been produced, the messages they convey and the assumptions they embody (Freeman, 2006, p 51). Since randomised controlled trials offer little insight into social interventions related to tackling health inequalities, the relationship between research and policy becomes even more critical (Elliott and Popay, 2000; Macintyre et al, 2001; Petticrew et al, 2004).

So, what does this evidence deficit tell us about public health, and how can such lessons be applied to tackling health inequalities? What are the limitations of translating evidence – of various kinds – into policy and everyday practice? We analyse these questions in relation to the impact of inquiries upon policy.

Impact of inquiries upon policy

Over the past 30 years, three seminal inquiries have been held – producing the Black Report (Black et al, 1980), the Acheson Report (1998) and the Marmot Report (2010). The name of the report refers to the inquiry's chair. In this chapter, we take these three reports as case studies. The cases are illustrations of the ways in which health inequalities have been variously defined, framed and tackled. The cases also consider the policy responses to such revelations of the 'problem'. Individually, they are mini-case studies, separated by 18 and 12 years respectively. However, we also consider the extent to which each builds on the previous one, synthesising extant knowledge.

> Any policy discussion of how to improve public health in general or how to influence the social distribution of health will be strongly influenced by prevailing ideas about what generates health and health inequalities. (Vagero and Illsley, 1995, p 219)

These 'prevailing ideas' have often been shaped by previous inquiry report(s).

For each report, we consider the policy background, the evidence and the policy impact. We review the primary arguments in each report, emphasising the socio-political context and recommendations, and noting the continuities and discontinuities between them. We explore the extent to which these inquiries reinvent the 'policy problem' through the compilation, synthesis and interpretation of evidence. Finally, we consider the impact of such evidence upon the policy process by applying analytical models.

The Black Report (1980)

Background

In an open letter to the magazine *New Society*, in the mid-1970s, Richard Wilkinson urged the Secretary of State for Social Services, David Ennals, to commission an inquiry to examine health inequalities, as inequalities in death rates by social class were then at their greatest since records began. Wilkinson recommended that remedial action should be taken. Ennals was not persuaded but subsequently changed his mind, in part as a result of the influence of his adviser, Brian Abel-Smith. In March 1977, Ennals noted that socio-economic differentials in health had widened since the inception of the welfare state. He announced that he was commissioning an independent inquiry into inequalities, to be chaired by Sir Douglas Black, then Chief Scientist at the Department of Health and Social Security. Abel-Smith was also the key player in recommending to Ennals to appoint to the committee figures such as the sociologist Peter Townsend and the epidemiologist Jerry Morris, colleagues who had shared his long-standing concern with inequalities in health.

The Black Report was released in 1980. It focused on evidence of the decades preceding the mid-1970s. It presented evidence of the poorer health experience of lower occupational groups at all ages, and that the difference between the lower and higher occupational groups was widening. The widening gap was attributed to social class inequalities in the social determinants of health. The Report argued that the healthcare services had a marginal effect in causing these inequalities, and made recommendations such as increases in child benefits, maternity grants, infant care allowances, disabled benefit allowances, sheltered housing and home improvement grants. It also argued for emphasis on prevention and primary healthcare.

By the time of its publication, there had been a change of government. The new Conservative government did not implement the findings of the Black Report, and indeed attempted to suppress its dissemination. Its release was scheduled for the August Bank Holiday, with only 260 copies being made available, which, it may have been hoped, would minimise interest in the report. In response, the authors held their own press conference. Media interest was thus sparked.

Evidence

The Black Report found large differences in morbidity and mortality between social classes, and that health services did not remedy such inequalities (Smith et al, 1990, p 373). It presented four explanations of health inequalities:

- artefactual explanations
- natural or social selection
- materialist or structuralist explanations and
- cultural or behavioural explanations.

However, the Black Report did not contain any discussion or review of research that would naturally lead to such conclusions (Vagero and Illsely, 1995; also Freeman, 2006). Nonetheless, Vagero and Illsely continue, these explanations came to dominate 'thinking, arguments and reviews' (1995, p 220) on health inequalities. The Report framed the 'problem' of health inequalities as 'an issue of the socio-economic determinants of morbidity and mortality rather than one of access to health services' (Freeman, 2006, p 60) and concluded that the weight of evidence pointed towards material factors for health inequalities.

Policy impact

To some extent, the Black Report has achieved its 'seminal status' (Freeman, 2006, p 52) and acquired its 'enormous symbolism' (Berridge, 2003, p 10) by virtue of its reception by the Conservative government. Arguably, it is best remembered in terms of the 'suppression of a politically sensitive report' (Berridge, 2003, p 10).

The Report was submitted in 1980 to the newly elected Conservative government, who rejected it on three counts: (i) the recommendations were too costly, (ii) there was political antipathy to tackling health inequalities through public policy and (iii) there was no evidence that the recommendations would work. (It was also acknowledged that the report was a 'difficult read' [Buller, quoted in Berridge and Blume, 2002, p 157; also Freeman, 2006, p 62].) The then Secretary of State, Patrick Jenkin, rejected the premise of the report:

> It will be seen that the Group has reached the view that the causes of health inequalities are so deep-rooted that only a major and wide-ranging programme of public expenditure is capable of altering this pattern ... I cannot ... endorse the Group's recommendation. I am making the report available for discussion but without any commitment by the government to its proposals. (Jenkin, 1980)

The authors of the Black Report denied that the costs were as high as Jenkin had intimated (Black et al, 1999).

Nonetheless, Richmond (2002) claims that the report had a 'huge impact on political thought' internationally. It prompted an Organisation for

Economic Co-operation and Development assessment of health inequalities in 13 countries, in sharp contrast to its reception in the UK.

The Black Report had no impact on UK policy for more than a decade (Smith et al, 1990; Berridge and Blume, 2002), and so it heralded a period of policy inaction during the 1980s and the early 1990s. Individual behavioural approaches dominated health policy during this period and none was framed in terms of health inequalities. However, the Black Report defined the agenda and stimulated further research into health inequalities in the 1980s:

> Most academic writing on health inequalities has subsequently tended to adopt its [Black Report] agenda, questions, concepts and definitions … (Vagero and Illsley, 1995, p 219)

For example, the *Health Divide* (Whitehead, 1987) updated much of the Black Report's analysis. Ten years after the publication of the report, Smith et al (1990) concluded that research evidence had provided a fuller picture of health inequalities (p 373). However, such new evidence offered little insight into strategies to reduce those inequalities.

By the early 1990s, signs of a policy shift were apparent in the publication of the *Health of the Nation* (DH, 1992). Although this consultation document did include 27 targets in areas of public health, they were not framed in ways that address inequalities (Harrison and McDonald, 2008, p 162). The shift in policy was perhaps most obvious in its use of the term 'health variations' (cf health inequalities), which, at best, denoted a neutral political stance. The policy shift in the 1990s was also evident in the research agenda. The Department of Health commissioned the University of York to examine the effectiveness of interventions to address health variations (Arblaster et al, 1995) and the ESRC commissioned a 'Health Variations Programme', directed by Professor Hilary Graham (www.lancs.ac.uk/fass/apsocsci/hvp/default.htm).

The Black Report was also significant for the way in which it was conducted and its relationship to policy makers. The research working group, Black himself claimed, was more concerned with 'getting it absolutely right with the long-term rather than with any political deadline' (Berridge, 2003, p 11). This approach differed from that of the civil servants who, cognisant of political timetables, did much to obstruct the publication of the Black Report.

The Acheson Report (1998)

The Labour Party resolved to engage with the issue of health inequalities on its return to government, but this was not to be until 1997. One of the first decisions that it took was to commission an 'independent inquiry' into inequalities in health, chaired by the former Chief Medical Officer, Sir Donald Acheson.

The Acheson Report was much less polished than the Black Report, possibly because the inquiry team was given only one year in which to complete its work. By presenting evidence up to the 1990s, the Acheson Report started from where the Black Report left off, and the former was an updated if less dense version of the latter (Exworthy, 2002). The Acheson Report concluded that socio-economic inequalities in health remained a significant problem. It made 39 recommendations that extended across the social determinants of health, with only three referring to healthcare services. The Report also transcended health inequalities by social class and income by looking at these across groups defined by, for example, level of education, gender and race.

Background

Although the independent inquiry commissioned in July 1997 was chaired by the former Chief Medical Officer, Sir Donald Acheson, it has been termed the 'second *Black Report*' (Exworthy, 2002) and a 'successor' to the Black Report (Freeman, 2006; see also Macintyre, 1997; Evans, 2002). Indeed, Smith et al (1998) specifically refer to the Black Report as the primary antecedent of the Acheson Report.

The inquiry team was asked to 'moderate a Department of Health review of the latest available information on inequalities of health' and 'to conduct – within the broad framework of the Government's overall financial strategy – an independent review to identify priority areas for future policy development, which scientific and expert evidence indicates are likely to offer opportunities for Government to develop beneficial, cost effective and affordable interventions to reduce health inequalities' (www.archive. official-documents.co.uk/document/doh/ih/anxb.htm).

Evidence

The inquiry amassed evidence of health inequalities across areas including poverty, education, employment and social groups including mothers, children and families, young people, older people, as well as gender and ethnicity. The Report ran to 164 pages (with 529 references), but only nine pages were devoted to the NHS. It made 39 main recommendations, three of which were claimed to be 'crucial', namely:

• 'All policies likely to have an impact on health should be evaluated in terms of their impact on health inequalities'

- 'A high priority should be given to the health of families with children', and
- 'Further steps should be taken to reduce income inequalities and improve the living standards of poor households' (p xi).

Overall, it is debatable how far these recommendations did offer 'opportunities for Government to develop … interventions to reduce health inequalities' (which the terms of reference sought). The Report made only three recommendations on healthcare, denoting its perceived contribution to tackling health inequalities (Exworthy et al, 2003, p 1909). Birch (1999) noted that 'the 39 steps [recommendations] for policy direction are remarkably similar in scope and content to the recommendations of the *Black Report*'.

Policy impact

As it is now over 12 years since its publication, it is possible to discern the short-term and long-term impact of the Acheson Report. Initially, the report was 'welcomed' by the government, which noted that it was already implementing some of the initiatives that the report would later recommend (DH, 1998).

> The outline of some of the most important policy developments was beginning to take shape by the time the Acheson report was published. (DH, 2009, p 9)

The report may thus have served the purpose of 'buying' the government more time to develop policy in this field. Also, academics and practitioners generally welcomed the report (including the authors of the Black Report [Black et al, 1999]), although this was not universal (for example, Birch, 1999).

Exworthy et al (2003) concluded that most of the inquiry's recommendations were associated with new or adapted policies (p 1910). They appraised the influence of the Acheson Report upon policy in four ways:

- it prompted new policies to tackle health inequalities
- it introduced a health inequality dimension to existing policies
- it encouraged or contributed to a climate of opinion in favour of tackling health inequalities
- it acted as a source-book or reference against which policies are examined and tested.

Exworthy (2002) explains that the Acheson Report has become something of a 'source-book ... part of the folk psychology by which some practitioners make decisions *apparently* based on evidence' (p 185).

It is difficult to ascertain the policy initiatives that were specifically informed by the Acheson Report, not least because the government would probably have introduced some policy initiatives that were consistent with the report even if it had not been written (Macintyre, 1997). Thus, in some cases, the report served to provide added justification for existing and impending policy initiatives. Nonetheless, one cannot deny that the Acheson Report had an influence: addressing health inequalities became a central part of the government's health policy rhetoric, and the report and its three crucial recommendations were cited in several official policy documents. Some potential policies (such as income redistribution) were not included in the Acheson Report or subsequent government policy (Pickett and Dorling, 2010).

Despite a generally positive reception, the critiques of the report fell into five areas (Exworthy et al, 2003):

1. *No priorities.* Illsley (1999) argued that the recommendations apparently carried equal weight, implying that the recommendations were a 'shopping-list', but Acheson (1998b) claimed that the first three recommendations were 'crucial'. They were, however, vague and general in nature.
2. *No mechanisms.* The policy mechanisms to translate recommendations into action were, it was argued, absent. Illsley (1999) described the recommendations as 'politically naive'. Yet, the inquiry's terms of reference did not specify targets, seeking only contributions 'to the development of a new strategy for health' and 'within the Government's overall financial strategy' (Acheson, 1998a, p iv). This remit was criticised by some practitioners (Macintyre, 1997).
3. *Evidence–policy mismatch.* Klein (2000) argued that the evidence that the report cited was poorly associated with some recommendations, a conclusion which echoes criticism of the Black Report. While some evidence did prompt specific recommendations (such as water fluoridation [Smith, 2001]), other evidence appeared weaker (for example, income inequality, Birch, 1999). The lack or weakness of evidence from 'well controlled studies designed to assess the effects of interventions on health inequalities' was not seen as an excuse for inaction (Macintyre et al, 2001). Also, many of the recommendations were really addressed to general health improvements, rather than reduction of inequalities.
4. *Specificity of recommendations.* Some recommendations (such as high priority to the health of families with children, or policies to reduce the fear of crime) were, according to some, too vague for policy makers (Smith

et al, 1998; Evans, 2002). However, other recommendations (such as 'fluoridation or the water supply') were considered too specific.

5. *Cost-effectiveness.* The paucity of evidence concerning the cost-effectiveness of policies to tackle health inequalities concerned some (Williams, 1999; Oliver, 2001). Although the terms of reference sought recommendations which were 'affordable', the inquiry team did not include a (health) economist. The Black Report was similarly rejected on the grounds that recommendations were too costly.

In its first term, the Labour government implemented a plethora of policies including (*inter alia*) the minimum wage, the 'New Deal' to assist the young and long-term unemployed into work, a 'Strategy for Neighbourhood Renewal' of run-down areas, 'Health Action Zones', 'Sure Start' and a fuel poverty strategy. With so many concurrent policies, there is inevitably an attribution problem: it is virtually impossible to separate the effect that each policy initiative has had on inequalities in health.

In February 2001, the then Secretary of State for Health, Alan Milburn, announced two health inequalities targets, the first time that such targets had been set in England. (The Acheson Report had not, however, recommended these [Marmot, 1999].) They were as follows:

1. By 2010 to reduce by at least 10% the gap in infant mortality between those engaged in manual work and the population as a whole.
2. By 2010 to reduce by at least 10% the gap between the fifth of areas with the lowest life expectancy at birth and the population as a whole.

Specifically, in relation to the life expectancy target, the Labour government identified the fifth of local authority areas with the poorest health indicators and categorised these authorities as the 'spearhead group'. Such areas, which comprise 28% of the population of England, are those in the bottom fifth nationally on three of the following five measures:

1. Male life expectancy at birth
2. Female life expectancy at birth
3. Cancer mortality rate for those aged under 75 years
4. Cardiovascular mortality rate for those aged under 75 years
5. Index of multiple deprivation.

The Acheson Report seems to have had an enduring effect on policy development in England. Freeman (2006) charts the report's influence across several official policy documents. It was claimed (mainly by the Department of Health itself) that the Acheson Report influenced or informed the following policy developments:

- White Paper on public health (DH, 1999a)
- action report on reducing health inequalities (DH, 1999b)
- NHS Plan (DH, 2000)
- national health inequalities targets
- public service agreements (DH, 2002) and
- consultation process on tackling health inequalities (DH, 2002).

Indeed, in an era of evidence-based policy, such evidential claims are necessary justifications for policy developments, irrespective of their actual impact. The plethora of reports and updates published in the years following the Acheson Report does not, of course, guarantee that Acheson's recommendations were specifically adopted.

During the Labour government's second term of office (2001–05), a notable shift in the focus of health policy was apparent. This shift comprised a reassertion of healthcare as the 'centre of gravity' in the Department of Health. Healthcare services (and especially the NHS), for example, became a more central agent in tackling health inequalities than hitherto. This development may have been more about NHS 'modernisation' than health inequalities and is most evident in *From vision to reality* (Department of Health, 2001). It presented 'progress' since Acheson and proposed a strategy for development. It referred to the Acheson Report but also drew heavily on the 'modernizing project' of the NHS Plan (Freeman, 2006).

At the same time, a cross-cutting review (led by the Treasury) was published in November 2002 (DH, 2002b) and reinforced by the Department of Health's *Programme for Action* (DH, 2003). The latter report cited the Acheson Report 10 times in 80 pages, 'for the most part to buttress the government's plans by reference to research' (Freeman, 2006, pp 63–4).

Subsequently, the Department of Health (2008) claimed that its 2003 *Programme for action* 'built on the work' of the Acheson Report (p 14). Indeed, Michael Marmot (writing the preface to this Department of Health document) claims that the influence of the Acheson Report 'conforms rather well to evidence-based policy-making' because its 'recommendations [were] a base to formulate policies' (p 5). More recently still, the Department of Health (2009) claims that its decennial review of health inequalities summarises developments in health inequalities 'from the publication of the *Acheson Report* on health inequalities in November 1998 to the announcement of the post-2010 strategic review of health inequalities in November 2008 [the Marmot Review; see below]' (www.dh.gov.uk/en/Publicationsandstatistics/Publications/PublicationsPolicyAndGuidance/DH_098936). In citing the Acheson Report 109 times in 140 pages, it claims that the report has been 'a cornerstone for action on health inequalities' (p 5).

However, such stated impacts of the Acheson Report may be at odds with its impact on practice because, as Exworthy et al (2003) suggest, some of the Acheson recommendations would have been implemented anyway, and many other policies did not seem to have been influenced by the recommendations or the intent of the report. Moreover, given the weak evidence–policy link, Department of Health claims of attribution to the Acheson Report may seem somewhat tendentious. In sum, claims that policy has been influenced by the report do not guarantee that policy will be implemented or indeed tackle health inequalities.

The Marmot Review (2009)

Background

The World Health Organisation's global Commission on the Social Determinants of Health (chaired by Professor Sir Michael Marmot) published its findings in 2008 and recommended that national government policy should adapt to the context of each country. In November 2008, the Department of Health commissioned a review (also chaired by Marmot) as 'a response to that recommendation and to the government's commitment to reducing health inequalities in England' (another report rather than action?) (www.ucl.ac.uk/gheg/marmotreview). The intention was to shape policy beyond 2010, when the then-current national targets for reducing health inequalities expired. Critics might claim that more action, rather than another review, was needed at this stage. The review may have been prompted because policies (recommended by Acheson) had not been implemented, the 'right' policies were not implemented (possibly because of a weak evidence base) and/or it was too soon to gauge the policy impacts. For example, evidence suggests that these targets have not been met (Table 19.1).

Table 19.1: National health inequality targets: evidence of progress?

	England	Spearhead areas	Difference
	Life expectancy, years	Life expectancy, years	%
Men			
1994–95	74.6	72.7	2.57%
2004–06	77.3	75.3	2.63%
Women			
1994–95	79.7	78.3	1.77%
2004–06	81.6	80.0	1.96%

Source: DH (2007)

The Marmot Review had four objectives:

1. '[T]o identify, for the health inequalities challenge facing England, the evidence most relevant to underpinning future policy and action'
2. '[T]o show how this evidence could be translated into practice'
3. '[T]to advise on possible objectives and measures, building on the experience of the current Public Service Agreement target on infant mortality and life expectancy'
4. '[T]o publish a report of the review's work that will contribute to the development of a post-2010 health inequalities strategy'.

Evidence

The collection, synthesis and interpretation of evidence were arguably more extensive than the Acheson Report, some 10 years earlier. A wide network of academics and others were involved in the process through 'Commissioners', 'Working Committees' and 'Task Groups', based on nine themes. These themes are similar to those of the Acheson Report (such as social groups, and topics such as education and employment). However, they also incorporated several new ones, such as 'built environment', 'sustainable development' and 'economics'. The former was not included in the previous reports and the latter was criticised for its omission in the Acheson Report.

Recommendations were grouped into the categories listed in Table 19.2, which did not necessarily match the thematic approach taken during its deliberations. The report made 20 recommendations across six main categories (Table 19.2).

However, it was also supplemented by 161 recommendations that were proposed in none of the groups. There was some duplication of recommendations between categories.

The agenda set by the Black and Acheson reports is apparent in the Marmot recommendations. It is therefore instructive to compare the (initial) reaction and analysis to the Marmot Review's report with the criticisms of the Acheson Report, some 12 years previous. To what extent did the Marmot Report address concerns that had been previously raised?

1. *No priorities.* The Marmot Report does not prioritise recommendations and indeed, with 161 recommendations, this may make implementation problematic.
2. *No mechanisms.* There appears to be more recognition of the mechanisms than in the Black or Acheson Reports, through the theme that addressed delivery systems and mechanisms. The Marmot Report also reflects the performance culture that has dominated the period since the Acheson Report (Greener, 2003). It adopts a technocratic approach by outlining,

Table 19.2: Marmot Report: policy objectives and recommendations

Policy objective	Recommendations
A: Give every child the best start in life	• Increased investment in early years • Supporting families to develop children's skills • Quality early years education and childcare
B: Enable all children, young people and adults to maximise their capabilities and have control over their lives	• Reduce the social gradient in educational outcomes • Reduce the social gradient in life-skills • Ongoing skills development through lifelong learning
C: Create fair employment and good work for all	• Active labour market programmes • Development of good quality work • Reducing physical and chemical hazards and injuries at work • Shift work and other work-time factors • Improving the psychosocial work environment
D: Ensure healthy standard of living for all	• Implement a minimum income for healthy living • Remove 'cliff edges' for those moving in and out of work and improve flexibility of employment • Review and implement systems of taxation, benefits, pensions and tax credits
E: Create and develop healthy and sustainable places and communities	• Prioritise policies and interventions that reduce health inequalities and mitigate climate change • Integrate planning, transport, housing and health policies to address the social determinants of health • Create and develop communities
F: Strengthen the role and impact of ill-health prevention	• Increased investment in prevention • Implement evidence-based ill-health preventive interventions • Public health to focus interventions to reduce the social gradient

Source: Marmot (2010, pp 94–148)

for each recommendation, the delivery mechanisms and interventions, process indicators, output indicators, outcome indicators and the responsible delivery agencies.

3. *Evidence–policy mismatch.* There is no unifying narrative about how health inequalities can be effectively reduced. Many of the recommendations are seemingly focused on general improvements rather than inequality reductions.

4. *Specificity of recommendations.* The Marmot Report offers both specific and highly general recommendations. General recommendations tend to predominate: for example, 'Create and develop communities' (p 136); while specific recommendations include 'providing paid parental leave in the first year of life with a minimum income for healthy living' (p 180).

5. *Cost-effectiveness.* The Marmot Report addressed economic issues in ways that the Acheson Report did not and for which it was criticised:

'His report concluded that inequality in illness accounted for annual productivity losses of £31bn–£33bn, lost taxes and higher welfare payments in the range of £20bn–£32bn per year. Additional NHS healthcare costs associated with inequality are in excess of £5.5bn per year' (Ford, 2010).

However, the report considers analysis of the cost burden, which bears little relation to cost-effectiveness. The burden of costs could be enormous and might be irrelevant unless there were cost-effective interventions to tackle the problem. Moreover, it is unclear how sensitive such analyses were in practice.

Given this analysis, it might appear that lessons from previous reports have only been partly learned. This might reflect the ways in which evidence is gathered, synthesised and communicated. The problem, Hunter (2009) claims, lies in 'the methods used to assemble it and the political context in which that evidence then gets deployed (or not) to inform policy and practice' (p 583).

Policy impact

As the review was published only in February 2010, it is too early to judge its full impact upon policy. Impacts of related policies can be gauged from evidence such as the National Equality Panel (Hills, 2010) and from the shift towards more individualistic approaches to health (Hunter, 2009). However, it is possible to gauge its likely impact through a conceptual approach that has been applied previously to health inequalities policy (Exworthy et al, 2002). This is explored in the next section. As with the Black and Acheson reports, criticisms of the Marmot Report 'focus on what is missing, rather than what the reports contains' (Whitehead and Popay, 2010).

Reflections on the case study: evidence into policy?

The adoption and implementation of the recommendations from these three reports can be assessed through the application of Kingdon's 'windows' model. This model argues that change will occur if three 'windows' are aligned, possibly with the aid of a 'policy entrepreneur' (Exworthy et al, 2002).

Problem window

The 'problem' of health inequalities continues to be reasserted over a period of 30 years. Following the Black Report, which rejected the individual/behaviourist framing of health inequalities, the problem was overlooked or even denied. Following the Acheson Report, health inequalities were defined more clearly (though in terms of the Black agenda). However, the government often found the shift from rhetoric to action problematic, and sought both individual and structural solutions, as illustrated by, for example, the choice agenda and bans on smoking in public places. More recently, the Marmot Report continues to define the problem conceptually in terms set out by Black and Acheson, though it does identify wider manifestations of the 'problem'. Common to all three reports is the neglect of the countervailing forces, notably the global economic system which is not framed as part of the problem (Whitehead and Popay, 2010).

However, this problem definition is set against a different contextual background. International comparisons (for example, note the US's, albeit limited, efforts to address racial and ethnic disparities; and EurohealthNet and Eurothine), new techniques (such as social marketing: www.dh.gov. uk/en/Publichealth/Choosinghealth/DH_066342) and new players in the policy network (for example the commercial sector; see www.bitc. org.uk/community/economic_renewal/health/index.html) point to such differences.

Policy window

The development and implementation of strategies have remained a stumbling block across all three inquiries. 'Wider-ranging programmes of public expenditure' were not deemed effective or acceptable strategies to solve the problem as defined by Black. By contrast, a plethora of policy initiatives were implemented by the Labour government in the wake of the Acheson Report. Given unprecedented policy efforts from 1997–2010, a favourable political climate and 'healthy' tax revenues (at least until 2008), it might be hard to understand why further progress was not made. Either the policy was wrong or the dose was insufficient. The answer is probably both. Many policies were initially short-term projects that did not challenge the mainstream service planning or provision. Latterly, mainstreaming did take place, but within a NHS-centric context. Also, the 'dose' may have been insufficient to remedy intractable 'wicked issues' like health inequalities. Some redistribution, for example, did take place, but this was largely outweighed by rising income inequality.

Politics window

The general reception for each report confirms Hunter's (2009) assertion that some researchers assume 'that merely publishing their work should constitute sufficient grounds for the take-up of their findings and recommendations' (p 583). As elsewhere, politics matter.

The political reception for the Black Report has been extensively covered (Berridge and Blume, 2002). Its failure to grapple with the political context was widely recognised and shaped the antecedents of the Acheson Report. Nonetheless, it is arguable whether the Acheson Report fully 'opened' the political window. There may have been an ambivalence about seriously tackling inequality in the Blair administration (Gray and Jenkins, 2001; Exworthy and Hunter, 2011). Marmot recommended cross-government action, but, as with previous policy initiatives, calls for joined-up government have not always been enacted (Exworthy and Hunter, 2011). Marmot balanced this call for cross-government action with one for the Department of Health to retain a central role (Ford, 2010).

With echoes of the Black Report and unlike Acheson, the Marmot Review was published shortly before the 2010 general election that resulted in the formation of the Conservative/Liberal Democrat Coalition government. Despite some reference to notions of fairness, and even to health inequality, in the Coalition's programme for government, it seems that the political priority remains the NHS, with its relatively protected budget. In an era of fiscal constraint and a government led by the Conservative Party, health inequalities may thus not be at the top of the political agenda. Health inequalities seem not to have become sufficiently established in policy networks to keep the 'political window' open. This may be (partly) due to the notion that tackling inequality is 'synonymous' with redistribution (Lawlor, 2010).

Policy entrepreneur

Each inquiry chair was a policy entrepreneur, with differing levels of success. However, Marmot played a pivotal role in two of the three case study reports, and also chaired the World Health Organisation Commission. As such, he can be classed as a long-standing advocate, but his entrepreneurial skills in policy have only been honed more recently as he has become more closely involved with policy development and not just research. Moreover, as the policy on health inequalities has sought to engage wider groups and stakeholders, the political and policy skills of entrepreneurs will need to adapt. The arguments and tactics used by such entrepreneurs within the health inequalities 'policy networks' may be less effective in the broader policy arenas (Exworthy, 2008); accurate diagnosis does not always ensure effective prescription.

In summary, the three documents each acts as an individual case study; but as a collective case study, they also demonstrate the way in which evidence has been assembled and the policy response that its publication has precipitated. They thus illustrate the variable and uncertain impact that inquiries of evidence can have on policy development. Indeed, it is difficult to trace the precise influence, because the link between research evidence and policy has disparate effects from a direct relationship upon policy to one of enlightenment (Weiss, 1977). Weiss suggests that policy makers tend to 'use research indirectly, as a source of ideas [and] information' (p 531); the effects of such research evidence upon policy are thus not 'easily discernible', but are nonetheless 'profound'. Yet, in other cases, evidence does not inform policy at all; for example, the House of Commons Health Select Committee (2009) was critical of the ways in which several policies were implemented without any evaluation. This may be because the willingness of some actors to take action influences their view of the evidence presented in reports (Hunter, 2009).

At a broader level, the effectiveness of translating evidence into policy and of policy learning can be seen in terms of the degree to which the 'equivalences between epidemiology and government are accepted by relevant actors on both sides of the research–policy equation' (Freeman, 2006, p 54). In other words, the uptake of evidence by policy makers often says less about the nature of the evidence (its presentation or its message) – since the nature of inequalities did not change dramatically between Black and Acheson or between Acheson and Marmot – than about the nature of government and policy making itself. Oliver and Nutbeam (2003) claim that the government's belief system did change, but Freeman (2006) suggests that it did not change enough to impact upon health inequalities (p 66). That said, Hunter (2009) also calls for changes in the ways in which research communities communicate their findings.

Despite the accumulation of evidence, and its synthesis in these three reports, there remains insufficient political and/or public will to shift from faith in the liberal market economy. It may be that such intent will never exist on the scale that is necessary. It may also be impossible to narrow inequalities effectively without doing that, unless some way can also be found to 'force' convergence in the cultural and behavioural habits across income groups.

References

Acheson, D. (1998a) *Independent inquiry into inequalities in health*, London: HMSO.

Acheson, D. (1998b) 'Letter: Report on Inequalities in Health Did Give Priority for Steps to Be Tackled', *British Medical Journal,* vol 317, no 12, p 1659.

Arblaster, L., Entwhistle, V., Lambert, M., Forster, M., Sheldon, T. and Watt, I. (1995) *Review of the research on the effectiveness of health service interventions to reduce variations in health*, CRD Report 3, York: Centre for Reviews and Dissemination, University of York.

Asthana, S. and Halliday, J. (2006) 'Developing an evidence base for policies and interventions to address health inequalities: the analysis of "public health regimes"', *Milbank Quarterly*, vol 84, no 3, pp 577–603.

Berridge, V. (2003) 'The Black Report: interpreting history', in A. Oliver and M. Exworthy (eds) *Health inequalities: Evidence, policy and implementation*, London: Nuffield Trust.

Berridge, V. and Blume, S. (eds) (2002) *Poor health: Social inequality before and after the Black Report*, London: Frank Cass.

Birch, S. (1999) '"The 39 steps": the mystery of health inequalities in the UK', *Health Economics*, vol 8, pp 301–8.

Black, D., Morris, J.N., Smith, C. and Townsend, P. (1980) *Inequalities in health: Report of a research working group*, London: Department of Health and Social Security.

Black, D., Morris, J.N., Smith, C. and Townsend, P. (1999) 'Better benefits for health: plan to implement the central recommendation of the Acheson Report', *British Medical Journal*, vol 318, pp 724–7.

DH (Department of Health) (1992) *Health of the nation*, London: HMSO.

DH (1998) *Our healthier nation*, Cm 3852, London: Department of Health.

DH (1999a) *Saving lives: Our healthier nation*, Cm 4386. London: The Stationery Office.

DH (2000) *The NHS plan*, London: DH.

DH (2001) *From vision to reality*, London: DH.

DH (2002) *Tackling health inequalities: The results of the consultation exercise*, London: Department of Health.

DH (2002b) *Tackling health inequalities: 2002 cross-cutting review,* London: DH.

DH (2003) *Tackling health inequalities: A programme for action*, London: HM Treasury/ DH.

DH (2007) *Tackling health inequalities: 2007 status report on the Programme for Action*, London: DH.

DH (2008) *Health inequalities: Progress and next steps*, London: DH.

DH (2009) *Tackling health inequalities: 10 years on*, London: Department of Health.

Elliott, H. and Popay, J. (2000) 'How are policy makers using evidence? Models of research utilisation and local NHS policy making', *Journal of Epidemiology and Community Health*, vol 54, pp 61–468.

Evans, R. (2002) *Interpreting and addressing inequalities in health: From Black to Acheson to Blair to …?*, London: Office of Health Economics.

Exworthy, M. (2002) 'The "second Black Report"? The Acheson Report as another opportunity to tackle health inequality', *Contemporary British History*, Special Issue: *Poor health*, vol 16, no 3, pp 175–97.

Exworthy, M. (2008) 'Policy to tackle the social determinants of health: using conceptual models to understand the policy process', *Health Policy and Planning*, vol 23, pp 318–27.

Exworthy, M. and Hunter, D.J. (2011) 'Tackling health inequalities in the UK: the role of joined-up government', *International Journal of Public Administration*, Special Issue: *Joined-up government*, vol 30, no 4, pp 201–12.

Exworthy, M., Berney, L. and Powell, M. (2002) '"How great expectations in Westminster may be dashed locally": the local implementation of national policy on health inequalities', *Policy and Politics*, vol 30, no 1, pp 79–96.

Exworthy, M., Blane, D. and Marmot, M. (2003) 'Tackling health inequalities in the UK: progress and pitfalls of policy', *Health Services Research*, Special Issue: *Social determinants of health*, part II, vol 38, no 6, pp 1905–21.

Exworthy, M., Bindman, A., Davies, H.T.O. and Washington, A.E. (2006) 'Evidence into policy and practice? Measuring the progress of policies to tackle health disparities and inequalities in the US and UK', *Milbank Quarterly*, vol 84, no 1, pp 75–109.

Ford, S. (2010) 'Marmot might be fair but will it be feasible?', *Health Service Journal*, vol 4, available at: www.hsj.co.uk/news/policy/marmot-might-be-fair-but-will-it-be-feasible/5012062.article.

Freeman, R. (2006) 'The work the document does: research, policy and equity in health', *Journal of Health Policy, Politics and Law*, vol 31, pp 51–70.

Graham, H. (2009) 'Health inequalities, social determinants and public health policy', *Policy & Politics*, vol 37, no 4, pp 463–79.

Gray, A. and Jenkins, B. (2001) 'Government and administration: the dilemmas of delivery', *Parliamentary Affairs*, vol 54, no 2, pp 206–22.

Greener, I. (2003) 'Performance in the NHS: insistence of measurement and confusion of content', *Public Performance and Management Review*, vol 26, pp 237–50.

Harrison, S. and McDonald, R. (2008) *The politics of healthcare in Britain*, London: Sage.

Hills, S. (chair) (2010) *An anatomy of economic inequality in the UK. Report of the National Equality Panel*, London: Government Equalities Office.

House of Commons Health Select Committee (2009) *Health inequalities. Third report of session 2008–09*, Volume 1. HC 286-1, London: The Stationery Office.

Hunter, D.J. (2009) 'Relationship between evidence and policy: a case of evidence-based policy or policy-based evidence?', *Public Health*, vol 123, no 9, pp 583–6.

Illsley, R. (1999) 'Reducing health inequalities: Britain's latest attempt', *Health Affairs*, vol 18, no 3, pp 45–6.

Jenkin, P. (1980) Foreword, in D. Black, *Inequalities in health: Report of a research working group*, London: DHSS.

Klein, R. (2000) 'From evidence-based medicine to evidence-based policy?', *Journal of Health Services Research and Policy*, vol 5, no 2, pp 65–6.

Klein, R. (2002) 'Making policy in a fog', in A.J. Oliver and M. Exworthy (eds) *Health inequalities: Evidence, policy and implementation*, London: Nuffield Trust, pp 55–7.

Lawlor, E. (2010) 'Investing in equality', *Guardian*, 12 February, available at: www.guardian.co.uk/commentisfree/2010/feb/12/marmot-social-inequality-improve.

Lewis, R.A. (1952) *Edwin Chadwick and the public health movement, 1832–1854*, London: Longmans, Green & Co.

Macintyre, S. (1997) 'The Black Report and beyond: what are the lessons?', *Social Science and Medicine*, vol 44, pp 723–45.

Macintyre, S., Chalmers, I., Horton, R. and Smith, R. (2001) 'Using evidence health policy: case study', *British Medical Journal*, vol 322, pp 222–5.

Marmot, M.G. (1999) 'Acting on the evidence to reduce inequalities in health', *Health Affairs*, vol 18, no 3, pp 42–4.

Marmot, M.G. (chair) (2010) *Fair society, healthy lives. Strategic review of health inequalities in England post-2010*, London: Department of Health.

Oliver, A. (2001) *Why care about health inequalities?*, London: Office of Health Economics.

Oliver, A.J. and Exworthy, M. (eds) (2003) *Health inequalities: Evidence, policy and implementation*, London: Nuffield Trust.

Oliver, A. and Nutbeam, D. (2003) 'Addressing health inequalities in the UK: a case study', paper presented at *Health equity research: Beyond the sound of one hand clapping*, Bellagio, Italy, 23–27 April.

Petticrew, M., Whitehead, M., Macintyre, S., Graham, H. and Egan, M. (2004) 'Evidence for public health policy on inequalities – 1: the reality according to policy-makers', *Journal of Epidemiology and Community Health*, vol 58, no 10, pp 811–16.

Pickett, K. and Dorling, D. (2010) 'Against the organization of misery? The Marmot Review of health inequalities', *Social Science and Medicine*, vol 71, no 7, pp 1231-3.

Richmond, C. (2002) 'Obituary: Professor Sir Douglas Black', *Independent*, 17 September, available at: www.independent.co.uk/news/obituaries/sir-douglas-black-643017.html.

Sanderson, I. (2002) 'Evaluation, policy learning and evidence-based policy-making', *Public Administration*, vol 80, no 1, pp 1–22.

Smith, G.D. (2001) 'How policy informs the evidence', *British Medical Journal*, vol 322, no 27, pp 1884–5.

Smith, G.D., Bartley, M. and Blane, D. (1990) 'The Black Report on socio-economic inequalities in health: ten years on', *British Medical Journal*, vol 301, pp 373–7.

Smith, G.D., Morris, J.N. and Shaw, M. (1998) 'The independent inquiry into inequalities in health', *British Medical Journal*, vol 317, no 28, pp 1465–6.

Vagero, D. and Illsley, R. (1995) 'Explaining health inequalities: beyond Black and Barker. A discussion of some issues emerging in the decade following the Black Report', *European Sociological Review*, vol 11, no 3, pp 219–41.

Weiss, C. (1977) 'Research for policy's sake: the enlightenment function of social research', *Policy Analysis*, vol 3, no 4, pp 531–45.

Whitehead, M. (1987) *The health divide*, London: Penguin.

Whitehead, M. and Popay, J. (2010) 'Swimming upstream? Taking action on the social determinants of health inequalities', *Social Science and Medicine*, vol 71, no 7, pp 1234-6.

Williams, A. (1999) 'Commentary on the Acheson Report', *Health Economics*, vol 8, pp 297–9.

World Health Organisation, Commission on Social Determinants of Health (2008) *Closing the gap in a generation: Health equity through action on the social determinants of health*, Geneva: WHO.

Part Five

twenty

Policy learning from case studies in health policy: taking forward the debate

Mark Exworthy and Stephen Peckham

The chapters in this book provide a range of observations about health policy in the UK. Each contribution presents a 'policy' case study but there is enormous variation in the scope, focus and methods of each case study. This chapter examines how practitioners and researchers can learn from these case studies, and indeed how we understand the learning process itself.

The first aim of this chapter is to trace the interconnections between case studies and policy learning in the context of health policy. We pose a series of questions concerning how the learning from case studies can be and is translated into policy and practice. How do policy makers or practitioners learn from case studies? How and what did they learn from previous efforts or from elsewhere? How did they accommodate the learning from these lessons into their day-to-day routines and practice? The second aim focuses on methodology, and we explore the ways in which the case study, as an approach to policy research, provides a useful methodological approach – both in terms of understanding policy and also in providing policy learning.

As Marinetto argues in Chapter Two, the 'policy case study is multi-dimensional beast which can, potentially, operate at different ontological levels of analysis'. The preceding chapters provide ample illustration of this 'beast', covering a range of policies and situations from the birth of the NHS (where both Marinetto and Powell agree that Eckstein is an important case study), policy blueprints such as the Hospital Plan (Mohan, Chapter Four) and system upheaval in the 1990s (Greener, Chapter Five and Allen, Chapter Eighteen) to current policy on patient choice, where policy is still developing (Peckham and Sanderson, Chapter Fourteen). The methods addressed in the chapters range from historical analysis to 'thick'. What they share is an illuminative quality (Illsley, 1975), shedding light on both methods for understanding policy and lessons for policy. In a sense, the chapters in this book provide us with both analysis of policy and analysis for policy (Gordon et al, 1977).

Is the case study a method?

In Chapter Two, Marinetto asks the question of whether a case study is a method or a design, or in fact, as Stake (2005) argues, neither, but rather, a choice of what is to be studied. However, as some of the chapters in this book show, choices about what is being studied are intrinsically connected to decisions made about the boundaries of the case, linked to methodological issues. A number of the case studies raise important questions about the time frame of the case study (for example, compare Higgins, Chapter Six with Paton, Chapter Sixteen). Others raise questions about definitional boundaries (identifying the policy) or substantive issues about the subject or activity (for example, Peckham and Sanderson, Chapter Fourteen). The subjects of these chapters themselves illustrate these problems. In Chapter Three, Powell discusses a number of historical accounts of the birth of the NHS, questioning whether these are 'case studies'. Similarly in Chapter Eight, Peckham and Willmott examine Alford's study of healthcare reform in which he himself discusses what constitutes his case, drawing, as he does, on a time frame of some 30 years and setting his study in a broad political context.

This suggests that a case study is more than simply choosing what to study. The case often emerges in analysis, with the 'case' being determined by both an understanding of the substantive nature of the case and also methodological consequences. Some of the chapters examine comparative studies where, clearly, the comparison is not just simply about choosing different cases, but the comparison of the cases is meant to further some understanding of the cases themselves. In this sense, a case study is certainly part of the research design – integral to the method. But, as Marinetto argues, there is no specific methodology that is used for case studies. While there has been a dominance of qualitative methods, quantitative methods are also used in case study research. This multiplicity of methods is amply demonstrated in the preceding chapters.

What constitutes a case study?

A recurring theme throughout the chapters in this book is the question of what constitutes the case. In Chapter Two, Marinetto discusses how case study research developed from psychotherapeutic, management, sociological and political analysis origins. Clearly, many writers on case studies (for example, Ragin and Becker, 1992; Yin, 2009) are concerned with case definition and there has been much debate about how to define the case and when this is done. The variety of pre- and post-definition of the case is amply shown in this text. If case study is simply the choice of the case – that is, of what to study – then presumably the definition of the case is made before studies commence, but clearly this is not represented well in the literature.

Often, the definition of the case occurs at some point during the research, and possibly retrospectively. However, some definitional framing of the case must take place before studies commence, otherwise all we are left with is Wittgenstein's observation that 'The world is all that is the case' (*Tractus Logicophilosophicus*).

So choosing a case study approach is not simply about choosing what to study, as choices about the nature and extent of the case are linked to methodological and conceptual issues. As many of the case studies in this book demonstrate, policy is itself sufficiently complex that the framing of the case will have direct and important consequences for the ensuing analysis, in much the same way that choice of methods will obtain different kinds of data that allow different analyses.

Which methods are employed in health policy analysis?

As with researchers undertaking case studies, the policy analyst employs a variety of disciplines, theories and methods to examine the policy process. Policy analysis draws on the disciplines of economics, sociology, politics and, increasingly, psychology to provide approaches to analyse the nature and purpose of policy and the way individuals and organisations develop and implement policy. The methodological 'toolbox' includes both quantitative and qualitative methods. It is also clear that the methodological toolbox is continuously expanding. Marinetto briefly discusses the history of case studies in Chapter Two and how disciplines have developed and refined both the way case studies have been used and also the methods applied in data collection and analysis.

The chapters in this book show how these methods are used to illuminate the conduct of policy making and offer theoretical insights into that process. Perhaps of specific interest is the way different methods are used and how methods develop. In his account of Berridge's study of the development of AIDS policy, Evans (Chapter Ten) characterises her approach as having a lack of methodology; he points out that there is no methodological discussion in her book:

> We learn little, for example, about recruitment and sampling of informants. How did Berridge decide whom to talk to? How many of the people she approached agreed or declined to be interviewed? Was there any systematic bias in non-respondents? Similarly, we know very little about the interview process. Were respondents asked open, semi-structured or structured questions? Were the questions based on pre-existing theories? Finally, we know little about the process of analysis. Were interviews analysed thematically?

Was the validity of the analysis tested in any way? Indeed, were the transcripts coded at all?

So does this invalidate her account? As Evans points out, this approach is not uncommon in historical analysis, even though to the social scientist failure to address these details would be seen to invalidate the data. Yet, does this mean that we should discount historical methods? This point is also discussed by Powell (Chapter Three) with reference to the 'birth' of the NHS. Yet much contemporary policy analysis is increasingly drawing on analytical approaches found in the humanities. The question of history is one that crops up in many of the case studies – usually addressed in terms of a discussion about setting contexts and time frames.

The role of case studies in policy learning

The approach in this book has been to explore policy through cases. While not a comprehensive collection of key policies or even policy cases, the chapters here do demonstrate the enormous variety in the way researchers have approached examining empirical and theoretical analysis of the policy process.

How can case studies support analysis for policy?

As important as understanding policies is, a key question for policy analysts and policy makers is: 'Can we learn from past policies, and if so what is it we can learn?' These questions are vital because, as Hunter (2003) argued, the way recent policy developments have taken place, the evidence of learning is scant. If future policies are going to be effective, there is a strong argument that they must learn lessons if previous shortcomings are not to be repeated.

Although disciplines such as educational theory, organisational sociology, the sociology of organisations and social psychology have addressed learning, the primary focus here is on 'policy learning', because for sure, there are important lessons to learned from previous experience. However, our understanding of methods cautions us to be wary of simply extrapolating lessons directly from these and other examples of previous policy.

With so much attention of the policy interventions, it is easy to lose sight of where the impetus for such initiatives arose, how the disparate influences were assimilated by policy makers and practitioners. These factors are important because, as will be discussed later in this chapter, there are important consequences for policy transfer and the degree to which this signifies greater convergence between places or organisations.

What is policy learning?

Freeman (2007) suggests that learning is a natural activity, done automatically, and that 'Thinking about learning is difficult at least in part because it is a matter of common sense' (p 477; see also Freeman, 2008). However, for clarity, he suggests that policy learning implies a degree of reflexivity in which individuals 'learn to learn differently' (p 478). This is similar to the definition offered by Helderman et al (2005):

> Policy learning denotes the process by which policy makers and stakeholders deliberately adjust the goals, rules, and techniques of a given policy in response to past experiences and new information. (p 189)

For Hall (1993), policy learning is 'A deliberate attempt to adjust the goals or techniques of policy in response to past experience or new information' (p 278).

Hall's definition points to two key ways of learning – from elsewhere (such as other countries or regions) and from the past (either one's own experience or others'). Freeman (2008) argues that policy learning is not simply about such reflection but is intrinsic to the policy process:

> Learning is not only the what and how of public policy but also its why. Public policy is an applied science and learning is much of its rationale. (p 368)

Adopting this definition helps in understanding that the process of policy formulation and implementation becomes a site of learning for policy makers.

In policy circles, 'learning' is widely seen as a good thing with positive overtones; how can one be against it? However, it is not always clear that policy makers or practitioners do actually learn. Day-to-day, practical concerns tend to dominate the minds of policy makers and practitioners. They are often concerned with how they can introduce new programmes or improve existing ones or why some interventions are not working as intended. They do not always enjoy the luxury of reflection or introspection upon the nature of the intervention itself. But, as evident in this book, policy is set within changing and different contexts. Thus, our understanding of how policy is made and implemented and what constitutes evidence in policy is also critical. Questions that need to be addressed are, therefore, not just whether policy makers learn, but what kinds of things they need to learn and what other or previous experience can bring to the process. As Weiss (1977) and Innvaer et al (2002) have shown, policy makers draw on a range of evidence and values to develop policy; learning from previous or other experiences will only ever be one such form of evidence.

There is an intense interest in how others have, or are tackling (apparently) the same or similar issues. These 'others' might be elsewhere in the UK or abroad. This interest has also tended to breed a degree of competition and rivalry in keeping abreast of the latest developments. Indeed, many academic and practitioner conferences specifically focus on the lessons to be learned from 'elsewhere'.

Greener (2002) argues that 'social learning' provides an 'index of the extent of policy change' (p 163), namely first order change, second order change and paradigm shift, the extent of change progressively becoming more extensive. Learning thus offers a contrast and assesses the 'coherence of the present paradigm' (p 163). The interest in policy learning has echoes of the 'evidence-based' policy and practice movement. There is an apparent intuitive appeal in ensuring that services are based upon the latest and most reliable (research) evidence.

As Marmor et al (2009) argue, learning about what happens elsewhere or previously is 'a pre-condition for understanding why change takes place or for learning from that experience' (p 13). Such learning is often enhanced by stories or vivid accounts, rather than dry prose or even research evidence (Marmor et al, 2009).

A concept closely associated with policy learning is 'lesson drawing'. How do individuals 'draw lessons' from the experience elsewhere? Rose (1991) notes that lesson drawing begins with a 'search', by noting differences and seeking to learn from others:

> The process of lesson-drawing starts with scanning programmes in effect elsewhere, and ends with the prospective evaluation of what would happen if a programme already in effect elsewhere were transferred here in future. (p 3)

The corollary of learning is also apparent in the form of non-learning or negative learning (Dolowitz, 2000) and unlearning (Pollitt, 2009). It does not simply follow that lessons will be learned, with consequences for policy development and implementation. Rather, exposure to experiences elsewhere may be rejected in favour of the *status quo*, as an explicit rejection of the 'other' or as the result of interests antithetical to the lesson. While non-learning and negative learning have similar connotations, 'unlearning' implies that the lessons learned previously have been forgotten, or even that non-decisions were involved. The loss of 'organisational memory' is significant if the knowledge acquired through experience is not transmitted over time and between individuals (DH, 2000) (see Higgins, Chapter Six). For example, individuals move jobs, taking with them their social capital.

Knowledge management systems cannot always capture the tacit, experiential knowledge required in increasingly complex systems and organisations (as in the cases of health and social care, for example) (Jashapara, 2004). Knowledge management systems (such as intranet, data warehouses and so on) cannot always distil the experience of individuals into knowledge for the organisation (Mallinson et al, 2006).

What learning takes place?

As the preceding discussion shows, learning is not a straightforward exercise in which the dissemination of knowledge (evidence, information and so on) takes place. Policy makers engage in 'collective puzzlement' as they come to terms with the uncertainty facing them (Heclo, 1974). To accommodate the relationships between non-rational actors and learning, and to understand the way in which they 'puzzle collectively', three different ways of conceiving learning can be identified, namely, rationalist, institutionalist and constructionist (Freeman, 2007). These ways have echoes of different ways of understanding the policy-making process: rational actor, organisational process and bureaucratic politics (Allinson, 1971; Ham, 1981).

The first – the rationalist mode – is, arguably, the one which is seen as the stereotypical approach to learning. It posits a simple cause and effect relationship whereby the production of knowledge, the verification of evidence and its dissemination is a linear, rational process. Failings in this approach require refinement in each stage. As such, the production of knowledge and its consumption/application in practice are distinct.

The second – the institutionalist mode – places the bureaucratic codes and regulations in a dominant position to influence the ability of organisational actors to learn. Hence, individuals with different professional or occupational backgrounds may struggle to adapt and apply the lessons from a different organisation because of differences in language and culture, for example. The institutionalist mode is inevitably incremental by nature, foreseeing no radical or dramatic changes over time but rather, slow, marginal reforms. This incrementalism may be heavily influenced by the (epistemic) communities which shape the knowledge relevant to that organisation (for example, healthcare as opposed to social care) (Dunlop, 2009). This learning by 'group-think' is integral to the organisational norms, routines and practices. This mode is commonly found in health policy case studies.

The third is the constructionist mode of learning, whereby learning draws on experience of day-to-day practice. The focus is thus on the meaning that individuals ascribe to learning. It is a collective activity in which new forms of learning are accommodated into existing ones. This mode is perhaps the way in which practitioners use their knowledge from case studies in their own learning.

Policy learning is evident in various forms. Marmor et al (2009) offer a taxonomy based on increasing conceptualisation of the learning. First, policy learning is often promoted through the medium of statistical documents and databases of comparisons between places (such as countries, localities) or organisations. In this case, learning takes place by appreciating 'what something is by reference to what it is like or unlike' (Marmor et al, 2009, p 10).

Learning may thus be implicit; appreciating the difference may not stimulate action to emulate or copy the other. This category tends to be the most common example of policy learning documents (see Macfarlane et al, Chapter Nine). Second, collections of comparative studies aid policy learning by presenting 'stapled' or 'parallel' case studies (Marmor et al, 2009, p 14) (see Exworthy and Oliver, Chapter Nineteen). Again, these case studies could be of places, organisations or activities or policies. They tend to be historical accounts of the development of services or systems. Third, some reports comprise collections of individual case studies with a common approach (see Powell, Chapter Three). The fourth offers the most conceptually robust example, where case studies are framed by a theoretical perspective upon a specific topic or theme.

How effective might policy learning be? Jenkins-Smith and Sabatier (1993) argue that the 'probability' of learning is a function of the level of conflict, the analytical tractability of the issue and the presence of a professionalised forum (p 48) (compare, for example, Keen, Chapter Seven with Exworthy and Oliver, Chapter Nineteen). Drawing on their own theory of advocacy coalitions, the level of conflict is, they claim, a reflection of the 'incompatibility' of beliefs within different coalitions. The second variable is the analytical intractability, which refers to the difficulty encountered in understanding and acting upon complex phenomena 'when causal relationships span several policy areas and when the issues concern conflicting policy objectives' (p 51) (see Hughes, Chapter Twelve; Peckham and Sanderson, Chapter Fourteen). Third, the nature of the 'professionalized forum', the arena within which debate takes place, is shaped by the discussion of 'policy-relevant facts and values, the number and kinds of people involved in the discussion' (p 53) (see Dowswell and Harrison, Chapter Seventeen).

How does policy learning take place?

The idea of a learning organisation draws attention to the ways in which structures and processes for individual development and team work are fostered within the organisation (Senge, 1992). Mallinson et al (2006) identified five components of organisational learning:

a. personal learning and development
b. mental models
c. team learning
d. shared vision
e. systems thinking (p 267).

Jenkins-Smith and Sabatier (1993) argue that learning occurs within and across jurisdictions, but it is arguable that most policy learning takes place at a local or regional level *within* countries rather than *between* countries. (Here, policy case studies focus on the UK only, so cross-national learning is limited; see Marmor et al, 2009.) Individuals are most familiar with developments that are intra-national rather than international. Despite the globalisation of public policy, most health systems remain largely local or even regional in character.

The UK experience of (political) devolution in the last decade or so is highly germane to the location of policy learning, as reflected in the chapter by Peckham and Sanderson (Chapter Fourteen). Each nation has been a natural experiment but has also had the opportunity of learning from other nations. How, if at all, have they learned about experience elsewhere?

Policy learning in practice?

Having discussed the approach to learning, the focus now shifts to how this learning is transferred between countries, organisations and individuals. It is crucial to understand why and when policy stakeholders engage in and apply their learning. The changing context of UK health policy following devolution provides a new context for policy analysis in the UK. This context is addressed in the chapter by Peckham and Sanderson (Chapter Fourteen), but, given the recent nature of this change, this is the only chapter to address this. Yet we now have four NHSs, not one. We are, therefore, interested in the 'patterns of adoption and adaptation' of policy learning which differ as a result of institutional structures and processes as well as local cultural meanings – of particular interest where there are shared institutional and policy developments within the UK since 1948 (Marmor et al, 2009). There are two broad ways of thinking about this. One is policy convergence and the other is policy transfer.

There has been a long-standing debate in social policy about whether national health systems are converging or diverging (Greener, 2002). This has assumed greater significance with the advent of increased internationalisation in health policy and, in the UK context, political devolution. One effect of this internationalisation has been the widespread claims of (apparent) convergence between health systems. Yet it also seems that national health systems have remained remarkably different during this period. In addition, the effect of international agencies on facilitating policy transfer is often uneven and indirect (Marmor et al, 2005, p 338) and most debates about healthcare and reform take place within a national context – hence the focus of this book (Marmor et al, 2009, p 8).

However, while important contextual factors are not deterministic (and the discussions in chapters here demonstrate concurrent convergence and divergence), contextual factors can describe and explain the pressures for change, but do not indicate whether change will take place or what form it might take.

The convergence debate at sub-national levels such as localities or regions is sometimes defined as isomorphism: '[a] constraining process that forces one unit in a population to resemble other units in it that face the same set of environmental conditions' (DiMaggio and Powell, 1983, p 147).

Whether this adequately describes the devolved policy context of the UK is not clear (Smith et al, 2009). The account of patient choice (Chapter Fourteen) suggests that organisations come to resemble each other in structure and form (mimetic isomorphism) but there are clear differences in beliefs at a policy level (normative isomorphism) and little attempt by a national government to impose policy (coercive isomorphism) (see Paton, Chapter Sixteen). If convergence becomes a coercive exercise, then isomorphism (rather than learning, for example) is likely to result because of the 'institutionally structured *fear* that politicians (and bureaucrats) have of "being left behind" in the international arena – a problem that has the potential to increase in the future as more organisations and institutions start to publish and publicise league table and benchmark performances across a range of comparison nations' (Dolowitz, 2009, p 322; original emphasis). In the UK context it would appear, however, that the need to address quality and waiting-list issues did create a pressure in the different health systems.

Drawing on historical institutionalism, the notion of path dependency has increasingly assumed an important conceptual approach to this debate. It posits that, as systems develop, an inertia sets in that limits the range of options available to policy makers (Exworthy and Freeman, 2009). Despite the radical change of the NHS since 1948, it continues to remain a potent symbol of policy making in the UK. Indeed, the purpose of this book has been to chart the ways in which interests, ideas and institutions have shaped the NHS over time and through the policy process. Offering multiple explanations of how health systems have maintained their path dependence and, on occasion, deviated from it, is an essential task for health policy analysis (Greener, 2005) and one well suited to the case study approach.

Policy transfer

Policy transfer refers to the exchange of knowledge (Dolowitz and Marsh, 2000, p 5) and can be defined as:

> the process by which the ideas (e.g. what is a problem, what is a success, how to frame an issue), policies (e.g. Earned Income Tax Credit, Workfare) and practices (e.g. how to measure success, what counts as evidence), in one political system are fed into (and used) in the policy-making arena of another political system. (Dolowitz, 2009, p 318)

In the UK context, policy transfer is potentially of increasing interest because of political devolution in the UK and increasing institutional links within the European Union. The extent and nature of what is transferred and the extent to which transfer is voluntary or enforced are central to discussions of policy transfer (Dolowitz and Marsh, 2000; Greener, 2002).

The extent to which the UK has emulated policy from other countries is not always clear. The influence of the US and European health systems and policy is apparent to some degree in relation to the internal market (Allen, Chapter Eighteen) and clinical guidelines (Dowswell and Harrison, Chapter Seventeen). On the other hand, it can be argued that the UK has predominantly forged its own policy path because of the uniqueness of the NHS. Dolowitz and Marsh (2000) argue that there are different degrees of transfer, in that it is not a case of either transfer or not, but that there are various possibilities which may be summarised into four stages ranging between copying and inspiration (Table 20.1).

It is notoriously difficult to disaggregate cause and effect in policy transfer, partly because accounts of transfer are often derived from proponents (or opponents) or particular policies and because of the difficulty in researching such transfers.

Success and failure of policy transfer may be in the 'eye of the beholder', depending on their interest in and the impact of the policy, and Dolowitz

Table 20.1: Types of policy transfer

Degree of transfer	Feature
Copying	Direct and complete transfer
Emulation	Transfer of ideas underpinning a policy
Combination	Mixtures of different policies
Inspiration	Policy in one area 'inspires' policy change elsewhere but does not 'draw upon' the original

Source: Dolowitz and Marsh (2000, p 13)

and Marsh (2000) suggest that failure can be because of uninformed transfer, incomplete transfer and inappropriate transfer (p 17). Much analysis of policy transfer highlights the iterative process involving ongoing interchange between interests, ideas and institutions. While some individuals are especially influential in the transfer process (Kingdon, 1995), the extent to which such policy entrepreneurs are reflected in the case studies in this book are, at best, limited. This is not to argue that the UK has been immune, but it may reflect the traditional inward focus of policy analysis in the UK until recent years and a shift in attention towards a focus on mechanisms and organisational and clinical aspects of healthcare since the 1970s, where more international exchange has occurred. Perhaps more important is the fact that transfer of policy is not necessarily the same as policy learning.

Dolowitz (2009) argues that the extent of learning depends crucially on the motivations underlying the policy transfer process (Figure 20.1; cf Freeman, 2006). If transfer is a voluntary exercise, then it can be argued that learning will be a 'rational' process, involving 'more complex forms of learning' (Dolowitz, 2009, p 320). By contrast, if transfer is coercive or mandatory, then 'softer forms of learning' will occur, the reason being that coercion relates more to 'force and power' than to learning. Here, hard forms of learning involve a more informed understanding of the importing and exporting (health) system.

Much hinges on the institutional culture within which the learning takes place, which leads Dolowitz (2009) to conclude that 'Policy makers consciously and unconsciously filter what they observe (or learn) to make it fit into existing solutions, understandings and situations' (p 321).

This process of aligning evidence and experience suggests a more pragmatic approach to policy transfer and learning, whereby practitioners go 'policy shopping' or 'on vacation' for ideas and strategies (Walshe, 2001; Freeman, 2007; Dolowitz, 2009). This is illustrated in encounters made through conferences, exchanges, study or work visits (which are increasingly international). Copying rather than learning is the dominant mode of transfer here. Freeman (2007) goes further and evokes the notion of the *bricoleur* to describe this process. Freeman's study of public health practitioners shows how they are heavily engaged in 'piecing together, assembling and literally making sense of different bits of information and experience, often creating something new from what they have acquired secondhand' (p 476).

Figure 20.1: Forms of policy learning

Purely voluntary ←——————————————————→ Purely coercive

*(harder forms
of learning*

*(softer forms
of learning*

[post transfer
learning]

Source: Dolowitz (2009, p 321)

They 'piece together' what they 'know' from various sources, presenting a plausible account. Often, they begin their search nearby because of closer 'subjective identification' with colleagues elsewhere (Rose, 1991, p 14). This is a different approach to the traditional scientific approach (which gathers evidence, appraises it and them disseminates it). By contrast, the *bricoleur* 'acquires and assembles tools and materials as he or she goes, keeping them until they might be used' (Freeman, 2007, p 486), and it is only in the process of assimilating these that their properties become manifested.

Freeman's notion of bricolage does not nullify the traditional accumulation of research evidence published in academic or professional media. He argues that this evidence 'generate[s] and report[s] what is taken to be established fact' (2007, p 482). Research evidence becomes one of the artefacts that practitioners gather, to be 'stored', and used (if at all) at a later date.

While practitioners collaborate and share knowledge about problems and policies that are similar enough to prompt that exchange (Freeman, 2008, p 380), the degree of transformation that is required to transfer a policy from one country to another might, it is argued, be significant in this field. This highlights further the motivation behind transfer, for, as Dolowitz (2009) argues, 'if uncertainty is the primary motivation for engaging in the policy transfer most policy transfer is likely to involve little more than emulation' (p 327).

Conclusions: evidence into policy?

The dramatic rise in the volume and extent of case studies relating to health policy makes a synthesis or even an illustration of such literature a daunting and inevitably fraught task. However, it is much less clear how far 'reflexive social learning' has taken place (Walshe, 2001, p 31). Have policy makers learned from these case studies?

Policy learning often takes place through the medium of reports and documents, which become the core material of many studies. The interface between research and policy illustrates the ways in which evidence is (or is not) translated into policy. As documents are the primary means of exercising the politics of health (Freeman, 2006), it is interesting to note that many of the chapters in this book focus on published books or inquiries (Powell, Chapter Three; Higgins, Chapter Six; Evans, Chapter Ten; Exworthy and Oliver, Chapter Nineteen) or the development and/or implementation of legislation (Wainwright and Calnan, Chapter Eleven; Peckham and Sanderson, Chapter Fourteen; Paton, Chapter Sixteen).

It is perhaps useful to ask, therefore, whether there is something intrinsically useful in a case study approach to policy analysis which supports policy learning. Learning from the past is an important aspect of analysis for and of policy. Much has been written about how policy makers use evidence and absorb new ideas. In this book, there are examples of how case studies have influenced future policy development and implementation (see Higgins, Chapter Six; Wainwright and Calnan, Chapter Eleven; Locock and Dopson, Chapter Thirteen; Allen, Chapter Eighteen; Exworthy and Oliver, Chapter Nineteen). However, these are limited examples and demonstrate the need to understand how policy learning is recontextualised in contemporary policy development. Without such context, it is difficult to identify real learning.

The strength of the case study is that it can illuminate a range of factors and that analysts should be encouraged to explore broadly the context and nature of their cases. The development of new approaches to evidence synthesis, research methods and analysis may be more influential in future than more traditional case study approaches. In a number of the chapters, history and narrative are key analytical approaches and there is some support for the idea that these approaches are more easily understood by policy makers.

Contextualisation by the case study is also critical to enable the understanding and enactment of the replication logic of the case (Yin, 2009). Equally, the collection of chapters here has shown how theory plays an important role in research, through empirical testing.

This chapter has outlined the ways in which policy makers and practitioners learn from their own experience, and from others locally, nationally or internationally. At one level, individuals simply see problems differently (Marmor et al, 2005, p 335). Difference and variation in policy approaches would seem to be inevitable. However, at another level, we might begin to see greater convergence between certain policy approaches. The internationalisation of evidence has made practitioners more aware of what is happening elsewhere. They are encouraged to adopt the best available evidence, conform to good/best practice and follow recommended guidelines. Case studies have played a role in that *apparent* convergence. The challenge of enacting and replicating the findings or lessons into a different context underlines the challenge for future health policy analysis. In short, the ideal of policy learning is often not realised because of the constraints within which policy makers operate.

References

Allinson, G.T. (1971) *Essence of decision*, Boston: Little Brown.

DH (Department of Health) (2000) *Organisation with a memory*, London: DH.

DiMaggio, P.J. and Powell, W.W. (1983) 'The iron cage revisited: institutional isomorphism and collective rationality in organizational fields', *American Sociological Review*, vol 48, pp 147–60.

Dolowitz, D.P. (2000) *Policy transfer and British social policy: Learning from the USA?*, Buckingham: Open University Press.

Dolowitz, D.P. (2009) 'Learning by observing: surveying the international arena', *Policy & Politics*, vol 37, no 3, pp 317-34.

Dolowitz, P. and Marsh, D. (2000) 'Learning from abroad: the role of policy transfer in contemporary policy-making', *Governance*, vol 13, no 1, pp 5–24.

Dunlop, C.A. (2009) 'Policy transfer as learning: capturing variation in what decision-makers learn from epistemic communities', *Policy Studies*, vol 30, no 2, pp 289–311.

Exworthy, M. and Freeman, R. (2009) 'The United Kingdom: health policy learning in the NHS', in T.R. Marmor, R. Freeman and K.G.H. Okma (eds) *Comparative studies and the politics of modern medical care*, New Haven, CT: Yale University Press, pp 153–79.

Freeman, R. (2006) 'The document does the work: research, policy and equity in health', *Journal of Health Politics, Policy and Law*, vol 31, no 1, pp 51–70.

Freeman, R. (2007) 'Epistemological bricolage: how practitioners make sense of learning', *Administration and Society*, vol 39, pp 476–95.

Freeman, R. (2008) 'Learning in public policy', in M. Moran, M. Rein, and R.E. Goodin (eds) *Oxford handbook of public policy*, Oxford: Oxford University Press, pp 365–86.

Gordon, I., Lewis, J. and Young, K. (1977) 'Perspectives on policy analysis', *Public Administration Bulletin*, December, p 25.

Greener, I. (2002) 'Understanding NHS reform: the policy-transfer, social learning and path dependency perspectives', *Governance*, vol 15, no 2, pp 161–83.

Greener, I. (2005) 'The potential of path dependence in political studies', *Politics*, vol 25, no 1, pp 62–72.

Hall, P. (1993) 'Policy paradigms, social learning and the state', *Comparative Politics*, vol 25, pp 275–96.

Ham, C.J. (1981) *Policy-making in the National Health Service*, Basingstoke: Macmillan.

Heclo, H. (1974) *Modern social politics in Britain and Sweden: From relief to income maintenance*, New Haven, CT: Yale University Press.

Helderman, J.-K., Schut, F.T., Van Der Grinten, T.E.D. and Van De Ven W.P.M.M. (2005) 'Market-oriented health-care reforms and policy learning in the Netherlands', *Journal of Health Policy, Politics and Law*, vol 30, nos 1–2, pp 189–209.

Hunter, D.J. (2003) *Public health policy*, Cambridge: Polity.

Illsley, R. (1975) 'Promotion to observer status', *Social Science and Medicine*, vol 9, pp 63–7.

Innvaer, S., Vist, G., Trommald, M. and Oxman, A. (2002) 'Health policy-makers' perceptions of their use of evidence: a systematic review', *Journal of Health Services Research and Policy*, vol 7, pp 239–44.

Jashapara, A. (2004) *Knowledge management: An integrated approach*, Harlow, Essex: Prentice Hall.

Jenkins-Smith, H.C. and Sabatier, P.A. (1993) 'The dynamics of policy-oriented learning', in P.A. Sabatier and H.C. Jenkins-Smith (eds) *Policy change and learning: An advocacy coalition approach*, Boulder, CO: Westview Press, pp 41–56.

Kingdon, J. (1995) *Agenda, alternatives and public policy*, 2nd edn, New York: Longmans.

Mallinson, S., Popay, J. and Kowarzik, U. (2006) 'Collaborative work in public health? Reflections on the experience of public health networks', *Critical Public Health*, vol 16, no 3, pp 259–65.

Marmor, T., Freeman, R. and Okma, K. (2005) 'Comparative perspectives and policy learning in the world of health care', *Journal of Comparative Policy Analysis*, vol 7, no 4, pp 311–48.

Marmor, T.R., Freeman, R., Okma, K.G.H. (eds) (2009) *Comparative studies and the politics of modern medical care*, New Haven, CT: Yale University Press.

Pollitt, C. (2009) 'Bureaucracies remember, post-bureaucratic organizations forget?', *Public Administration*, vol 87, no 2, pp 98–218.

Ragin, C. and Becker, S. (1992) *What is a case? Exploring the foundations of social inquiry*, Cambridge: Cambridge University Press.

Rose, R. (1991) 'What is lesson drawing?', *Journal of Public Policy*, vol 11, no 1, pp 3–30.

Senge, P.M. (1992) *The fifth discipline: The art and practice of the learning organization*, London: Century.

Smith, K.E., Hunter, D.J., Blackman, T. et al (2009) 'Divergence or convergence? Health inequalities and policy in a devolved Britain', *Critical Social Policy*, vol 29, no 2, pp 216–42.

Stake, R.E. (2005) 'Qualitative case studies', in N.K. Denzin and Y.S. Lincoln (eds) *The Sage handbook of qualitative research*, 3rd edn, Thousand Oaks, CA: Sage, pp 443–66.

Walshe, K. (2001) 'Don't try this at home: health policy lessons for the NHS from the United States', *Economic Affairs*, vol 21, no 4, pp 31–5.

Weiss, C.H. (1977) 'Research for policy's sake: the enlightenment function of social research', *Policy Analysis*, vol 3, no 4, pp 531–45.

Yin, R.K. (2009) *Case study research: Design and methods*, 4th edn, London: Sage.

twenty-one

Case studies in health policy: concluding remarks

Mark Exworthy and Martin Powell

In Chapter One, we set out the aims of the book. In this chapter, we review those aims in the light of the intervening chapters, enabling us to draw conclusions about the role of case studies in health policy and the methodological and analytical challenges that they present. At the outset, we sought to explore the conceptualisation, design, practice and impact of case studies in health policy in the UK. In more detail, these aims were: to raise awareness of case study as a technique for scholarly inquiry; to provide an accessible resource; to identify the value of exploring health policy in the UK; to reflect upon the value of case studies for contemporary health policy; and to assess the ways in which case studies have enabled policy learning.

The collection of chapters has shown case studies as a 'flexible research tool' (Marinetto, 1999, p 64) available to social scientists. This flexibility is evident through its adaptability and its inclusiveness, but also its potential for ambiguity. It thus shows the need for clarity in the ways and settings in which case studies are deployed.

Methodologically, the chapters have been diverse in their use of evidence and their interrogation of it. Either directly or indirectly, the chapters rely heavily on qualitative methods, notably the secondary sources, including historical analysis of documentary evidence (for example, Powell, Chapter Three; Mohan, Chapter Four). Other Chapters have drawn on analysis of secondary sources from a key text (such as Higgins, Chapter Six; Evans, Chapter Ten; Allen, Chapter Eighteen) or from official reports (such as Wainwright and Calnan, Chapter Eleven; Exworthy and Oliver, Chapter Nineteen).

Whichever methods have been deployed, the explanatory power of case studies has also been evident. All the case studies reported here display this power by offering 'thick description' of the policy process (for example, Paton, Chapter Sixteen), drawing on 'multiple variables' in an 'array of scenarios' (for example, Dowswell and Harrison, Chapter Seventeen) and exploring 'further theoretical statements' (for example, Hughes, Chapter Twelve) (cf Marinetto, 1999, p 66).

Nonetheless, there is a continuum of case studies, in terms of scope/ definition, method and analysis. Case studies, as displayed here (and indeed elsewhere), are a 'broad church.' Certainly, there is an emphasis on process. In policy studies, however, this 'process' focus is necessarily problematic; policy has no 'start' or 'end', only 'middle' (John, 2000, p 26). Although detailed description is the mainstay of all case studies (and policy research), this has, arguably, been to the detriment of assessment of policy outcomes. Nonetheless, most case studies have ventured into the development or application of theoretical perspectives.

As discussed in Chapter One, the temporal perspective of case studies appears to continue to present a challenge (at least, in terms of Yin's 2009 criteria of case studies): how far should case studies address only contemporary policy issues? The chapters in this collection all consider the extent to which the 'original' case study has permeated the ideology, interests or institutions of contemporary health policy in the UK. Such 'infiltration' has been more and less explicit, and has operated over differing lengths of time. Take, for example, the theme of patient safety, which has taken years, if not decades, to shape the agenda of health policy and to become implemented in practice (see Higgins, Chapter Six, and Keen, Chapter Seven). Arguably, these two case studies have had specific and profound impacts by permeating clinical and policy domains. By contrast, case studies of current policies such as patient choice (Peckham and Sanderson, Chapter Fourteen) or the market mechanisms (Allen, Chapter Eighteen) can work backwards, tracing their historical antecedents. Likewise, Exworthy and Oliver (Chapter Nineteen) explore this explicitly by comparing the ways in which evidence from three inquiries about health inequalities have been influenced by previous inquiries and, in turn, have shaped subsequent health policy.

Valuing the 'emergent' case study

From the collective analysis presented in the preceding chapters, we argue that case studies are not a pauper's choice, to be used when experiments cannot be conducted. Rather, they fulfil a different and complementary role. They contribute to the bridging process between science and common-sense practice, helping practitioners to frame their thinking and to make sense of more detailed findings. Equally, they play a role in developing and testing theories against empirical evidence. As such, we may view them as emergent, reflecting the way in which they evolve in response to empirical data and theoretical perspectives.

However, questions remain, not least about the nature of case studies themselves and their unclear definition. For sure, definitions of case studies commonly repeat the types of topics to which studies have been applied (Yin, 2009, pp 16–18). Yin's definition and features of case studies are complex and demanding. As we saw in Chapter One, Yin (2009, pp 185–90) writes that 'exemplary' case studies should have the following characteristics: be significant, be complete, consider alternative perspectives, display sufficient evidence and be composed in an engaging manner. Furthermore, Yin (2009) presents, *inter alia*, six sources of evidence, three principles of data collection and five analytical techniques. In short, 'good case studies are still difficult to do' (Yin, 2009, p 16). Faced with such a counsel of perfection, it is likely that all case studies will fall short to some extent. It is hard to imagine a case study that satisfies all of Yin's criteria. Indeed, perhaps Yin and others have set the standard so high that all of the ideal-type criteria may never be met. It remains unclear, however, whether all such criteria are required in order to meet the standard, or whether they are necessary *and* sufficient. Moreover, if we remain unclear about what comprises a case study, then it becomes nigh impossible to determine whether the criteria can ever be satisfied.

In some cases, the case under investigation 'emerges' during the course of the study (Ragin and Becker, 1992; see Mohan, Chapter Four). Particularly in the case of qualitative research, analysis and writing up are the creative acts that help to define and give form to the case. This is especially pertinent in (health) policy studies where the policy process is dynamic and in flux. Policy processes are, by their nature, liable to 'adaptation, transformation and implementation', reflecting the shifting 'constellation of ideas, institutions and interests' (Klein and Marmor, 2008, pp 907, 908) (see Hughes, Chapter Twelve and Paton, Chapter Sixteen). Some definitions of 'cases', for example, stress the importance of clear boundaries of the case, but often such boundaries are malleable and ill defined, adapting to forces acting within the policy sphere. It therefore makes some sense to live with the uncertainty and lack of clarity. This apparent latitude reinforces the role of theory in guiding and providing coherence to the study as empirical events shape the course of the investigation.

The shifting governance within publicly funded health systems in recent years has also meant that the clear boundaries of the 'case' (the decision, the site or the event) seem to be 'disintegrating'. Greater complexity in the congested state might imply that the policy process is becoming 'messier' than ever (Exworthy and Powell, 2004). Hollowing out (upwards to supra-national agencies, downwards to locality and regions, and outwards to markets) adds dubiety to the nature of the policy field itself (Skelcher, 2000). As the policy process is only 'middle', the temporal and institutional boundaries of policy case studies will inevitably reflect contextual characteristics.

Mohan (Chapter Four) illustrates the inherent difficulty of defining precisely the nature of the case study with reference to 'hunting the Snark'. If, Mohan argues, the boundaries of the case are liable to interpretation, then it points to a wider issue about the degree of precision that might be expected from any case study. The notion of 'clear' boundaries around such processes is not only over-ambitious but also unhelpful.

> It is very difficult to classify (or anatomise) public policy. What counts as an issue, or what similar 'issues' evoke, depends on context which in turn is filtered through mental models of actors and audiences. (Klein and Marmor, 2008, p 902)

It may therefore be better, for example, to consider framing case studies around thematic approaches instead or in addition. Some of the chapters in this book illustrate how this flexibility might be deployed. For instance, Justin Keen (Chapter Seven) shows how ideas from Perrow's study were translated into healthcare settings. Likewise, Macfarlane et al (Chapter Nine) and Peckham and Sanderson (Chapter Fourteen) show how multiple influences have acted upon the nature of the policy itself and its subsequent (and ongoing) implementation. Moreover, within each chapter the contemporary reflections upon the original case study demonstrate the disparate influence of the original policy or study. So, rather than just becoming preoccupied with the boundaries of the case (important though this indeed is), more attention should also be devoted to analysis.

The case studies in this book reflect the rich variety of different case study research methods (see Marinetto, Chapter Two). Paton (Chapter Sixteen) favours the 'Harvard' study, which tells a punctuated chronological story. Dissatisfaction with some existing case studies set him in search of case studies which seek to combine case studies of policy with theoretical concerns such as the theory of the state (Paton, 1990; Paton and Bach, 1990; see also Marinetto, Chapter Two). Hughes (Chapter Twelve) favours Hunter's simple yet effective strategy of combining in-depth case studies with wider survey data. As Hughes points out, too many researchers opt instead to combine a survey with an excessive number of small, truncated case studies. Where small research teams present 8, 10 or even more case studies within the constraints of a three-year study, the adequacy of observations and understanding of social processes inevitably suffers. (Arguably, these matters are being exacerbated by current funding regimes within UK health research.) Similarly, Locock and Dopson (Chapter Thirteen) support the Pettigrew et al model, which has parallels with the approach taken by David Hunter (see Hughes, Chapter Twelve). It is invidious to arbitrate between these 'competing' or alternative approaches to defining and studying case studies. Rather than choose one 'best' method, Marinetto (Chapter Two) and Klein (1974) recognise the value of 'methodological and intellectual pluralism'.

Health policy in context

We now move on to consider the implications and impact of the featured case studies for health policy. How does the nature and content of health policy shape the design, execution and interpretation of case studies?

There certainly appears to be a collection of 'academic' case studies which have shaped health policy. Though it is somewhat invidious (and misleading) to focus on a selection, the classic and highly cited case studies include Alford (1975; Peckham and Willmott, Chapter Eight), Hunter (1980; Hughes, Chapter Twelve) and Pettigrew et al (1992; Locock and Dopson, Chapter Thirteen). We focus on these to illustrate points about case study methods and analysis.

Although Alford (1975) is frequently cited (there are mentions of dominant, challenging and repressed interests in many health policy texts, for example), there have been few detailed analyses of drawing on or extending Alford's thesis in relation to the UK (Peckham and Willmott, Chapter Eight). Yet, power is an endemic theme in public policy and is appropriate to explaining intra- and inter-professional relations in healthcare.

Hughes (Chapter Twelve) claims that, although probably unknown to many of today's younger generation of researchers, Hunter's (1980) study can be seen as the prototype for an important stream of qualitative case studies of NHS management, based on intensive fieldwork in chosen organisational settings, that continues to the present time. Hughes cites Illsley (1980), who regarded Hunter's study as leading the way to a more 'process' form of evaluation that was needed to supplement other forms of evaluation such as randomised controlled trials. Writing in the Silver Anniversary issue of the journal *Sociology of Health & Illness*, Lesley Griffiths (2003) traces Hunter's influence on a series of more sociologically influenced studies in this domain.

Locock and Dopson (Chapter Thirteen) write that Pettigrew et al (1992) firmly placed case study method as a rigorous design option in healthcare organisational studies. It was, and remains, one of the largest in-depth comparative case study research projects in the NHS. They state that there exist a cohort of context-sensitive and theoretically informed health service researchers who would trace their intellectual antecedents to this key text, among others. In particular, it is their examination of the role of context (and its interaction with content and process) which is perhaps their most significant contribution. They championed the search for 'receptive contexts' through research that is historical, processual in character. Although not discussed by Yin, the approach to context adopted by Pettigrew et al (1992) has resonances with the search for context–mechanism–outcome configurations, advocated by Pawson and Tilley (1997) in 'realistic evaluation'. In other words, a rich description of 'context' is important in order to determine whether processes are universalistic or contingent. Case studies are thus able to handle diverse contexts as the setting for and agency in shaping health policy.

However, others have more specific impacts in terms of shaping health policy in particular domains/fields. These might include Berridge (1996; Evans, Chapter Ten), Martin (1984; Higgins, Chapter Six) and Perrow (1999; Keen, Chapter Seven) and Tuohy (1999; Allen, Chapter Eighteen). Of course, the longer-term impacts of more recent case studies have yet to emerge.

The impacts of these 'policy' case studies are qualitatively distinct. The case studies themselves seek to ascertain the multifarious impacts of such policies. The task of tracing such 'outcomes' is always complex, as it seeks to attribute policy cause and effect. As authors in this book such as Macfarlane et al (Chapter Nine) or Hann (Chapter Fifteen) demonstrate, this is not straightforward. It is contingent upon the definition of the case in the first place, and choices about methodology and theory.

The role of theoretical generalisation has been posited as a key contribution of case studies, as this seeks to link data to propositions. (By contrast, case studies contribute poorly to empirical generalisation.) We certainly agree with Yin (2009, p 35) that the role of theory development, prior to the conducting of any data collection, is one point of difference between case studies and related methods. For case studies, prior theory development as part of the design phase is essential, whether the ensuing case study's purpose is to develop or to test theory.

However, we disagree with Yin (2009) on the need for a focus on 'contemporary events'. Rather, we include 'historical case studies', as Yin's condition would exclude some of the narrative descriptions such as many of the individual accounts of the creation of the NHS. However, examination of the accumulated studies does provide some theory development, as Martin Powell demonstrates in Chapter Three, for example.

Generalisation involves 'replication logic' rather than 'sampling logic'. This relates to the theoretical framework, which needs to state the conditions under which a particular phenomenon is likely to be found (a literal replication) as well as the conditions when it is not likely to be found (a theoretical replication) (Yin, 2009, p 54).

Case studies as a tool for health policy learning

The value of case studies is both to shed light on an empirical phenomenon and to offer insights into theoretical statements. However, as case studies illustrate policy evolution and change over time, they can also provide opportunities for learning – the way in which we understand learning in theory and in practice (Exworthy and Peckham, Chapter Twenty).

As learning takes place through a myriad of ways, including uptake of research evidence and findings from inquiries, communities of practice, international comparisons and isomorphism, this book was only able to look at some of them as examples of case studies. For example, Keen (Chapter Seven) argues that inquiries into high-profile tragedies, such as the Bristol (Kennedy, 2001) and Laming (2003) inquiries, are 'case studies in all but name'. The precise impacts of the inquiries featured elsewhere in the text are unclear (Chapters Six and Nineteen). Evidence is often contested, equivocal and thereby facilitates a struggle between the competing interests of stakeholders. Evidence is thus not always easily translated into policy; indeed, the impact might be much more diffuse, 'enlightening' policy makers and practitioners rather than presenting specific courses of action (Weiss, 1977).

If inquiries specifically set up to produce recommendations do not have clear outcomes (apart from the formulaic 'Mistakes have been made; no one is to blame; measures will be put in place; we will learn from this; this must never happen again'), it is difficult to determine the learning impact of case studies on policy (Klein and Marmor, 2008). Such impacts will, for example, vary according to the type of learning. The task of tracing policy impacts requires multiple sources of evidence, longitudinal data collection with a focus on process; in fact, an exercise that case studies are well placed to deliver. However, evidence from this book and elsewhere suggests that the ideal of case studies is rarely (if ever) achieved; researchers have not always executed case studies with such precision.

Earlier, in Chapter One, we identified the current features of contemporary health policy research in the UK. In short, these were described thus:

- short-term approaches are favoured ahead of longitudinal ones;
- local case studies are favoured ahead of those with a central government or supra-national focus;
- theoretical approaches are evident but could be emphasised further.

We also noted areas of health policy that have often been relatively absent from academic inquiry (such as the involvement of the independent sector in shaping health policy and the ways in which public and patients are engaged in policy making); no doubt, other health policy areas are also missing. One could argue that the dominance of market-based approaches to healthcare in recent years has skewed scholarly enquiry away from other areas – an illustration of non-decisions, perhaps!

So, given our 'learning' thus far in this book, what can be deciphered about the future? Speculations for future (research) agenda are fraught with uncertainty and are invariably proved wrong and/or misguided. Notwithstanding these comments, we do consider the drivers that shaped the emerging health policy research agenda. Two primary drivers are evident currently (as of summer 2011). The first is the reform programme (*Equity and excellence: Liberating the NHS*, Cm 7881, July 2010, and the Health and

Social Care Bill, January 2011). The reform programme emphasises still further the role of GPs in commissioning care, abolishing Strategic Health Authorities and Primary Care Trusts, advancing the Foundation Trust model and opening up opportunities for 'any willing provider'. As a result, the Coalition government is embarking upon the largest-scale reform (in scope and content) since the inception of the NHS. Although the direction of travel is clear, these proposals remain as such until they are implemented. The second is the UK fiscal crisis. The Spending Review (October 2010) indicates that the coming decade will be one of austerity, even though the NHS's funding has been 'protected'. Yet, operational and demographic pressures continue to loom large (some of which are exacerbated by the reforms themselves). It is certain that the NHS will undergo major change as a result of the combination of these two drivers.

In turn, for the future, the analysis of such health policy changes needs to be reframed so as to address extant shortcomings of the case study method, and to both reflect and shape the policy under implementation. Health policy research needs to aid policy learning within and by the academic and policy communities. As many familiar policy themes continue to reappear, it might be argued that little policy learning has taken place. This might also denote the extent of path dependency: How do actors shape, and how are they shaped by, the pre-existing context (Pierson, 1997; Greener, 2002)? Arguably, it reflects a propensity for ideological solutions in the absence of evidence. Many have noted the growing rapidity of 'major' reform programmes in the NHS. Note, for example, that between 1997 and 2010 the NHS was subject to 26 Green and White Papers and 14 Acts of Parliament (Thorlby and Maybin, 2010, p 8). Walshe (2010) makes a similar argument: 'Reorganisation has happened frequently – with at least 15 identifiable major structural changes in three decades, or one every two years or so.'

The consequence for policy learning is that reorganisations hamper such learning by reducing the organisational memory (Pollitt, 2009), as well as costing significant amounts and distracting effort from the NHS's core purpose (Walshe, 2010). The conduct of health policy research is also affected because studies are rarely completed before another reform is implemented; researchers are left to hope that their findings may 'enlighten' policy makers. In these ways, analysis of policy *and* analysis for policy is becoming increasingly hard to perform, a situation not made easier by the system of research ethical approval, which is largely inappropriate to the nature of the studies being conducted. So, there is a pressing need for longitudinal case study research, possibly published in a book-length format, which incorporates opportunities for learning and theory development.

Conclusions

Case studies come in all shapes and sizes. There is certainly not one 'size' of study that fits all situations. Moreover, methodological pluralism is essential to capture the diversity within and between cases. Likewise, theoretical plurality offers multiple perspectives, potentially on apparently similar phenomena. Methodologically and theoretically, case studies are valuable precisely because of their flexibility both in the field and in the researcher's office.

While we were somewhat agnostic in defining case studies at the outset and we still recognise the value of diversity, it is hard to point to many case studies that satisfy all of Yin's (2009) criteria; some studies might not even be considered case studies in his terms. We have, however, taken a more minimalist approach which draws on the advice of Pettigrew and colleagues that research should be processual, comparative, pluralist, contextual and historical. To achieve this, there needs to be a 'continual interplay' between the context, process and content of change (Locock and Dopson, Chapter Thirteen). We might also add two further necessary 'interactions'. The first is between process and action, at different levels (local, national and global) (Shore and Wright, 1997, p 14). The second is between extant knowledge and theory building. While acknowledging this agenda, we also note that policy case studies are especially challenging, given the ways in which 'the constellation of ideas, institutions and interests ... converge in any policy activity' (Klein and Marmor, 2008, p 908).

In summary, case studies reflect the 'best and worst' of health policy research in terms of theoretical development, empirical investigation and the research–policy interface. The future of case studies offers huge potential. Their value will reflect the ways in which advocates and exponents of the case study method interpret and enact the case study. In turn, health policy makers and health practitioners will continue to derive learning from them. Hence, case studies will undoubtedly continue to shape health policy. The task for both producers and consumers of case studies is therefore to improve the art of creating them and of applying them.

References

Alford, R. (1975) *Health care politics. Ideological and interest group barriers to reform*, London: University of Chicago Press.

Berridge, V. (1996) *AIDS in the UK: The making of policy, 1981–1994*, Oxford: Oxford University Press.

Exworthy, M. and Powell, M. (2004) 'Big windows and little windows: implementation in the congested state', *Public Administration*, vol 82, no 2, pp 263–81.

Greener, I. (2002) 'Understanding NHS reform: the policy-transfer, social learning and path dependency perspectives', *Governance*, vol 15, no 2, pp 161–83.

Griffiths, L. (2003) 'Making connections: studies in the social organisation of health care', *Sociology of Health & Illness* (Silver Anniversary Issue), vol 25, pp 155–71.

Hunter, D.J. (1980) *Coping with uncertainty: Policy and politics in the National Health Service*, Letchworth: Research Studies Press.

Illsley, R. (1980) *Professional or public health? Sociology in health and medicine* (Rock Carling Monograph), London: Nuffield Provincial Hospitals Trust.

John, P. (2000) *Analysing public policy*, London: Continuum.

Kennedy, I. (2001) *Learning from Bristol: The report of the public inquiry into children's heart surgery at the Bristol Royal Infirmary 1984–1995*, Cm 5207, London: TSO.

Klein, R. (1974) 'Policy problems and policy perceptions in the National Health Service', *Policy & Politics*, vol 2, no 3, pp 219–36.

Klein, R. and Marmor, T.R. (2008) 'Reflections on policy analysis: putting it together again', in M. Moran, M. Rein and R.E. Goodin (eds) *Oxford handbook of public policy*, Oxford: Oxford University Press, pp 892–912.

Laming, Lord (2003) *The Victoria Climbié Inquiry*, Cm 5730, London: TSO.

Marinetto, M. (1999) *Studies of the policy process: A case analysis*, London: Prentice Hall.

Martin, J.P. (1984) *Hospitals in trouble*, Oxford: Basil Blackwell.

Paton, C. (1990) *US health politics*, Aldershot: Gower.

Paton, C. and Bach, S. (1990) *Case studies in health policy and management*, London: Nuffield Provincial Hospital Trust.

Pawson, R. and Tilley, N. (1997) *Realistic evaluation*, London: Sage.

Perrow, C. (1999) *Normal accidents: Living with high risk technologies*, Princeton, NJ: Princeton University Press.

Pettigrew, A.M., Ferlie, E. and McKee, L. (1992) *Shaping strategic change: Making change in large organizations: The case of the National Health Service*, London: Sage.

Pierson, P. (1997) *Path dependence, increasing returns, and the study of politics*, Cambridge, MA: Harvard University Center for European Studies.

Pollitt, C. (2009) 'Bureaucracies remember, post-bureaucratic organizations forget?', *Public Administration*, vol 87, no 2, pp 198–218.

Ragin, C. and Becker, S. (1992) *What is a case? Exploring the foundations of social inquiry*, Cambridge: Cambridge University Press.

Shore, C. and Wright, S. (eds) (1997) *Anthropology of policy: Critical perspectives on governance and power*, London: Routledge.

Skelcher, C. (2000) 'Changing images of the state: overloaded, hollowed out and congested', *Public Administration*, vol 15, pp 3–19.

Thorlby, R. and Maybin, J. (eds) (2010) *A high performing NHS? A review of progress 1997–2010*, London: King's Fund.

Tuohy, C. (1999) *Accidental logics: The dynamics of change in the health care arena in the United States, Britain and Canada*, Oxford: Oxford University Press.

Walshe, K. (2010) 'Reorganisation of the NHS in England', *British Medical Journal*, vol 341, no 3843, p 341.

Weiss, C. (1977) 'Research for policy's sake: the enlightenment function of social research', *Policy Analysis*, vol 3, no 4, pp.531-45.

Yin, R.K. (2009) *Case study research: Design and methods*, 4th edn, London: Sage.

Index

Note: Page numbers in *italics* indicate figures.